HEALTH AND HEALING IN THE EARLY MODERN IBERIAN WORLD

Health and Healing in the Early Modern Iberian World

A Gendered Perspective

EDITED BY MARGARET E. BOYLE
AND SARAH E. OWENS

UNIVERSITY OF TORONTO PRESS
Toronto Buffalo London

Toronto Buffalo London
utorontopress.com
Printed in the U.S.A.

ISBN 978-1-4875-0518-9 (cloth)
ISBN 978-1-4875-3171-3 (EPUB)
ISBN 978-1-4875-3170-6 (PDF)

Library and Archives Canada Cataloguing in Publication

Title: Health and healing in the early modern Iberian world : a gendered perspective / edited by Margaret E. Boyle and Sarah E. Owens.
Names: Boyle, Margaret E., 1983– editor. | Owens, Sarah E., 1969– editor.
Series: Toronto Iberic ; 57.
Description: Series statement: Toronto Iberic series ; 57 | Includes index.
Identifiers: Canadiana (print) 20210118482 | Canadiana (ebook) 20210119160 | ISBN 9781487505189 (hardcover) | ISBN 9781487531713 (EPUB) | ISBN 9781487531706 (PDF)
Subjects: LCSH: Medical care – Sex differences – Spain – History. | LCSH: Medical care – Sex differences – Latin America – History. | LCSH: Health – Sex differences – Spain – History. | LCSH: Health – Sex differences – Latin America – History. | LCSH: Social medicine – Spain – History. | LCSH: Social medicine – Latin America – History. | LCSH: Sex factors in disease – Spain – History. | LCSH: Sex factors in disease – Latin America – History. | LCSH: Spain – Social conditions – To 1800. | LCSH: Latin America – Social conditions.
Classification: LCC RA427 .H43 2021 | DDC 362.1—dc23

University of Toronto Press acknowledges the financial assistance to its publishing program of the Canada Council for the Arts and the Ontario Arts Council, an agency of the Government of Ontario.

Canada Council for the Arts   Conseil des Arts du Canada

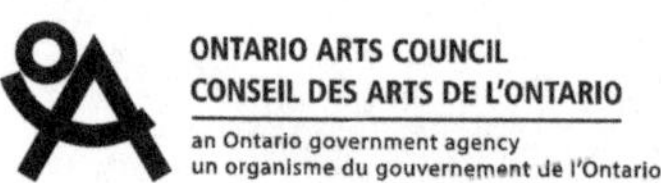

Funded by the Government of Canada   Financé par le gouvernement du Canada   Canadä

In Memory of Dr. Amy Williamsen

Contents

Illustrations and Tables

Illustrations

Tables

Acknowledgments

Over the last several years this volume has been shaped by the thoughtful contributions and excellent questions of many colleagues across our disciplines. We are especially grateful to the participants of various seminars and symposia hosted by the Renaissance Society of America, the Massachusetts Center for Interdisciplinary Renaissance Studies, the Modern Languages Association, and the Grupo de Estudios de la Mujer en España y Las Americas dedicated to topics around health and healing in the early modern world. We are grateful to be part of the Iberic Series at University of Toronto Press, and extend our gratitude especially to Suzanne Rancourt, Barb Porter, Charles Stuart, Carla DeSantis, and the editorial board of the series. We wholeheartedly thank the contributors of this volume as well as the anonymous reviewers of this manuscript for their collaborative spirit and rigorous commitment to the project.

Margaret Boyle expresses her gratitude to Bowdoin College, and particularly to the Fletcher Family research award for supporting for this book. She is grateful to her colleagues across the college, especially her fellow early modernists. Extra thanks to the departments of Romance Languages and Literatures, and Gender, Sexuality and Women's Studies, and of course to the dedicated cohort of students from her fall 2017 seminar on health and healing. The ongoing energy coming out of this class as well as the conversations that semester with Pablo Gómez, Alisha Rankin, and especially Sarah Owens led to the creation of this volume. Academic research and writing wouldn't be possible without the support of her family – with love to Andrew, Nora, and Beatrice.

Sarah Owens is indebted to the College of Charleston and the Department of Hispanic Studies for their generous support of her research. With some extra funding and time, she was able to travel to Arequipa, Peru, and become inspired by the health care provided in colonial convents. This never would have happened without the insight and help from Kathryn Santer and Jane Mangan, both experts on Arequipa. She is most appreciative of her collaborative work with Margaret Boyle, who signed onto this project without hesitation. It has been a true pleasure to work with her. Like always, she is grateful for her family's unconditional support, especially from her parents Miriam and Raymond Owens.

HEALTH AND HEALING IN THE EARLY MODERN IBERIAN WORLD

Introduction

Why Gendered Health and Healing?

MARGARET E. BOYLE AND SARAH E. OWENS

This edited volume recognizes the variety of health experiences across geographical borders and the ways these experiences change over time. The ten essays here interrogate the concepts of "health" and "healing" from a gendered perspective within the early modern Iberian world between 1500 and 1800. Our contributors bring together innovative and cross-disciplinary explorations of healers and patients. These essays explore topics related to the creation and circulation of drugs and herbal remedies; religious and magical practices; the status and representation of herbalists and apothecaries; geography, climate, and places of healing; the professionalization of medicine and gendered divisions of labour and care; recipe books, diet practices, and access to food. Through a systematic focus on women and gender in early modern Iberia and its global territories, this collection of essays engages with a series of enduring questions raised by the history of health and medicine, though seldom addressed in these geographic contexts.

An underlying theme in this volume is the confluence of the healer-witch, an icon unearthed by the second wave of feminist history and more recently reconfigured by contemporary scholarship in gender that attends to the historical and legal ramifications of the construct while problematizing the lasting impact of its fictional imprint. Certainly, in the context of the Spanish Inquisition, accusations of sorcery and witchcraft often intersected with practices of health, medicine, and contradictions of gender norms. Still, this volume does work to dispel commonly held beliefs around early modern gender and health: witchy women are not the only category of healers to be found, just as pregnancy and childrearing are not the only medical events that shaped women's lives.

Similarly, the volume considers how medical practice has been shaped by prayer and mystical experience particularly within gender-segregated environments, attending to health expectations for both men and women and the ways in which they impact spiritual life. Finally, several essays in this volume make space to examine the ways diagnoses and treatments of diseases are gendered – for example, in the specific instance of disease as a moral punishment for illicit sexuality and the ways these beliefs impact medical treatment and outcomes.

Several essays in the volume attend to health and healing practices in the changing context of Galenic medicine. Medical practice in the early modern period relied extensively on the writings of the Roman physician Galen (129–201?) and his contemporaries. According to Galenic medicine, the healthy body was thought to depend on a balance of its humours, that is, the bodily fluids: blood, yellow bile, black bile, and phlegm. The humours were one of the seven "naturals" required for health; the others were spirits, elements, complexions, members, virtues, and operations. The six non-naturals were meant to be regulated: air, food and drink, motion and rest, sleep and waking, repletion and evacuation (including sexual emissions), and emotions or passions. As Jennifer Evans and Sara Read explain, "The flexibility of the framework was useful because these factors would affect different bodily constitutions in different ways" (xiii).

Medical humanists took up the work of Galen and Hippocrates and revived them in the context of the university, though these were certainly not the only theories to impact medical practice. Paracelsianism too impacted a variety of health practices across early modern Spain and colonial Latin America, though as many chapters in this book demonstrate the connections to the supernatural and occult made this work more contested. Although rates of illiteracy were high, knowledge of Galenic theory and its changing landscape was widespread. As anatomical treatises began to be published at the start of the sixteenth century, including the work of Andreas Vesalius (1514–64), the study of anatomy slowly and dramatically changed medical practice. As several chapters in this volume demonstrate, conversations about these medical theories reached the populace through frequent references in literature, theatre, proverbs, and songs. While humoralism seemed to be everywhere, healthcare practices varied greatly. The processes of healing and the ways in which medical ideas were implemented differed tremendously according to geographic location, race, social status, ability, and, as this collection abundantly documents, gender.

Through an interdisciplinary approach to medical history, women's history, and early modern Atlantic history, this volume points to ways in which the practice of medicine, the delivery of health care, and the experiences of disease and health are gendered. From the early 1500s to the late 1800s we see how the medical profession tried to exert its power over patients, determining standards that impacted conceptions of self and body. At the same time, we see how this influence was uneven. The essays build from wide-ranging source material and reveal the multiple and sometimes contradictory ways early modern health and healing discourse intersected with gender and sexuality, as well as the ties to interconnected and multiply situated ethical, racial, and class-driven concerns.

As a way to introduce a volume centred on the keywords of "health" and "healing," we turn to contemporary definitions of the terms as a kind of road map for the volume, demonstrating the reach and use of these terms. In his 1611 dictionary, Spanish lexicographer Sebastián de Covarrubias defines the words *salud* (health) and *sano* (healthy), a set of words with unique valences for the early modern period but with compelling contemporary resonance. When defining *salud*, for example, Covarrubias equates the concept of health (here *sanidad*, pointing to larger structures of health over individual experiences) with physical fitness ("sandidad y entereza del cuerpo"); in his definition of healthy, he addresses the relationship between food, medicine, and morality.[1] Both of these definitions highlight topics for further investigation, including relationships between mind and body, the implementation and use of diet regimens, the manufacturing of medicine, and the influence of religion or other belief systems on health and wellness. The eighteenth-century *Diccionario de autoridades* defines healing in relationship to caregiving, citing the Latin *curare* alongside the Spanish *cuidar*, pointing us to the ways in which the study of health and healing practices are not studies of individual patients or ailments but patients in communication with caregivers. That is to say, the study of health and healing are not studies of individuals in isolation but studies of dynamic relationships.

More than four hundred years later, conversations around health and wellness endure. We find ourselves again grappling with mutable definitions of health alongside the proliferations of both novel and well-worn healing and wellness practices. The consumption of evolving and wearable fitness trackers provides evidence for the monetization and quantification of the body; along with the widespread popularity of mind-body practices in home, work, and leisure spaces. These include both ancient and novel yoga practices, apps for meditation and mindfulness, various other modes of secular spirituality, and the extensive dissemination of personal transformations. Consider the variety of wellness corporations marketing their own brand of health and healing products and practices; alternative food movements and fitness regimes; and the proliferation of herbal supplements and essential oils with strong global markets, including reach in Latin America and Spain. Contemporary US polemicist Barbara Ehrenreich has recently described annual physical exams as a "high-stress hurdle in the life of any health-conscious medical consumer, a trial, so to speak, to determine innocence (health) or guilt (disease)" (19). Many of these practices force a kind of reckoning with the notion of responsibility for predictable health outcomes as well as the anxieties circulating around these assorted and sometimes messy categories of being: disability, chronic illness, aging, and mortality. Our current cultural moment has allowed us greater insight into how definitions of health and wellness reflect everyday lived experiences and their underlying social values in addition to the ways these definitions are shaped by race, class, ability, and gender. A return to the early modern conversations around health allows contemporary readers to better engage with their current historical moment, understanding some of the historical legacies that have shaped practices of health care, the delivery of medicine, and the gendered implications of these conversations.

The topic of the 2018 NEH Jefferson lecture, provocatively titled "How the Humanities Have What Medicine Needs," further highlights the relevance and urgency of interdisciplinary approaches to health. Rita Charon's framework of narrative medicine argues that the tools of the humanities are what best prepare physicians to broaden their view of the patients from simple metrics to real human beings with stories to tell: perceiving and incorporating patients' personal experiences, valuing the narration of the past, and recognizing the significance of the encounter between doctor and patient. As Charon argues, "At the core of the concepts of narrative medicine ... is our framing principle that the central events of health care are the giving and receiving of accounts of self ... the teller requires a listener to register that a story has been told" (286). In this cultural and political moment where humanities scholars once again find themselves justifying the existence of their field and sometimes even their profession, it is worthwhile to highlight the powerful relationships between medical practice, health experiences (literary and historical), and the critical tools of the humanities, widely defined and interdisciplinary as reflected by the essays in this volume. This interdependent and reflexive approach to our collection emphasizes early modern health and healing practices as relational and dynamic. While our project does not cater directly to physicians or medical students, it is deeply invested in the relevance and ongoing practice of critical thinking about medicine and health care across the curriculum and the ability of these histories to shape our current values and practices.

The ten innovative essays collected in this volume represent emerging scholarship in feminist and critical race theories along with disability studies that attend to pressing questions surrounding early modern health.[2] It is the first collection of its kind to highlight the prominent role of gender and its relationship to health and medicine in the early modern Iberian world. This volume builds on the solid ground recently established by scholars in the history of science and medicine that has done significant corrective work to put Iberian science and medicine back on the map.[3] This project follows John Slater et al.'s excellent 2014 volume, which argues persuasively for the plurality of medical culture, insisting on the "many medical cultures of the early modern Spanish empire" (13). It likewise recognizes and seeks to highlight the variety of medical experiences that emerged from the "tension between global ambition and local control" (16).[4] We also heed Linda Newson's cogent reminder that "Western science was not the product of a one-way process, but that colonial practices were forged through interactions and exchanges with local scientists within both the colonies and Europe, and that they varied according to different cultural, social, political and geographical settings" (11).[5] With these varied contexts in mind, this volume attends to a range of health practitioners, both professional and non-professional, and sheds light on how practices of medical pluralism and hybridity move indigenous, African, and European health and medical traditions into conversation with one another.

This volume breaks new ground in the field through its systematic focus on gender and sexuality as they relate to the delivery of health care, the practice of medicine, and the experiences of health and healing across early modern Spain and colonial Latin America. Feminist criticism has relied steadily on the expansiveness of the category of gender, assuring ongoing interdisciplinarity and applicability.[6] In particular, the volume builds upon and engages with the excellent work on early modern gender and history of science and medicine in a transnational context and attempts to fill some of the gaps raised by Alisha Rankin's comprehensive overview of women in science and medicine, citing "very little research thus far on continuities and differences between women scientists and healers in Europe and the New World" (*Panaceia's Daughters* 415) and calling for gender-focused scholarship in "transatlantic studies of Spanish and Portuguese colonies" (416).[7] Certainly the volume benefits from the boom in scholarship over the last twenty-five years on women and gender in early modern Spain and colonial Latin America, exploring what Harold E. Braun and Lisa Vollendorf have named "the Atlantic Turn" (6) or what Mónica Díaz and Stephanie Kirk describe as the "the transatlantic paradigm" (56), although few of these studies have focused on health and medicine.[8] We take as a point of departure Allyson M. Poska's case for "agentic gender norms" ("The Case for Agentic Gender Norms for Women in Early Modern Europe") decentring views of women's activities as reactive to or exceptional from a patriarchal context, recognizing the nuances of gendered behaviour and expectation in the health and healing roles of both men and women. These lines of scholarship pave the way for new generations of research informed by the intersection of gender with sexuality, social class, race, geography, and ability.

Understanding the nuances of health and healing in the early modern Iberian world is not an easy task, although as this collection makes clear, these questions are rich and urgent.[9] The ten essays presented here provide evidence for the dynamic roles of gender and its impact on health experience and medical practice across early modern Spain and colonial Latin America. The collection weaves together an interdisciplinary approach to the gendered uses of foods, herbs, medicines, and healing techniques and provides a framework for future scholarship not only in early modern health and medicine, but also broadly about science. We have intentionally brought together a diverse group of scholars from varying disciplines, from the history of medicine to literature and theatre studies. The essays on the whole take the reader across the Spanish Empire and weave together experiences of illness, faith, religion, art, and the theatrical representations of health.

In order to guide the reader and to help tease out the experiences of health care we have divided our book into three sections: "Treatment Models," "Representing Health," and "Faith and Illness." The first section, "Treatment Models," sheds light on different types of treatments and implementation, incorporation of local ingredients, and racial and gendered components of drugs. Based on meticulous archival research, Carolin Schmitz and Maríaluz López-Terrada's first essay in the collection, "Healing across Ideological Boundaries in Late Seventeenth-Century Madrid," launches the topic of treatment models. Their study explores the healing practices of a mother and daughter, including the making of medicines and the purchasing of medical recipes, before being prosecuted by the Inquisition. In addition to reconstructing the biographies of these two urban women healers for the first time, Schmitz and López-Terrada also describe and analyse the inventory of medicinal products kept at their home, providing insight into the belongings and working conditions of urban empirical healers.

The following three essays under the category of "Treatment Models" take us from Peru to Mexico. Kathleen M. Kole de Peralta's "Killer Skin

Care: Gender and Venereal Disease Experiences in Colonial Lima" negotiates gender, sex, and treatment of venereal disease in sixteenth-century Lima, Peru. As argued by Peralta, fewer women checked into hospitals than men for *bubas* due to the gendered implications of the disease, which stigmatized women for promiscuity. Her study analyses how women, to their detriment, circumnavigated hospitals and purchased toxic remedies such as mercury paste directly from pharmacies.

Sarah E. Owens's "Convent Medicine, Healing, and Hierarchy in Arequipa, Peru" also looks at women's medical care but moves from the space of Lima's working-class women to that of religious women in three convents of late eighteenth-century Arequipa, Peru. Owens combines information gleaned from convent ledgers about medicinal items purchased for the convents' medicine cabinets with letters written by the abbess of the Convent of Santa Catalina to the bishop of Arequipa requesting medical care for nuns and servants. In the case of Arequipa, we also see how the nuns fought against the strict reforms of the Bourbon Crown. The abbess's letters bring to life an attempt to maintain a lifestyle that emphasized hierarchy and still relied on servants to care for upper-class nuns.

From the convents of Arequipa, Peru, we next turn to Karen Stolley's insightful essay "*Leche* and *lagartijas*: Injecting the Local into Eighteenth-Century Spanish American Medical Discourse." This study highlights fascinating debates regarding the effects of ingested lizard meat and breast milk on the body. Among different sources, Stolley draws from newspaper articles and pamphlets published by *criollo* authors in Lima and Mexico City in the late 1700s. Naturalists and enlightened colonial elites negotiated what they considered traditional versus modern knowledge in lively debates such as the consumption of lizard meat as the cure for cancer or the quality of breast milk depending on the race of the wet nurse. What stands out from these chapters is the idea that medicine was largely the same from place to place, whether in the imperial metropolis or in the American territories. As Owens's chapter 3 points out, for example, many of the same medicines could be found in convents in Mexico and Peru.

The second section of our book, "Representing Health," turns to visual, theatrical, and textual representation to elucidate gendered health concerns and practices. Emily Colbert Cairns in "Breastfeeding in Public? Representations of Breastfeeding in Early Modern Spain" takes a fresh look at images of the Virgin Mary breastfeeding in the medieval Spanish text *Cantigas de Santa María* and compares them to early modern paintings of the *virgo lactans* and also to Pedro de Luján's *Coloquios matrimoniales* (1571). Her study delves into how these medieval texts not only racialized early modern wet nurses but also helped shape the importance of breast milk as part of maternal care.

Although it is certain that religious paintings, like those of the *virgo lactans*, shaped how early modern society viewed miraculous breast milk, it is also true that the vast majority of subjects around the Spanish Empire never saw those works with their own eyes. In contrast, the genre of early modern theatre engaged more directly with Spanish people. A variety of playwrights wrote about subjects that tapped in directly to gendered health issues. Sherry Velasco's chapter "The Queer (Evil) Eye and Deviant Healing on the Early Modern Stage" provides salient examples of the evil eye and its representation on the early modern stage. In particular, her study analyses the anonymous one-act comedy *Entremés de los aojados* (*Victims of the Evil Eye*, published in 1680). This anonymous entremés speaks to anxieties regarding men's failed masculinity and transgressive sexuality and the varying culpability of those casting and healing the evil eye.

Margaret E. Boyle's "Staging Women's Healing: Theory and Practice" complements Velasco's essay, as she describes the representation of gendered health questions staged in a number of plays by Tirso de Molina, including his three-act comedy *El amor médico* (*Love, the Doctor*). Early in this play Tirso mocks the play's heroine: "Why should a woman study medicine?" – the perfect stepping stone for Boyle's study of the significance of the woman as medical practitioner, one related to both theatrical fiction and contested social reality. Both essays enlighten the reader on the fluid definitions of the gendered work of healers and patients and speak to the relationship between medical practice and theatre.

The third section of this book, "Faith and Illness," tackles the complex experiences of illness and disability and draws connections between religion and health. Patricia W. Manning's "Work and Health in the Jesuit Province of Aragon (1617–1667)" offers a much-needed analysis of health care pertaining to male religious. Juxtaposed with Bárbara Mujica's essay in this section, Manning's study helps provide texture to the gendered differences between men and women of the cloth. Work, both physical and mental, defined the Society of Jesus, and in order to carry out the peripatetic lifestyle Jesuits needed to stay healthy. Based on these precepts, the Jesuits crafted their own definition of masculinity.

Religious women viewed bouts of illness quite differently from the Jesuits. In "Chronicles of Pain: Carmelite Women and Galenism," Bárbara Mujica examines how Carmelites often embraced illness as a way to imitate Jesus's suffering and therefore come closer to God. Mujica's fine-tuned analysis of melancholy – a catch-all phrase that could define a wide variety of illnesses – demonstrates gendered differences between the treatment of patients. Combined with Manning's analysis of the Jesuits, Mujica's chapter adds another layer of differences between male and female religious orders. In general, melancholy was associated with hysteria in women, while in men it could be interpreted as a sign of genius. But on the other hand, the Society of Jesus would often expel young men for melancholy because it could detract from travel and the mission of the order.

George A. Klaeren in "Sacred Embryology: Intrauterine Baptisms and the Negotiation of Theology and Health Sciences across the Eighteenth-Century Spanish Empire" addresses a topic quite different from that of Mujica and Manning, but it brings to the fore another issue of gender and religion, one that deals with the spiritual health of the unborn fetus. After providing a general overview of obstetrics in the late eighteenth-century Hispanic world, Klaeren delves into an analysis of sacred embryology and the debates over intrauterine baptisms. Ultimately, his study teases out gendered implications of pregnancy and how theological debates over ensoulment can help enrich our understanding of how medical knowledge and science could have serious implications for Hispanic women, especially those undergoing caesarean sections.

In conclusion, our ten essays build from wide-ranging source material and reveal the multiple and sometimes contradictory ways early modern health and healing discourse intersected with the topics of ethics, race, class, ability, and gender. This book postulates that we must take a multidisciplinary approach to engage with gendered healing. To be sure, even late eighteenth-century intellectuals viewed women as physically, spiritually, and intellectually inferior (Jaffe and Lewis 5), but that only tells one side of the story. Men and women across the Spanish Empire in Spain and Latin America found different ways to circumvent strict norms imposed on them by the church and their families. Women's work in medical professions required them to engage in a broad array of healing practices and occupations. In some cases, women found agency due to these unique circumstances; in other cases, they experienced repression.

Most likely, their contemporaries (such as Spanish playwrights) sensed these cultural continuities and disjunctures and imbued them in their writings. Their dramatic portrayals of the quotidian lives of men and women indicate a desire to present subverted alternatives of health and healing to the general public. From archival documents gleaned from hospitals, apothecary inventories, and convent ledgers, to first-hand accounts of pain contained in letters and life stories, to debates about the spiritual health of fetuses in religious treaties and anatomical articles, to visual representations of miraculous breast milk, to playwrights who used the pen to bring alive the pulse of early modern medicine, this book foregrounds the centrality of gender in the early modern Iberian global world, and demonstrates how our understanding of early modern health is ever expanding.

NOTES

1 "Sano: *Latine sanus, a, um; integer, incorruptus, bene hablens, prospera utens valetudine vuiusque partes omnes probe suas obeunt functiones, transfertur ad animum*, y decimos hombre sano, *id est*, bien intencionado; y por analogía decimos medicina sana y comida sana, porque acarrea salud" (1428).

2 For a compelling example of theoretical framework integrating disability studies and critical race theory, see Subini Annamma et al.

3 When Jorge Cañizares-Esguerra authored the essay "Iberian Science in the Renaissance: Ignored How Much Longer?," a wave of scholarship responded with corrective fury. We highlight some of the major contributors to this wave of criticism here: Victor Navarro Brotons and William Eamon; Daniela Bleichmar; Alexandra Parma Cook and Noble David Cook; Michele Clouse; Noemí Quezada; Martha Few; Teresa Huguet-Termes et al.; Laura A. Lewis; Pablo Gómez; María M. Portuondo; Antonio Barrera-Osorio; Cristian Berco; Michael Soloman; Carolyn Nadeau; and Marcy Norton.

4 For an extended discussion on plurality in this context, see Pamela H. Smith's "Science on the Move."

5 Matthew James Crawford's study of cinchona bark provides a compelling model for ways to trace objects and their competing uses and interpretations. As he persuasively argues, "By working from the perspective of an itinerant object defined by many bodies of knowledge beyond European science, we reduce the risk of reinscribing an imperial politics of knowledge in which European ways of knowing nature are implicitly labelled 'science,' while other (i.e., non-European) ways of knowing are labelled 'non-science' or 'superstition'" (Crawford 19). The argument underscores coexistence across multiple geographic and ideological contexts in our discussion of early scientific and medical practices.

6 We of course owe a debt of gratitude to Joan Wallace Scott's seminal article "Gender: A Useful Category of Historical Analysis" (1986). In her words, historical analysis of gender "provides a way to decode meaning and to understand the complex connections among various forms of human interaction" (1070). Merry Wiesner-Hanks stands out as a pioneer in the field for her work moving the category of "gender" into conversation with "the

global turn," ushering in new waves of scholarship that would transform the study of women, gender, and sexuality across multiple cultural and geographic contexts.

7 See Alisha Rankin's "Women in Science and Medicine, 1400–1800" for a survey of scholarly trends within the field from the 1970s through 2013. We also highlight some outstanding resources here, including landmark works in gender and early modern medicine by Montserrat Cabré, Mary Fissell, Laura Gowing, Monica H. Green, Kathleen Long, Alisha Rankin, Londa Schiebinger, Sharon Strocchia, and Olivia Weisser.

8 We offer a sampling of recent work attending to the cultural and literary history of women in early modern Spain and/or colonial Latin America, highlighting main sources for scholarly reference as well as anthologies that could be easily used in a classroom setting. See Nieves Baranda and Anne J. Cruz, as well as the online database *Bibliografía de Escritoras Españolas* (BIESES) (bieses.net); Nora E. Jaffary and Jane E. Mangan; Mar Rey Bueno; Allyson Poska; Nieves Romero-Díaz and Lisa Vollendorf; Margaret E. Boyle; Sarah E. Owens and Jane E. Mangan; Sherry Velasco; Anne J. Cruz and Rosilie Hernández; María M. Carrión; Catherine M. Jaffe and Elizabeth Franklin Lewis; Nora Jaffary, Lisa Vollendorf and Daniella Kostroun; Lisa Vollendorf and Grady C. Wray; Elizabeth Lehfeldt; Bárbara Mujica; Helen Nader; Martha Few; Georgina Dopico Black; Valerie Hegstrom and Amy Williamsen; Teresa Ortiz Gómez and Montserrat Cabré; Jodi Bilinkoff; Mary E. Giles; Magdalena S. Sánchez; Susan Migden Socolow; Teresa Scott Soufas; and Amy Katz Kaminsky.

9 As Rebecca Earle demonstrated in *The Body of the Conquistador*, linking food practices to colonization, "We do well to attend to the immense importance of such ordinary human activities in our attempts to understand the past" (219).

WORKS CITED

Annamma, Subini, et al. "Cultivating and Expanding Disability Critical Race Theory (DisCrit)." *Manifestos for the Future of Critical Disability Studies*, edited by Katie Ellis, Rosemarie Garland-Thomson, Mike Kent, and Rachel Robertson, Routledge, 2019, pp. 230–8.

Baranda, Nieves, and Anne J. Cruz. *Routledge Research Companion to Early Modern Spanish Women Writers*. Routledge, 2017.

Barrera-Osorio, Antonio. *Experiencing Nature: The Spanish American Empire and the Early Scientific Revolution*. U of Texas P, 2006.

Berco, Cristian. *From Body to Community: Venereal Disease and Society in Baroque Spain*. U of Toronto P, 2016.

Bilinkoff, Jodi. *Related Lives: Confessors and Their Female Penitents*. Cornell UP, 2005.

Bleichmar, Daniela. *Visual Empire: Botanical Expeditions & Visual Culture in the Hispanic Enlightenment*. U of Chicago P, 2012.

Bleichmar, Daniela, et al., editors. *Science in the Spanish and Portuguese Empires, 1500–1800*. Stanford UP, 2009.

Boyle, Margaret. *Unruly Women: Performance, Penitence and Punishment in Early Modern Spain*. U of Toronto P, 2014.

Braun, Harold E. and Lisa Vollendorf, editors. *Theorising the Ibero-American Atlantic*. Brill, 2013.

Bueno, Mar Rey. *Evas Alquímicas*. Glyphos Publicaciones, 2017.

Cabré, Montserrat. "Women or Healers? Household Practices and the Categories of Health Care in Late Medieval Iberia." *Bulletin of the History of Medicine*, vol. 82, no. 1, 2008, pp. 18–51.

Cañizares-Esguerra, Jorge. "Iberian Science in the Renaissance: Ignored How Much Longer?" *Perspectives on Science*, vol. 12, no. 1, 2004, pp. 86–124.

Carrión, María M. *Subject Stages: Marriage, Theater and the Law in Early Modern Spain*. U of Toronto P, 2010.

Charon, Rita, et al. *The Principles and Practice of Narrative Medicine*. Oxford UP, 2017.

Clouse, Michele. *Medicine, Government and Public Health in Philip II's Spain: Shared Interests, Competing Authorities*. Routledge, 2011.

Cook, Alexandra Parma, and Noble David Cook. *The Plague Files: Crisis Management in Sixteenth-Century Seville*. Louisiana State UP, 2009.

Covarrubias, Sebastián de. *Tesoro de la lengua castellana o española. 1611*. Iberoamericana, 2006.

Crawford, Matthew James. *The Andean Wonder Drug: Cinchona Bark and Imperial Science in the Spanish Atlantic, 1630–1800*. U of Pittsburgh P, 2016.

Cruz, Anne J., and Rosilie Hernández, editors. *Women's Literacy in Early Modern Spain and the New World*. Ashgate, 2011.

Díaz, Mónica, and Stephanie Kirk. "Theorizing Transatlantic Women's Writing: Imperial Crossings and the Production of Knowledge." *Early Modern Women*, vol. 8, 2013, pp. 53–84.

Dopico Black, Georgina. *Perfect Wives, Other Women: Adultery and Inquisition in Early Modern Spain*. Duke UP, 2001.

Earle, Rebecca. *The Body of the Conquistador: Food, Race and the Colonial Experience in Spanish America, 1492–1700*. Cambridge UP, 2012.

Ehrenreich, Barbara. *Natural Causes: An Epidemic of Wellness, the Certainty of Dying, and Killing Ourselves to Live Longer*. Twelve Press, 2018.

Evans, Jennifer, and Sara Read. *Maladies and Medicine: Exploring Health and Healing, 1540–1740*. Pen & Sword Books, 2017.

Few, Martha. *For All of Humanity: Mesoamerican and Colonial Medicine in Enlightenment Guatemala*. U of Arizona P, 2015.

– *Women Who Live Evil Lives: Gender, Religion, and the Politics of Power in Colonial Guatemala*. U of Texas P, 2002.

Fissell, Mary. "Introduction: Women, Health and Healing in Early Modern Europe." *Bulletin of the History of Medicine*, vol. 82, Spring 2008, pp. 1–17.

Giles, Mary E., editor. *Women in the Inquisition: Spain and the New World*. Johns Hopkins UP, 1998.

Gómez, Pablo F. *The Experiential Caribbean: Creating Knowledge and Healing in the Early Modern Atlantic*. U of North Carolina P, 2017.

Gowing, Laura. *Common Bodies: Women, Touch and Power in Seventeenth-Century England*. Yale UP, 2013.

Green, Monica H. "Caring for Gendered Bodies." *Oxford Handbook of Women and Gender in Medieval Europe*. Oxford UP, 2013.

– "Gendering the History of Women's Healthcare." *Gender & History*, vol. 20, no. 3, 2008, pp. 487–518.

Hegstrom, Valerie, and Amy Williamsen. *Engendering the Early Modern Stage: Women Playwrights in the Spanish Empire*. UP of the South, 1999.

Huguet-Termes, Teresa, et al. *Health and Medicine in Haspburg Spain: Agents, Practices Representations*. Wellcome Trust Centre for the History of Medicine at UCL, 2009.

Jaffary, Nora, editor. *Gender, Race and Religion in the Colonization of the Americas*. Ashgate, 2007.

Jaffary, Nora, and Jane Mangan, editors. *Women in Colonial Latin America: Texts and Contexts*. Hackett Publishing Company, 2017.

Jaffe, Catherine M., and Elizabeth Franklin Lewis. *Eve's Enlightenment in Spain and Spanish America, 1726–1839*. Louisiana State UP, 2009.

Kaminsky, Amy Katz. *Water Lilies/Flores del agua*. U of Minnesota P, 1995.

Lehfeldt, Elizabeth A. *Religious Women in Golden Age Spain: The Permeable Cloister*. Routledge, 2005.

Lewis, Laura A. *Hall of Mirrors: Power, Witchcraft and Caste in Colonial Mexico*. Duke UP, 2003.

Long, Kathleen. *Gender and Scientific Discourse in Early Modern Culture*. Ashgate, 2010.

Mujica, Bárbara. *Women Writers of Early Modern Spain: Sophia's Daughters*. Yale UP, 2004.

Nader, Helen, editor. *Power and Gender in Renaissance Spain: Eight Women of the Mendoza Family, 1450–1650*. U of Illinois P, 2004.

Nadeau, Carolyn. *Food Matters: Alonso Quijano's Diet and the Discourse of Food in Early Modern Spain*. U of Toronto P, 2016.

Navarro Brotons, Victor, and William Eamon, editors. *Más allá de la Leyenda Negra: España y la Revolución Científica*. Instituto de Historia de la Ciencia y Documentación López Piñero, 2007.

Newson, Linda A. *Making Medicines in Early Colonial Lima: Apothecaries, Science and Society*. Brill, 2017.

Norton, Marcy. *Sacred Gifts, Profane Pleasures: A History of Tobacco and Chocolate in the Atlantic World*. Cornell UP, 2010.

Ortiz Gómez, Teresa, and Montserrat Cabré. "Mujeres y salud: Prácticas y saberes." *Dynamis*, vol. 19, 1999, pp. 17–24.

Owens, Sarah E., and Jane E. Mangan, editors. *Women of the Iberian Atlantic*. U of Louisiana P, 2012.

Portuondo, María M. *Secret Science: Spanish Cosmography and the New World*. U of Chicago P, 2009.

Poska, Allyson M. "The Case for Agentic Gender Norms for Women in Early Modern Europe." *Gender & History*, vol. 30, no. 2, 2018, pp. 354–65.

– *Gendered Crossings: Women and Migration in the Spanish Empire*. U of New Mexico P, 2016.

– *Women and Authority in Early Modern Spain: The Peasants of Galicia*. Oxford UP, 2006.

– Quezada, Noemí. *Enfermedad y maleficio: el curandero en el México colonial*. Universidad Nacional Autonoma de Mexico, 2000.

Rankin, Alisha. *Panaceia's Daughters: Noblewomen as Healers in Early Modern Germany*. U of Chicago P, 2013.

– "Women in Science and Medicine, 1400–1800." *The Ashgate Research Companion to Women and Gender in Early Modern Europe*, edited by Allyson M. Poska et al., Ashgate, 2013, 407–21.

Romero-Díaz, Nieves, and Lisa Vollendorf, editors. *Women Playwrights of Early Modern Spain*. Translated by Harley Erdman, AMCRS Publications, 2016.

Sánchez, Magdalena S. *The Empress, the Queen and the Nun: Women and Power at the Court of Philip III of Spain*. Johns Hopkins UP, 1998.

Schiebinger, Londa. *Plants and Empire: Colonial Bioprospecting in the Atlantic World*. Harvard UP, 2007.

Scott, Joan Wallach. "Gender: A Useful Category of Historical Analysis." *American Historical* Review, vol. 91, no. 5, 1986, pp. 1053–75.

Slater, John, et al., editors. *Medical Cultures of the Early Modern Spanish Empire*. Ashgate, 2014.

Smith, Pamela H. "Science on the Move: Recent Trends in the History of Early Modern Science." *Renaissance Quarterly*, vol. 62, no. 2, 2009, pp. 345–75.

Socolow, Susan Migden. *The Women of Colonial Latin America*. Cambridge UP, 2000.

Soloman, Michael. *Fictions of Well Being: Sickly Reading and Vernacular Medical Writing in Late Medieval and Early Modern Spain*. U of Pennsylvania P, 2010.

Soufas, Teresa Scott. *Women's Acts: Plays by Women Dramatists of Spain's Golden Age*. UP of Kentucky, 1996.

Strocchia, Sharon. "The Nun Apothecaries of Renaissance Florence: Marketing Medicines in the Convent." *Renaissance Studies*, vol. 25, 2011, pp. 627–47.

– "Women and Healthcare in Early Modern Europe." *Renaissance Studies*, vol. 28, no. 4, 2014, pp. 496–514.

Velasco, Sherry. *Lesbians in Early Modern Spain*. Vanderbilt UP, 2011.

– *Male Delivery: Reproduction, Effeminacy and Pregnant Men in Early Modern Spain*. Vanderbilt UP, 2011.

Vollendorf, Lisa. *The Lives of Women: A New History of Inquisitional Spain*. Vanderbilt UP, 2007.

Vollendorf, Lisa, and Daniella Kostroun. *Women, Religion & the Atlantic World, 1600–1800*. U of Toronto P, 2009.

Vollendorf, Lisa, and Grady C. Wray. "Gender in the Atlantic World: Women's Writing in Iberia and Latin America." *Theorising the Ibero-American Atlantic*, Brill, 2013, pp. 99–116.

Weisser, Olivia. *Ill Composed: Sickness, Gender, and Belief in Early Modern England*. Yale UP, 2015.

Wiesner-Hanks, Merry E. "Early Modern Gender and the Global Turn." *Mapping Gendered Routes and Spaces in the Early Modern World*. Ashgate, 2015.

– editor. *Women and Gender in the Early Modern World: Critical Concepts in Women's History*. 4 vols., Routledge, 2015.

– "World History and the History of Women, Gender, and Sexuality." *Journal of World History*, vol. 18, no. 1, 2007, pp. 53–67.

PART ONE

Treatment Models

Chapter One

Healing across Ideological Boundaries in Late Seventeenth-Century Madrid

CAROLIN SCHMITZ AND MARÍALUZ LÓPEZ-TERRADA

María Sánchez de la Rosa (ca. 1642–1717), known since childhood as "La Rosa," spent at least thirty years of her life in Madrid: time enough to build up a solid reputation as a healer of various forms of illnesses. Her healing activities lasted until 1696, the year when she was first accused of witchcraft. The same allegation was expanded three years later to also implicate her daughter, Elena de Tordesillas (born ca. 1659). This episode led to a series of encounters with different courts of justice across Spain. Based on the documentation produced by the judicial proceedings, the objective of this essay is to reconstruct a crucial part of the medical culture of early modern Europe by giving voice to previously silenced subjects. That is, through the medium of fragmented and sometimes distorted documentation, we will examine ordinary women healers and their medical practices. Although the starting point of this study is based on individual experiences, in-depth biographical analyses allow for tackling a general series of historiographical questions that point to changes and contestations concerning ways of healing and general ideas surrounding health and illness at the end of the seventeenth century and the beginning of the eighteenth century.

In recent decades, scholarship on the social history of medicine has increasingly produced important accounts of women and their role in medical practice. Scholars have revised traditional medical historiography, which had focused more or less exclusively on university-trained physicians and the tripartite model that structured the regulated medical system in Europe.[1] Since women were excluded from universities and professional guilds that would train barber-surgeons and apothecaries (Fissell), they did not often figure in these historiographical narratives. As the introduction to this volume has already demonstrated, this monolithic historiographical picture has changed substantially, thanks to the thriving scholarship within women's history and gender studies, but also due to the attempts to widen the perspective of what entails the history of medicine,[2] including the processes related to health and illness as well as the broad field of care or bodywork (Fissell 10–11). Margaret Pelling and others have demonstrated that women in the early modern period were central providers of health and healing, and that considerable numbers of women were totally integrated members of their communities, both urban and rural, practising successfully and in a position of relative protection and acceptance within their social surroundings (Harkness; Leong, "Making Medicines"; Pelling, "Older Women"; Rankin). A range of studies in different European settings has shown how women operated in and outside the domestic sphere as midwives, empiric healers, caregivers, and experts in magic-religious cures (Broomhall; Kinzelbach; Whaley; Strocchia).

At the same time, the category of "women healers" is challenging and broad, as the types of individuals it includes run the gamut from German and English noblewomen (Leong, "Making Medicines"; Rankin; see also Leong, *Recipes*), to midwives as recognized practitioners with their own empiric knowledge often transmitted orally (Ortiz), to the illiterate and poor female healers, put on trial by courts of justice (Storey). Therefore, as various scholars have argued, it would be inappropriate to analyse the "healing women" in a homogenous manner (Pelling; see also López Terrada and Schmitz). Furthermore, as Alisha Rankin describes, women find themselves in complex situations that encompass "an uneasy compromise between utility as practitioners and their perceived threat to professional medicine" (7).Within this context, this chapter focuses on one particular type of woman healer: the urban empirical healer. That is, the common working woman who lived with her family in the metropolis and who used the domestic space for several purposes – including the making of medicine – but who was not confined to it, as she attended to her patients in various settings in the urban community.

Through examination of the biographical vicissitudes of two women who lived in Madrid at the end of the seventeenth century, this chapter situates their stories in a context that renders their existence plausible and therefore normal.[3] In this sense, the biographies of María and her daughter Elena do not represent the socially excluded; rather, their biographies include a set of characteristics common to a certain group of individuals who engaged in healing in the Spanish monarchy. Analyses of similar cases suggest that these two women were by no means exceptional, but common figures among providers of medical services in the urban landscape of European cities.[4] Reconstructing biographies within the context of illiteracy is a particular challenge, as the protagonists of these life stories are difficult to define, since they did not leave behind autobiographies, letters, or other forms of personal accounts.[5] If we are to explore the lives of these ordinary women – that is, often illiterate or semi-literate women – we are bound, as in the present case, to work with a "self" filtered through the surviving records of judicial proceedings.[6] The source material used for this study is mainly drawn from four inquisitorial trial records (Tribunal de la Inquisición de la Corte [Madrid] y de Toledo). One of them included a judicial proceeding held at a criminal court of justice in Madrid (La Sala de Alcaldes de Casa y Corte), and, in addition, another record of a litigation proceeded at the Royal Appeals Court in Valladolid (Real Chancillería de Valladolid). These records allow us to trace the work and life of María Sánchez de la Rosa, the protagonist of this essay, and her daughter Elena de Tordesillas.

In line with the medical culture of the period, the healer María Sánchez de la Rosa offered a diversified therapeutic service, ranging from supernatural means to chymical preparations, depending on the patient's demand and the nature of the illness.[7] Her case is therefore ideal to explore the eclectic use of therapeutic options available in the capital of the Spanish Empire at the turn of the seventeenth century, taking into account a joint perspective of practitioners and patients. This chapter explores the extent to which the belief in the supernatural continued to be an intrinsic part of Spanish society, in particular when it came to searching for the cause of an illness. It also aims to shed light on the understudied subject of how chymical medicine was produced and purchased by female healers.[8] Chymical medicine, or iatrochemistry – that is, the application of chemical ingredients in the preparation of medicaments – was praised for its mild effects, and became increasingly popular, particularly among court patients. Considered by contemporaries as the "modern medicine," iatrochemistry was practised among influential royal physicians of this time, such as Juan de Cabriada, Juan Muñoz y Peralta, and Diego Mateo Zapata,[9] by which it gained acceptance at the court in Madrid during the initial years of the eighteenth century.[10] María's preparation of pills composed of chymical ingredients invites us to examine the social spaces of their use and application. Based on her story, it is clear that chymical medicine was not only in use among circles of the academic elite but was shared and used by ordinary women healers without regulated training or licence, yet thrived for attending to the needs of both courtiers and commoners in Madrid.

The essay is structured in three parts, each focusing on a different aspect of María and Elena's story. First, we approach María's biography, starting with her origin, family background, move to Madrid, and her living and working conditions in the capital. We pay special attention to her multiple residencies and occupations as well as a detailed analysis of her healing knowledge and practices. Second, we explore how these developments led to the accusation of witchcraft and their following involvement in legal proceedings. Within this legal setting, the final part of the essay explores a specialized inventory created by a contemporary apothecary in order to provide an expert testimony on the nature and use of the materials owned by María and Elena. This document provides very rare insight into the belongings and working conditions of an empiric female healer.

Biography of a Female Empiric Healer in Madrid

María Sánchez de la Rosa was born around 1642 in the town of Torrijos, about thirty kilometres northwest of Toledo, to the town's governor (*regidor*),[11] Pedro Sánchez de la Rosa and his wife María de Illescas. Upon her mother's early death, María, age four, was brought by her father to live with her aunt in the village of Getafe, within the jurisdiction of Madrid (just fifteen kilometres south) and about eighty kilometres away from Torrijos.[12] Crucial for the development of her future interests in healing, María was raised by a family of apothecaries, putting her into contact at a young age with medicinal and pharmaceutical practice. Her aunt's husband, Juan de Torres, ran the village's apothecary in the mid-seventeenth century, later to be taken over by their son. While María was growing up in Getafe, her father, in the meantime, started a new family. Shortly after his first wife's death, he married María Rica, and together they had six children. María's relationship to her new stepfamily was not without its complications. In fact, it came close, as a later civil law trial over her father's inheritance reveals, to a late seventeenth-century Cinderella story. When María was thirteen years old, her father Pedro Sánchez arranged for her marriage to the tanner Juan de Tordesillas, of Getafe. Once married, María joined her husband in the business of the tannery and after four years gave birth to their first child, Elena de Tordesillas (1659), followed by their other children, María and Pedro de Tordesillas. In the years to follow, financial hardship befell her husband, leading him to borrow money from his wealthy father-in-law, Pedro Sánchez.[13] Since these debts were never covered, after Pedro's death in 1667, the new family systematically denied María's access to the considerable inheritance her father gave to her.[14] Given the troubling financial situation and the absence of family support, María and Juan decided to move with their children to Madrid in the search for new opportunities.[15]

Living and Working in Madrid

In the mid-1670s, the family settled down in a rental home in Madrid, on the Calle de los Preciados, in the vicinity of the famous Puerta del Sol.[16] There they would live for a period of seventeen years and engage in different types of occupations. As María explains, healing was just one among several jobs she had in Madrid, which included working with chickens and pigeons, manufacturing buttons and ribbons, and selling wine in their home tavern. Such flexibility was essential for working city people in general, and even more so for women, who did not experience the rigidity and formality tied to identification with a profession (Zemon Davis; see also Lanza). This, however, is not to say that occupational diversity was a solely female experience.[17] For example, consider the case of María's husband, Juan: his activity as a tanner was no longer mentioned in the accounts after moving to Madrid, as he instead engaged in the various family businesses. The phenomenon of labour flexibility should be taken into consideration when encountering the variety of occupations employed by María, and considered broadly as a shared trait among female healers.[18]

When the Count of Mora, whose property they were renting, claimed the need of the house for his private use, the family moved to the Calle del Codo (near Plaza Mayor), where they continued to specialize in the sale of wine. By that time, all three children had reached adulthood. In 1684, Elena de Tordesillas, the eldest daughter, married her second husband Diego de Burgos, a silversmith, and gave birth in 1689 and 1690 to their two children. María de Tordesillas, who had learned to read and write, married Antonio de Zafra, a well-known printer in Madrid.[19] Pedro de Tordesillas worked as a parish servant in the district of Lavapies and would later marry Isidra Suárez. During this period there is evidence that both generations had achieved social stability at that time. It is also worth noting that since the early 1680s the family employed a servant, Juan Rubio, an older man originally from the town of Colmenar de Oreja (near Madrid), who would stay with them for over twenty years, indicating improved financial stability.[20] After moving to Calle del Codo, the family again moved, though not for financial reasons: partly by choice and partly because their presence had started to raise conflicts of competition with the owner of the winery run by the nearby convent of Encarnación Real de Religiosas Agustinas Descalzas (Discalced Augustinian nuns). When settled into their new home at the Caballerizas de su Magestad – the royal stable of horses, a complex that included both housing and shops – they continued to run the wine business and tavern, but after some time eventually had to leave again, this time provoked by the owner's half-yearly raising of the rent. Their next residence was located on the Calle de Alcalá, where María added yet additional occupations to her list: she offered a washing service and also worked as a seamstress. It appears that the type of occupations performed, and as such stated in María's testimony in later years, were crucial to maintain her reputation. Working women in early modern Madrid, especially of lower social groups, were often at risk for being labelled as *vagabunda* (vagabond), a category that included not only vagrancy and beggary but also extended to unlicensed street trading, and violating the moral or matrimonial order, all crimes that would face judicial prosecution (López Barahona, "La caza de vagabundas" 3; see also *Las trabajadoras*). In this vein, public discourse and legal consequences established that women were expected to primarily engage in activities that would maintain a "protected and reputable" household. Domestic service in general, or associated tasks such as laundry or seamstress services, as well as the domestic manufacturing of goods, were considered, in the eyes of the authorities, appropriate jobs for working women as they were conducted within a more or less a controlled space (López Barahona, "La caza de vagabundas" 7).

This relatively stable domestic situation changed drastically yet again after a series of events in the early 1690s. Elena's husband died in 1693, followed by the death of the family's father, Juan de Tordesillas, in 1696. Later that same year María was tried and imprisoned for the first time by the Inquisition for witchcraft and illicit healing. The two widows could no longer afford their long-time servant Juan Rubio, which led to his dismissal. Also, the rent on the Calle de Alcalá became so costly following María's release from prison that she and Elena and her two grandchildren were forced to move to a new home on the Calle de las Infantas. There, they maintained a yard with 150 chickens, engaged in chocolate making, and worked as seamstresses.[21] These diverse occupations, however, did not spare them from poverty. In testimonies, their neighbours confirmed their neediness and reported how María would go regularly to the nearby convents of San Jerónimo and Recoletos Agustinos to receive alms for food (*alimentación*) for herself, her daughter, and her grandchildren.[22]

To sum up, over a period of about twenty-five years, María Sánchez de la Rosa and her family lived in five different locations (Calle de los Preciados, Calle del Codo, Caballerizas de su Magestad, Calle de Alcalá, Calle de las Infantas; see figure 1). Their moves were prompted by private needs of the landlord, issues of competition with other merchants, rising rental costs, or unexpected health events. Alongside a changing variety of occupations (trading animals, manufacturing buttons and ribbons, selling wine, running a tavern, making chocolate, working as

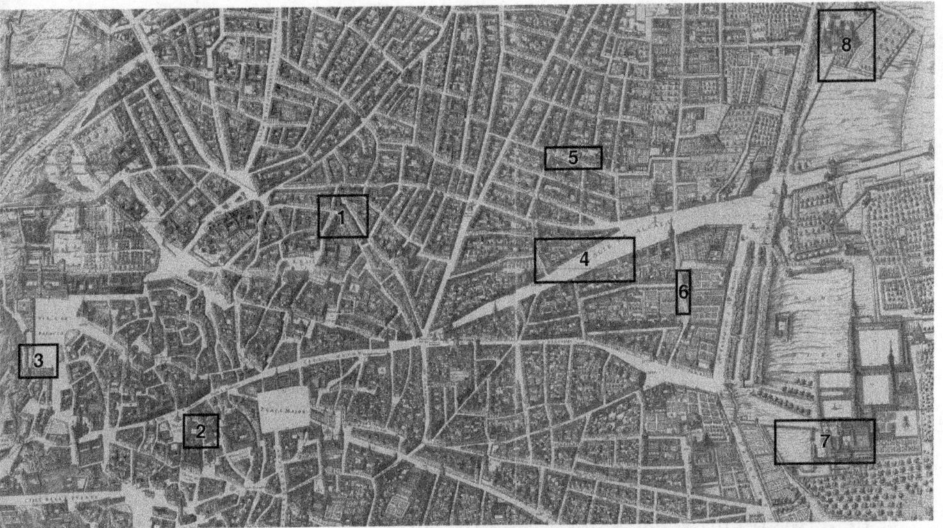

Figure 1. Map of Madrid, Pedro de Texeira, 1665, illustrating María's and Elena's housing. Key: 1. Calle de los Preciados; 2. Calle del Codo; 3. Caballerizas de su Magestad; 4. Calle de Alcalá; 5. Calle de las Infantas; 6. House of Juan de Ochoa; 7. Convento de San Jeronimo; 8. Convento Recoletos Agustinos.

a washwoman and seamstress), María maintained a relationship with healing practices. The variety in occupations and housing is worth highlighting, as it provides a compelling picture of the dynamic living and working conditions for women in the early modern period. Here, María's family history challenges the idea of one permanent home during a lifetime. Instead, it shows how housing needs and standards changed frequently due to a diverse set of social and economic conditions. In addition, it illustrates in detail the extent to which the variety of occupations could be part of women healers' reality during this period.

Healing in Madrid

María Sánchez de la Rosa's interest in healing and composing medicines can likely be traced to the fact that she was raised by a family of apothecaries. The importance of the household, for both training and engaging in healing activities, is highlighted by a number of prominent scholars including Mary Fissell, when she states, for example, that "the household, rather than the individual, was often the productive unit in medieval and early modern Europe. The family business, be that bleeding ... making medicines ... was structured in such a way that we often cannot know which person was doing exactly what work" (15). When María later married Juan de Tordesillas and continued to stay with him in Getafe, she likely began to build her reputation as a healer. This is supported by testimony given by a former servant, who reports about a male client who came from Getafe to Madrid precisely to be treated by María – "La Rosa" – as he heard that she had cured a man from *hechizos* (spells).[23] According to her own declaration, María's healing specialized in curing men and women of the "French disease" or the "great pox" (*humor gálico, mal francés*), sometimes for money. Most frequently, she cured the disease through the production of pills she manufactured at home.

María did not learn about this specific medicament from her uncle the apothecary but from her own personal experience and use. When struck by the great pox herself, a healer from Alicante named Marcedonio Galindo provided this cure to her. After the successful treatment, she asked for the recipe, which the man sold to her for "42 doblones de a dos escudos cada uno, antes de la bajada de la moneda" (42 doubloons each worth two Spanish escudos).[24] This particular way of knowledge transfer formed part of María's informal training. Although scholarship frequently shows that transmission of medical knowledge often occurred within the household or between generations, this case reminds us that women's medical knowledge could also be enriched by sources that originated from outside the family or domestic realm – that is, by travellers. The fact that María paid for the recipe also sheds light on the often overlooked economics related to the acquisition of knowledge.[25]

A more detailed composition of these pills is provided by María on two occasions: first, within the inquisitorial trial from 1696, in which she stated that she made her pills by combining sweet mercury, colocynth, senna leaves, anise, and a paste made of wheat flour with yeast.[26] In the later criminal law trial from 1699,[27] she gives a slightly modified account of the ingredients – colocynth and wheat flour do not figure but *azíbar* (aloe) does – and, importantly, details also the procedure, stating that sweet mercury[28] is itself composed of one ounce of *azogue* (mercury) and another ounce of *agua fuerte* (*aqua fortis*).[29] This mixture soaks in water for several days until the strength of the *agua fuerte* has diminished and it becomes *quajada* (thickened, set, coagulated). Then anise, aloe, and senna leaves are added to form a paste to create the pills.

The pills were not the only form María used to treat bodily manifestations of the French disease. She would also regularly induce artificial salivation using a prepared mercurial unction (*ungüento de unciones*),[30] which she would collect from the Hospital Antón Martín, a welfare and health-care institution that specialized in the cure of the great pox. She would apply this ointment particularly on "sobrehuesos,"[31] a type of hard tumour located above the bone,[32] which, as Juan Fragoso mentioned in his *Cirugía universal*, is a common ailment among poxed patients.[33] Together with her pills, these remedies proved effective not only on herself but also on other patients, and boosted her reputation as a skilful healer among a diverse clientele.[34]

Another one of her patients was don Francisco de la Fuente,[35] almoner and confessor to the renowned Cardinal Portocarrero (Luis Manuel Fernández de Portocarrero y Guzmán), cardinal archbishop of Toledo and regent of Spain during the interim time of the dynastic change from the House of Habsburg to the House of Bourbon. Portocarrero's choice of personal medical assistance fell to the physician Diego Mateo Zapata, who himself was one of the chief promoters of the modernization of medicine and the use of chemical remedies in therapeutic practice (Pardo Tomás, *El médico*). Similarly, the Duke of Osuna, whose indirect involvement in María and Elena's case will be seen shortly, had Juan Muñoz y Peralta as his personal physician, another high-ranking defender of chymical medicine (Pardo Tomás and Martínez Vidal, "Stories of Disease").[36] This network sheds light on the general arena of medicine practised in María's vicinity at that time in Madrid. Some additional examples of her patients include doña María Jargo, the porter of the Royal Council of the Military Orders and Dominga Peláez, the daughter of Domingo Peláez de Castro, bishop of Oviedo. According to the last patient, large bumps had appeared on her head, shoulder, and breast, the bodily outer signs of the French disease.[37] She consulted different surgeons and *químicos* without relief. It was after Dominga Peláez had learned of the success of her neighbour María Sánchez in curing similar ailments that she approached María and negotiated the remedy for the cure. Once agreed, María gave out her pills along with dietary instructions on what to eat and drink during the therapy, as was customary with all her patients. Apparently, Dominga Peláez was freed of the bumps after seven days. Considering the access this patient had to experts in surgery and modern medicine (*químicos*), the contracting of María Sánchez cannot simply be explained as the absence of a "proper" medical provision. Her decision was informed by multiple factors, including recommendation or reputation, hope, and proximity.

As is apparent across testimonies, María's healing practices were diverse. When living in the Caballerizas de su Magestad, she was called upon by a lady to cure a boy with a hernia. As it turns out, this boy was one of the two illegitimate sons of the Duke of Camiña (Pedro Damián Portocarrero y Meneses Noronha, 1640–1704), who lived with and were raised by their mother, doña Ana. Upon her arrival, María explained that she was not capable of healing the hernia, as a surgeon was needed for the intervention. In the duke's testimony – who appears as one of the witnesses in her favour – he confirms María's assistance in another illness of one of his sons, who experienced a severe case of *mal de orina* (urinary malady).[38] María was called in after physicians and surgeons were consulted. While the duke's testimony does not reveal much about the specific treatment, the inventory of products kept at her house lists *sebo de cabrito*, a tallow made of goat kid, which María claimed to have applied to cure these kinds of ailments.[39]

Apart from healing on her own, María also made use of collaborations with others, both laypersons and professionals. Within her direct network, most noteworthy is the support she received from her husband, Juan de Tordesillas, and, to a lesser extent, from her daughter Elena. María's husband accompanied her on at least one occasion when she travelled to the town of Escalona, about eighty kilometres southwest of Madrid, where she was called to treat the abbess of the Convento de la Concepción.[40] Juan de Tordesillas was also involved in manufacturing medicine.[41] According to Elena, Juan often helped compose pills and had an interest in collecting medical recipes.[42] In more professional collaborations, María worked with a surgeon, Cristóbal de León.[43] They came to know each other while both assisted Calleja y Clemente, the chaplain of the Holy Cross Church. When the surgeon's wife fell ill, he called in María to treat her as well as to purchase her recipe. Instead, María suggested collaborative work, under the condition that the payment be shared equally between the two.[44] María's decision to not sell or reveal the composition of her pills shows how much the recipe functioned as her "social capital," which enabled her to be in the position to negotiate with the surgeon (Leong and Pennell 148). From then on, Cristóbal de León and María would often visit patients together.

Prosecution of a Healer

The healing activities described above took place before 1696, and, as María assured the Inquisition that year, she did not return to the art of healing, a promise she seemingly kept for the years to follow. As a suspected collaborator in another bewitchment trial, she was also accused of illicit healing and sentenced to two years of prison and two hundred lashes. The records produced in this first inquisitorial trial are those that provide most of the information on María's healing activities, outlined above. Once sentenced and after she was whipped in the street, María, aged fifty-four by that time, was sent to the prison of "La Galera," a house of confinement especially dedicated to the punishment and correction of women.[45] During the time of her imprisonment, her daughters Elena and María were active in trying to secure a pardon for their mother, or at least a shorter prison sentence. While the literate María de Tordesillas petitioned the court to have mercy on her mother as she suffered in prison from physical and mental illnesses, Elena recruited help from her social network.[46] Together with their former servant Juan Rubio, Elena approached the clergyman Juan de Ochoa, who as the chaplain to the Duke of Osuna was an influential person in the court with promising contacts to the legal authorities. When he signalled his willingness to help, both Elena and Juan Rubio frequently appeared at the house of the chaplain, in the hope of good news. However, their presence soon triggered a serious disturbance at the chaplain's house. First, rumours reached Juan de Ochoa about the "true" motives behind his regular visitors when a neighbour revealed to him that Elena was the daughter of "La Rosa, the greatest witch known in these centuries, who at the present finds herself in the 'galera' [a women's prison], and was punished by the Holy Tribunal" and that "the older man [Juan Rubio] is her servant, helping to cover up all her misdeeds."[47] Second, disappointed at realizing that the chaplain did not live up to his promise to help, Juan Rubio expressed his anger – apparently with a threat on the household once his mistress was freed – upon which both were expelled from the house and barred to enter again in the future. Finally, these events coincided with a sudden and inexplicable illness that struck the chaplain himself as well as his cousin, Ana Sainz de la Barrera. Ana Sainz suffered dramatically, and there is evidence of household members increasingly concerned about her deteriorating health. She describes excessive pains in the whole body, "Parecía excesivos dolores en todo el cuerpo, y en ocasiones parecen la pican con lesnas, sin poder comer, dormir ni sosegar, con un disgusto inexplicable" ("Which occasionally feel as if someone would stitch her with an awl, without being able to eat, sleep nor rest, accompanied by an inexplicable disgust").[48] These pains developed over time into a chronic disfunction of the digestive system, enhanced by the applied purgatives.[49]

When María Sánchez de la Rosa was released from prison after only ten months of her two-year sentence – perhaps her daughter's petition had its intended effect – Ana Sainz's health declined steadily. This coincidence further fostered the suspicion of a bewitchment cast by María and Elena, and led the chaplain to approach María and Elena on repeated occasions, asking them for her cure. The apparent paradox can be explained by the widely held belief that the same person who causes the harm is often the most suited to heal or cure (Tausiet

452–5). This was not the case for María. When she was brought to Juan de Ochoa's house on the Calle de los Jardines she provided several reasons to prove why she was not the appropriate healer to cure this illness. First, she claimed that she and her daughter were not responsible for the spell. Second, she explained that these supernatural causes exceeded her realm of expertise; she only knew how to cure the "four humours." Even if she knew the necessary cure, she would not agree to any treatment after she had only recently been absolved from a sentence for the very same charge by the Inquisition. Although she denied having the skills to engage in an activity to undo a spell, her allusion to the supernatural is noteworthy. This fine distinction made by María is mirrored in the attendance of other medical practitioners who were called in to the home. Among the witnesses to testify in the case, the physician Francisco Rodríguez was one of the first employed for treatment. According to his report, to relieve the patient from her "thousands of pains, with fading episodes, and the whole body contaminated with thousands of ailments,"[50] he applied a series of Galenic remedies, which all remained ineffective. He determined that it was in vain to continue the treatment. After the doctor learned from the other priests present in the sickroom that the patient might be a victim of a spell, and coupled with his own uncertainty about the real cause of this illness, he saw himself limited to a single recommendation: bless all food or drink before introducing it to her body. The exorcist, who took over from that point, confirmed after several sessions of prayers that the illness continued to be a manifestation of a profound curse.

During these different therapeutic attempts, Juan de Ochoa had started to pursue legal prosecution against María, Elena, and their servant Juan. If María was released from prison in November 1698, it was only three months later, in February 1699, that the chaplain first launched his accusation of sorcery against the three to the Tribunal of the Inquisition. However, despite his numerous letters and petitions, the inquisitors did not consider his suspicion to be sufficient to file a case against the two women. Juan Rubio, the third suspect, had already fled by that time to the southern city of Puerto de Santa María. As a result of this inactivity, the chaplain decided to take action himself, and locked them up in his house. There, the mother and daughter were physically abused and tortured; they were forced to admit they were responsible for the spell and begin healing. This episode is described in detail by several witnesses, and accepted by the court of justice as matter of fact. Since María and Elena did not agree to either of the two conditions, Juan de Ochoa made use of his contacts he maintained with both the Duke of Osuna and the mayor of the city, resulting in their eventual arrest by the civil authorities on 2 May 1699. Set on trial at La

Sala de los Alcaldes – a tribunal of criminal and civil justice responsible for judicial matters of the royal court – the accusation formulated against them was modified slightly.[51] Instead of a focus on sorcery, the allegations included running a covert brothel and accusations of unorthodoxy. While María and Elena were put in the royal prison, the proceedings of the civil case continued, testimonies were collected, and an inventory of their house was ordered. To properly identify the nature and use of the many products stored at their house, another more specific examination was ordered, which in fact required the expertise of an apothecary due to the many medicinal items they kept. Starting in May, the trial of the civil/criminal court of justice proceeded until the end of the year, and involved a transfer of the two to another prison – namely, the newly founded place of confinement for women, Colegio de San Nicolás, designed for more reputable female delinquents of Madrid's society (López Barahona, "La caza vagabundas").

In the meantime, the chaplain continued to insist that their case should be judged by the Holy Office, arguing that since his cousin's health had not improved but instead developed into a life-threatening state, this crime called for a thorough investigation of the supernatural and malicious scheming of the two women. With the supernatural cause confirmed by the physician and the exorcist and possibly pushed by the eventual death of Ana Sainz in the second half of 1699, the relentless petitions of the chaplain were "finally" heard: the Inquisition of the Court, the local tribunal situated in Madrid, covertly started to call those involved to testify before the court. With enough evidence gathered, the trial was officially opened and on 27 January 1700, the Inquisition's order was given to move María and Elena from the Colegio de San Nicólas to prison, although the physical move itself took more than a month's time: 2 March. This case demonstrates how legal pluralism was practised and of how the existence of an overlapping court system allowed for an indictment of the same individuals before two different tribunals: the criminal and civil court of justice of the Sala de Alcalades and the tribunal of the Inquisition. The ease of difficulty of having someone imprisoned or having the same case move from one court to another depended on a series of factors, such as the persistence of the litigant, personal contacts to the authorities, and the appropriate formulation or framing of the charges.

Before 1698, María was well known as a healer among a highly diversified clientele in the central districts of Madrid. It was from this year forward that her reputation began to quickly deteriorate, starting with the first inquisitorial trial. This also coincided with the death of her husband, which left her financially and socially vulnerable. Poverty, widowhood, a previous inquisitorial sentence, and her age are all ingredients that made it relatively easy for her opponents to construct a plausible suspicion of witchcraft and to turn her into a culprit, who allegedly out of revenge caused a woman's illness and her eventual death. If this were not enough, Joan de Ochoa, as well as several witnesses who declared on his behalf, introduced additional elements to support the notion of supernatural forces at play. For example, one particular episode of an oversized black cat ("del tamaño de un carnero" ["size of a ram"]) appears frequently in these declarations. Apparently, its mysterious and frightening appearance coincided with the dispute that caused the servant and Elena to be thrown out of the chaplain's house.[52]

Inventories of a Female Healer's Home

As part of the criminal court proceeding, we have access to the home inventory on Calle de los Infantas (see figure 2), together with an expert examination by Armunia. Both inventories were not only relevant for the criminal trial but also important pieces of evidence for the inquisitorial trial. To allow for the examination to be conducted under proper conditions, Armunia suggested the objects in question be numbered and brought to his apothecary shop. There, he identified the nature of the items and substances, and explained in a written statement how these objects were commonly used.

During the hearings, María and Elena were confronted with selected items from the inventory. While María often gave a coherent explanation of their use, Elena stated her ignorance regarding many of the items and referred instead to her mother's expertise in healing. To gain a better understanding of the objects and substances used in the home and to infer María's knowledge and practices of healing, it is necessary to provide a more detailed analysis of the inventory's contents. Based on the general inventory as well as on the specified examination by the apothecary Juan de Armunia, the included objects can be divided into four categories: 1) clear medical use; 2) multipurpose items, including medical use; 3) work-related objects, such as silk yarn; and 4) devotional objects.

Within Armunia's report, he established the following items to be of clear medical use due to their frequent appearance in medical texts: goat's tallow (*sebo de cabrito*) and mercurial unction (*ungüento de unciones*) with an iron nail inside, nigella seeds (*simientes de neguilla*) and hemp seeds (*cañamones*), a pot full of starch (*almidón*), lodestone (*calamita, piedra imán*), betony (*betónica*), and senna leaves (*hojas de sen*). When asked about the ways in which María employed these products, she often cited their medical use and referred to her earlier practices of healing. For example, she explained that she used the goat's tallow for

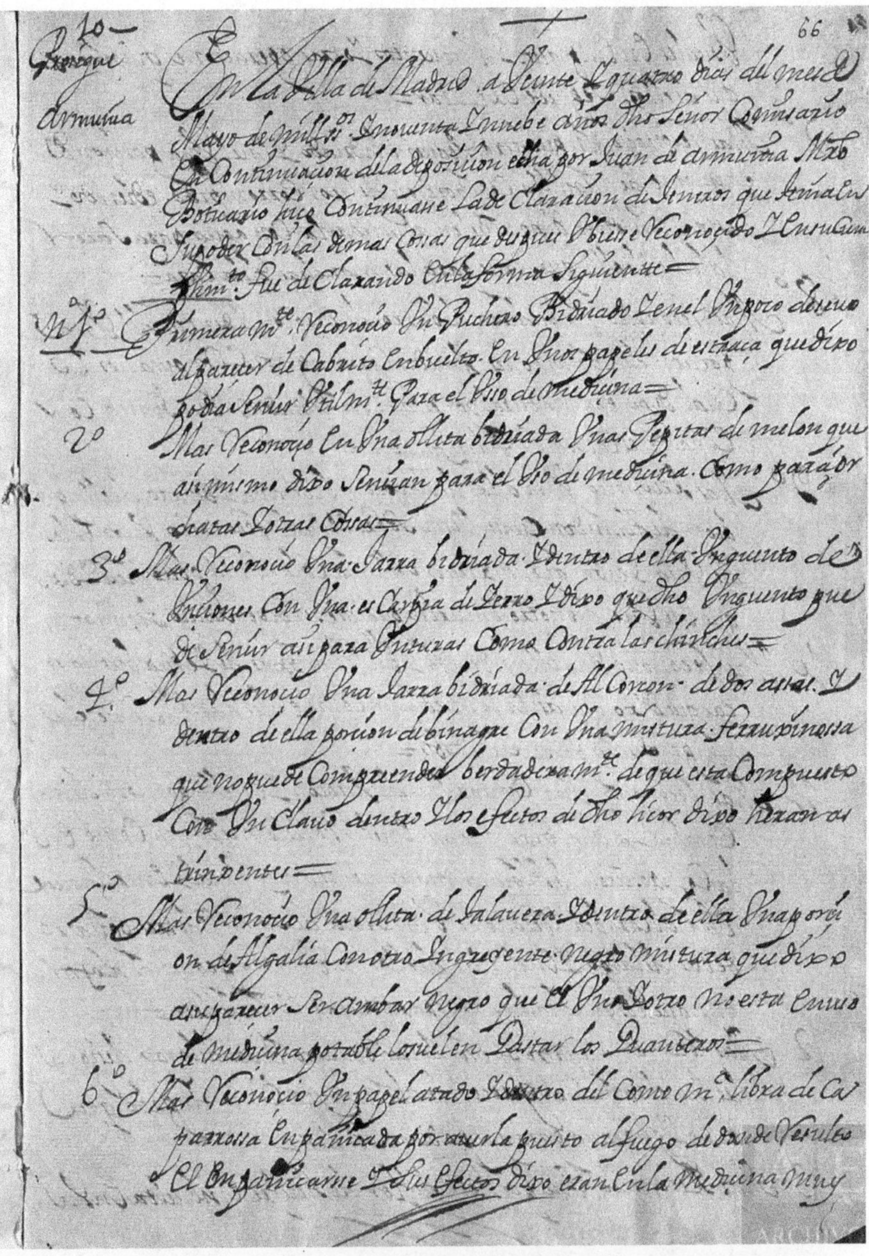

Figure 2. First page of the apothecary Juan de Armunia's inventory. Archivo Histórico Nacional.

urine maladies, or that she extracted milky liquids out of nigella and hemp seeds and combined them to produce a remedy for eye afflictions and skin impurities, a usage that coincides with the apothecary's observation. This applies similarly to the mercury ointment and pills. While the exact composition of the uncoated pills could not be determined by the apothecary, María clarified that these were pills she had fabricated many years ago, and due to their age, she expected that they would be ineffective.

In the context of chymical remedies and their handling by female healers, it is important to highlight that these pills, a composed preparation of mercury and colocynth, were not the only chymical product found in the house. In fact, the inventory features a series of other substances and minerals that were commonly applied both within chymical medicine and artisanal practices.

This is the case, among others, of marcasite (*marquesita de oro*), a mineral similar to pyrite, identified by the apothecary as used in medicine and "chymical arts,"[53] as well as for vitriol (*caparrosa empanizada*).[54] Armunia states that vitriol is used in medicine for poultices and ointments, particularly within chymical preparations. As an alternative use, María explained that, following the instructions of an artist, she had boiled it to produce paints, which she then sold to him.[55] This logic applies to a similar product, a vinegar liquor with a ferrous mixture made of vitriol and a nail inside. According to the apothecary, this substance has an astringent effect[56] and is of medical use, but María relates it to the sphere of paints and inks, claiming that she used it to make an ink for the frames of some paintings she intended to sell.[57] Also, she explains that vitriol (*caparrosa*) serves to dye objects black and that the nail was simply a tool for stirring. The dual use of vitriol vinegar manifests itself in its appearance in texts related to both the "art of dyeing" (including hair)[58] and to chymical medicine (Arredondo 128; see also de Villa).

In addition, contemporary medical texts can help contextualize the apothecary's expertise. For example, other items of medical use fit into the category of chymical medicine, such as flowers of sulphur (*flor de azufre*) or powder of raw antimony (*polvos de antimonio crudo*). The latter was classified by Armunia to be a common ingredient in medicinal treatment, without omitting, however, that it can be harmful if taken internally. This behaviour typifies the differing attitudes surrounding its application in medical practice. While also in use among Galenic physicians, though always mindful towards safe handling,[59] the antimony was a very prominent mineral in chymical medicine, and it became a protagonist in the polemic discussions that took place around 1700 between the defenders of iatrochemistry and its opponents, such as in texts authored by Juan de Cabriada and Diego Mateo Zapata. María herself presented contradictory explanations for its use on different occasions, ranging from buying it for a painter, to belonging to her son-in-law (the silversmith, who used it for his profession), to being left over from a medicine that had been made for her.

Another example of multipurpose substances is highlighted by Armunia himself, as depicted by the case of artificial cinnabar (*cinabrio artificial*). According to the apothecary, it can have an alchemical use in the transmutation of metals, and it is used by painters to fabricate the colour crimson (*carmesí*). As a medical substance, it can appear as a result of the sublimation of sulphur and mercury – that is, a chymical procedure – which with caution was used internally for the treatment of the great pox.[60]

Among the objects related to medical and chymical matters also figured a leather-bound portfolio filled with a collection of handwritten recipes to cure illnesses as well as a manuscript book, quarto sized, of medicines.[61] Although María and Elena claimed these notes on medical knowledge and practice could only belong to the recently deceased father of the family, Juan de Tordesillas, affirming his place as a *curioso*, a person eager for knowledge, they also distanced themselves from this work.[62] These claims concerning illiteracy can in principle be confirmed by an earlier document from 1667, where María confirmed receipt of goods without signing, since as stated by the notary, "she does not know how to write."[63] This, however, does not exclude a possible development in the following thirty years towards a basic knowledge in reading and it is worth speculating on their ability to interact with these documents. In this regard, the inventories also included a handwritten paper on the alchemist Ysaac Hollandus and the purification of the earth[64] as well as a notebook on "works of particular metallics and other metal mutations."[65] Although the interrogations on these texts did not lead to further explanations, they contribute to the picture of a household that shared an interest in chymical procedures.

Similarly, while it is impossible to verify the "real" use of the substances found in María's house, this inventory showcases the various and overlapping application of chemicals in an early eighteenth-century urban household, including medicine, arts, and other artisanal or craft professions. Furthermore, its presence in María and Elena's house attests to a wider and socially diversified public that engaged with chymistry and iatrochemistry in Madrid at the turn of the century.

The inventory also reveals a household interest in culinary arts and health care. As for the dry leaves of spearmint (*yerbabuena*), the caraway seeds (*aclaravea*), and the melon seeds (*pepitas de melón*), Armunia found for all three of them both a medical and culinary use,[66] while María and Elena declared to have used them only for seasoning, cooking, and for making a plant-based milk beverage (*horchata*).[67] The aspect of multi-usage applies in a similar vein to two distinctive items – namely, jet (*azabache o ámbar negro*), a gemstone; and algalia, known as civet musk, a glandular secretion produced by civets and used in perfumery. Stored in a small pot, Armunia identified its contents as a portion of algalia mixed together with black ambar and denied their use as internal remedies; instead, he informed that both were common products among glovers.[68] Among medical texts, one of the most noteworthy is the comment given by Andrés de Laguna, who in his *Pedacio Dioscorides Anazarbeo* treats algalia and ambar in tandem, alluding to their respective virtues and application in certain maladies. He also provided a recipe of both for a *poma*[69] against the pestilence (Laguna 61–2). Although María denied that she owned any of the items, it should be stated that the report of the expert in general does coincide in many ways with María's and Elena's explanations – in particular, when it comes to those products of a clear medical use. On a few occasions, however, due to the inherent multiuse of these substances, María finds reasonable explanations for a diversified professional application, allowing her to distance herself from the art of healing and at the same time to normalize suspicious items, which in the legal setting could be played out against her.

The latter strategy holds particularly true when their case was taken to the Tribunal of the Inquisition of the Court of Madrid. Close readings of trial proceedings reveal, although not very surprisingly, that the same body of evidence outlined above assumes now a different interpretation and focus. Whereas the apothecary could not find any harmful or suspicious objects, the definition of their usage experiences a notable shift towards a possible misuse in occult sciences when examined by the inquisitors:

> Having seen *la relación de todos los votos* and the declaration given by the master apothecary on all of these, we are of the opinion, that although most of them, according to the declaration of the said master, may be useful in medicine for medical and salutary purposes, but seen all together and having in mind the person in question, as well as the objects the said master declared not to know their utility and purpose, and particularly the two items in which iron nails were found, and those that had feathers inside, the loadstone and the antimony, all this together makes it extremely suspicious to have been captured for the use of curses and enchantments, and other superstitious works. This is how we think about it, in the monastery de la Victoria in Madrid, 27 January 1700.[70]

It seems whenever something undeterminable was combined with another item that did not normally belong – like an iron nail in a dark liquid matter – it was quickly associated with the supernatural. With the focus set on a collection of similar items within this new context of inexplicable episodes, including supersized cats and strange objects found in the bed of the bewitched patient,[71] the inquisitional narrative was increasingly informed by the belief in supernatural forces combined with a maleficent scheming that culminated in the death of the chaplain's cousin. Despite these charges, the lengthy interrogations and corresponding answers in the now two separated trials of María Sánchez de la Rosa and Elena de Tordesillas produced a coherent set of declarations on the side of the accused, resulting in suspension of the case on 23 November 1700, which became effective on 7 January 1701.

Conclusion

María Sánchez de la Rosa, once a respected healer in the central urban districts of Madrid, after three judicial trials within a short period of time (1696–8, 1699–1700, 1700–1), now faced a period of damaged reputation and exclusion. Although her case was dropped, she was sentenced to serve six months in a hospital and was banished from Madrid for four years. She died sometime before 1717.[72]

Despite this grim ending, the extraordinarily detailed accounts from her trial records – in particular, those produced by the Inquisition – allow us to go beyond the mere confirmation of the presence of urban women healers in the capital of the Spanish monarchy. These details reveal the general conditions that structured María's life, as well as information about her medical knowledge and practices. María's case reveals a accumulative form of training, in and out of the domestic setting, which prepared her for a diversified expertise in healing, of both physical ailments such as the great pox as well as more abstract spells. While healing was not her only occupation – rather, it was another element that added to the flexible combination of varied types of skills – her collaboration with a surgeon of the city, as well as her heterogeneous clientele of patients, testifies to a well-established reputation as a skilled healer in the capital.

The coexistence of natural and supernatural explanations for the cause of illness continues to be relevant in Madrid at the start of the eighteenth century. This social reality provides a window into a situation of extraordinary recognition and anguish. While María was recognized for her talent in healing evil spells, this same reputation led to an accusation against her and her daughter Elena, pulling both women into a complex entanglement of academic medicine, exorcism, pledges to undo the spell, and physical abuse, all taking place at the prominent house of the chaplain of the Duke of Osuna. This turn of fate underscores another aspect particular to the situation of urban women healers – that is, the precarious condition of a working woman increasing substantially when widowed and at an older age. Prior to the events of incrimination and the loss of their spouses, the family managed to endure and adapt to the changing working and housing situations; however, now María and Elena experienced extreme hardships. After years of success in performing a sought-after medical service to the urban public, María's case shows how quickly women healers could face an inverse situation: being defamed and expelled from the community.

The apothecary's inventory of María and her family's home provides rare insight into the existence of substances typical to the elaboration of chymical medicine in an ordinary household of a worker's and artisan's family, the manufacture of mercury-based pills, and the possession of texts and recipes related to healing and metal transformation. Such a finding confirms once more how chymistry, in its broad area of application, has become a standard feature not only in elite households but also in crafts households and among specialized healers, including "older bread-winning women" like María, who populated the urban districts of Madrid (Pelling 76). Chymical remedies were the subject of controversies among learned physicians; they were also widely available, and their elaboration and usage were common among a diversified public.

While María's case has generated fascinating material, she is far from an exceptional figure within the early modern urban landscape. Like other city-working women ascribed to the artisanal sector, over time she came to appropriate a set of practical craft knowledge and skills, ranging from the tannery business and laundry service to manufacturing chocolate, ribbons, and inks for painters. Healing is yet another skill that smoothly fits into the mix. Medical activities that involved the preparation of chymical remedies do not come as a surprise in this context but almost as a logical sequence, a coherent progression given María's involvement in a range of artisanal techniques that demanded a similar knowledge of substances and procedures of fabrication. Much of María's case can be extrapolated to other early modern regions, and it can propel further exploration of the connections between medical practice, urban crafts, and the women whose empirical knowledge and experience equipped them to work as healers and remedy makers.

NOTES

1 The tripartite model traditionally includes the regulated professions of medical practice, with university-trained and therefore learned physicians at the top of the hierarchy, followed by barber-surgeons and apothecaries, who received a more practical training by a master of their arts. For a critical revision of the tripartite model, see Mary Lindemann (especially chapter 7; 235–80) and Jennifer Evans and Sara Read (xix–xxi).

2 Important contributions to the broadening of health-care activities performed by women have been gathered in recent years in a series of special issues. See *Women, Health, and Healing in Early Modern Europe*, a special issue of *Bulletin of the History of Medicine*, edited by Mary Fissell. See also *Women and Health Care in Early Modern Europe*, a special issue of *Renaissance Studies*, edited by Sharon T. Strocchia. For an outstanding global approach, see *Mujeres y Salud: Prácticas y Saberes/Women and Health: Practices and Knowledges*, a special issue of *Dynamis*, edited by Montserrat Cabré and Teresa Ortiz-Gómez. Selected papers of this last volume were later published in Spanish together with a new introduction; see Montserrat Cabré and Teresa Ortiz-Gómez (*Sanadoras, matronas y médicas en Europa*). For pioneering works, see Margaret Pelling (*Common Lot* and *Medical Conflicts*, chapter 6).

3 A similar case of normalizing the individual can be seen in Daniel Roche.

4 Tessa Storey, for example, reconstructed in detail the practice of making and selling medicinal waters and oils of "Maddalena, the weaver," an ordinary working woman in Rome at the beginning of the seventeenth century. See also the Parisian healer Madeleine Colombier, a widow who illegally prepared chymical drugs in 1704, briefly portrayed in Leigh Whaley (137). Further, Pelling lists female practitioners from late sixteenth- and early seventeenth-century London who applied remedies based on chymical ingredients, such as mercury or antimony ("Older Women" 74–5).

5 For cases of literate women and the reconstruction of their biographies, see Natalie Zemon Davis.

6 For semi-literacy among Spanish women, see Anne Cruz and Rosalie Hernández. For a methodological and critical reflection on the nature of legal records, particularly testimonies, as historical sources, see Elizabeth S. Cohen.

7 Instead of maintaining a rather presentist separation in the meanings of "chemistry" and "alchemy" that would not hold true for the long seventeenth century, for this essay we adopt William Newman and Lawrence Principe's suggestion to use the inclusive term "chymistry" and its adjective "chymical" whenever we refer to the various subsets of chemical operations, such as alchemy, iatrochemistry, or spagyria.

8 There has been scholarly attention given to noblewomen, such as Anna Zieglerin, who practiced alchemy, or others who expressed at least an interest in the application of chymistry in medicine. See the works by Tara Nummedal; Meredith Ray; Rankin (152–3); Leong ("Herbals She Peruseth"). However, so far ordinary working women have not been included in the narrative of production and consumption of chymical medicine.

9 On the defence of these physicians regarding the use of chymical remedies, such as quina (cinchona bark) and antimony, see Àlvar Martínez Vidal and José Pardo Tomás.

10 An (institutional) expression of this acceptance can be seen in the royal approval of the first Spanish scientific academy, the Royal Society of Medicine and Other Sciences of Seville in 1700 and 1701; their principal goal was to defend iatrochemistry against traditional approaches to medical practice; see José Pardo Tomás and Àlvar Martínez Vidal ("Medicine and the Spanish Novator Movement").

11 "Regidor" means "a Ruler, a Governour, an Alderman of a City" (Stevens 332); or "Se llama también la persona destinada en las Ciudades, Villas o Lugares para el gobierno económico" (*Diccionario de Autoridades* 544; hereafter *Dicc. Aut.*).

12 Most of the biographical data on Maria's early life is gleaned from the information given in the inquisitorial trial records (Archivo Histórico Nacional [hereafter AHN], INQUISICIÓN, 96, exp. 1–3).

13 In 1665 and 1667, Juan de Tordesilllas borrowed considerable amounts of money from María's father, totalling over 90,000 *reales* (Archivo de la Real Chancillería de Valladolid [hereafter ARCHV], REGISTRO DE EJECUTORIAS, CAJA 3146,19).

14 Although María was initially entitled to to approximately 62,000 *reales*, according to the attorney, "it was on the instructions of her grandmother and her family members, that the accountants covered the distribution or awarding of inheritance with such diligence that there was no surplus of *maravedis*, in order for Maria to not receive anything, all in an unjust and wrongful manner" ("los contadores, a disposición de la abuela y parientes de la contraria, cubrieron dicha adjudicación con tal cuidado que no ay exceso de maravedis para que no consiguiese nada, todo injuste e ynordinadamente"); ARCHV, EJECUTORIAS, C. 3146,19, p. 24. This handling was disputed in later years by María's daughters, María and Elena de Tordesillas, first at a local court and later brought to the Royal Appeal Court in Valladolid. With the result, in the 1718 issued sentence, the daughters were awarded the sum of 28,020 *reales*; ARCHV, EJECUTORIAS, C. 3146,19.

15 AHN, INQ, 96, exp. 1, fol. 30r.

16 Renting was a common way to live for the majority of the population, especially in urban centres; see Raffaella Sarti (24). For Madrid, see Victoria López Barahona (*Las trabajadoras* 101).

17 For example, Pelling finds differing results, at least for late sixteenth- and early seventeenth-century England, where she ascertains that occupational diversity was also common among barber-surgeons (*Common Lot* 203–29).

18 See a similar case of a female practitioner with plural occupations, in Tessa Storey (143), where the author efficiently explains this phenomenon by alluding to Olwen Huften's coined term of "economy of makeshifts."

19 María de Tordesilla's husband was Antonio Francisco de Zafra, a Madrid-based publisher by whom more than seventy books are listed in the catalogue of the Patrimonio Bibliográfico Español. He started publishing in 1675 and had a particular interest in religious texts and in the history of religion, although his printing included other scientific topics.

20 INQ, 96, exp. 1. A letter from María de Tordesillas tells of Juan Rubio's roles; cf. INQ, 96, exp. 3, fol. 52r.

21 AHN, INQ, Exp. 3, fol. 72r–72v. This is the house in which the inventory took place.

22 AHN, INQ, Exp. 2, fol. 28r–29v.

23 Testimony by Domingo Pelarte, served to don Francisco de los Ríos; AHN, INQ, 96, exp. 1, fol. 2r.

24 AHN, INQ, 96, exp. 1, fol. 30v. Stevens writes in 1706, a doblón "is now generally taken for a Spanish Pistole, worth 17s. 6d." (155).

25 An exception to this lack of attention can be found in Elaine Leong and Sarah Pennell, who underline the "social capital" tied to recipes.

26 AHN, INQ, 96, exp. 1, fol. 30v.

27 AHN, INQ, 96, exp. 2, fol. 8v–9r.

28 On "sweet mercury," see the difference and more beneficial qualities as compared to "*mercurio crudo*" in Miguel Marcelino Boix y Moliner (101–2).

29 A distilled product in use since the Middle Ages, and popular with contemporary alchemists, this ingredient also appears in pharmacy manuals and other recipe books from the period.

30 "Unciones, is commonly taken for a Flux, or Salivation, because they us'd to anoint their Joynts with Mercury" (Stevens 399). Salivation refers to the effect that mercury provoked on the body and was a common treatment to cure the great pox, as explained in the later dated *Encyclopædia Britannica*: "The fastest and most commodious method of salivation is by mercurius dulcis six times sublimed, given inwardly in the milder pox; or by mercurial unction, when the disease is got into the bones"; Society of Gentlemen in Scotland (134). This explanation coincides with the logic behind the treatments applied by María Sánchez de la Rosa.

31 AHN, INQ, 96, exp. 3, fol. 84r–v.

32 "sobrehuesso: tumor duro que está sobre los huessos, el qual suele causar grandes dolores, Lat. Tumor super os. Quevedo, Casa de locos, Otros querían enamorar por lo lindo, muy preciados de tufos, y guedejas, manos blancas, y pies chicos con zapatos romos, grandes encubridores de juanetes y sobrehuesos" (*Dicc. Aut.* 128).

33 "De suerte que hazerse tumores en los huesos (que llamamos gomas o sobrehuesos) como vemos comúnmente en los que padecen mal francés no es cosa de admiración, más me admira dezir Galeno que se curen esos huesos apostemados como se curan los phlegmones" (Fragoso 258).

34 The importance of constructing a legible identity, especially for women healers who do not possess a licence, has been recently explored in María Luz López Terrada and Carolin Schmitz ("Licencias sociales para sanar").

35 AHN, INQ, 96, exp. 1, fol. 31r.

36 Also his father, the fifth Duke of Osuna, was patient to Juan de Cabriada, who set the tone for the movement of "renovation" with his *Carta phylosophica médica chymica* (1687); see Àlvar Martínez Vidal and José Pardo Tomás ("Un siglo de controversias" 114–16).

37 AHN, INQ, 96, exp. 2. Testimony by Dominga Peláez, thirty-two years old, fol. 11v–12r. Also, María Sánchez confirms this treatment and provides a concurrent, although less detailed, account of it; see AHN, INQ, 96, exp. 3, fol. 82r.

38 AHN, INQ, 96, exp. 1. Testimony of the Duke of Camiña.

39 "Que es cierto que entre los demás trastos que tenía en su casa tenía diferentes vasijas varias cosas, en unas, sebo de carnero derretido para untarse para el mal de urina"; AHN, INQ, 96, exp. 3, fol. 84r.

40 AHN, INQ, 96, exp. 1, fol. 34r.

41 AHN, INQ, 96, exp. 14, fol. 8v.

42 The existence of certain medical recipes and books were attributed by both María and Elena to the husband/father Juan de Tordesillas, claiming that he had always been a "curioso" and interested and eager to learn person, in addition to the fact that both mother and daughter were illiterate. In Elena's words, her father "era tan curioso que qualquiera cosa sentaba y sería muy posible tenerlos por esta razón en dicha su casa"; INQ, 96, exp. 14, fol. 15v.; INQ, 96, exp. 2, fol. 22v.

43 The certain extent of openness among regular medical practitioners to consider the help or advice of irregular healers has been highlighted by Michael Stolberg.

44 For other forms of collaboration between regular practitioners and irregular female healers, see Deborah Harkness and Sabrina Minuzzi.

45 Established in 1610, this prison for women was under the authority of the Consejo de Castilla and the Sala de Alcaldes. For further information on

Madrid's first female prison, see Margaret E. Boyle (in particular "Part One"); see also López Barahona (90–1); and Gema Martínez Galindo.

46 AHN, INQ, 96, exp. 1.

47 "La Rosa, la mayor bruja que es conocida en estos siglos, la qual está en la galera, y fue castigada por el Santo Tribunal, y este viejo es su criado encubridor en todas sus maldades"; AHN, INQ, 96, Exp. 3, fol. 7r.

48 Testimony by Ana Sainz de la Barrera, Madrid, March 15, 1699, AHN, INQ, 96, Exp. 3, fol. 18r.

49 The consequences are described vividly by María Sánchez de la Rosa, as she had heard that the patient was going through malignant purging, causing the bedsheets to have to be changed two or three times a day, and that she was vomiting; AHN, INQ, 96, Exp. 2, fol. 6r.

50 "Aberla allado con mil dolores, desbanissimientos de cabeza y todo su cuerpo contaminado de mil accidentes y dolores." Testimony by Francisco Rodríguez, Madrid, March 2, 1699; AHN, INQ, 96, Exp. 3, fol. 38v.

51 As its location was linked to the residency of the former itinerant royal court, upon its permanent location in Madrid the Sala de Alcaldes often entered conflicts of competence with the municipal court of justice of the City of Madrid. Cf. Carmen de la Guardia Herrero; see also José Luis de Pablo Gafas.

52 According to Juan de Ochoa's own declaration, he, his sister, and his cousin witnessed the appearance of "un gato de disforme cuerpo que sería como un carnero con diferentes manchas y dando bramidos como toro, que les causo orror y miedo grande, volvió la cara dicha doña Ana y biendole se quedo desmayada, y biendole el declarante començo a dar voces diciendo Jesus repetidas veces. Y dicho gato tan orrible se fue muy poco a poco, repitiendo bramidos, dejándoles a los tres con gran pavor y miedo. Y lo referido fue al poco tiempo de echar a los acusados de su casa"; AHN, INQ, 96, exp. 3, fol. 12v.

53 "Marquesita de oro, de plata, de cobre. Las dos primeras sin unas bolas como una nuez de gruesas, casi redondas y pesadas, morenas por fuera, y por dentro unas tienen el color de oro, y otras de plata, y todas brillantes y hermosas ... Las Marquesitas que se sacan de las minas metálicas contienen mucho azufre, y sal vitriólico, especialmente las de cobre" (de Terreros y Pando 534). Also, "Marcasita" is included as a metal in *Universale theatro farmaceutico*, which includes insights from the spagyric arts, and it says under its entry that while it is not common to apply it solely internally, it does figure together with other ingredients in prepared compounds, and its virtue corresponds to those similar of *Recremento piombino* (de Sgobbi 703).

54 "Genero u casta de sal mineral congelada de un agua verde, que destilan las minas del cobre, y que tiene en si alguna virtud metálica. Comun y vulgarmente se llama Flor de Cobre." (*Dicc. Aut.* 139,1). According to an entry in *Dictionary of Medical Vocabulary in English, 1375–1550: Body Parts, Sicknesses, Instruments, and Medicinal Preparations*, *caparrosa* is defined as vitriol, which "signified a variety of chemical substances, including colcothar, a reddish-brown oxide of iron" (Norri 2320).

55 On the multiuse of raw materials and chemical substances in medicine, craft and arts, see Ursula Klein and Emma C. Spary; and Ursula Klein and Wolfgang Lefèvre.

56 Astringent: "medicines to repel harmful substances by compressing them (astringency)" (Norri 124).

57 In the list of dual-use items can be included the bone of the cuttlefish in powder (*hueso de la jibia en polvo*), identified by the apothecary to be of medical use, as it is often applied to cure cataracts in the eyes (*nubes en los ojos*), although María claimed that it belonged to her son-in-law, who was a silversmith and used it for his profession, a usage that is confirmed by contemporary dictionaries (*Dicc. Aut.* 539,1).

58 Using a citation of Razhes, the first-century Persian physician and alchemist, Arredondo describes how he successfully changed a friend's grey hair back to its natural colour by giving him a dosis of "*caparrosa*" (vitriol).

59 For the physician Mercado, the antimony was a highly efficient medicine; he argued that if Spanish physicians do not apply it more often, it was because of concerns with preparation and expertise: "praeparatum aestivium : quod medicamentum nisi rustica quaedam timiditas impediret, plurimùm foret ex usu" (Mercado 276).

60 As an internal remedy it is attested by Andrés de Laguna (64–5).

61 AHN, INQ, 96, exp. 2, fol. 33r.

62 María further clarified that her husband had been in contact with the aforementioned surgeon, which made it plausible in her understanding that they exchanged recipes; AHN, INQ, 96, exp. 2, fol. 22v. Elena confirms her father's curiosity, saying that "su padre era tan curioso que cualquiera cosa sentaba"; AHN, INQ, 96, exp. 14, fol. 15v.

63 María Sánchez de la Rosa and Juan de Tordesillas confirmed the acceptance of the heritage of Pedro Sánchez de la Rosa before a notary in Getafe, October 24, 1667: "y firmó el dicho Juan de Tordesillas y la dicha María Rosa no sabe firmar, de ello doi fee"; ARCHV, EJECUTORIAS, C. 3146,19, p. 10.

64 On Isaac Hollandus, see Annelies van Gijsen.

65 Included in the general inventory and the in apothecary's, AHN, INQ, 96, exp. 2, fol. 32r, fol. 38v–39r.

66 For example, melon seeds appear as a component of sweet electuaries (Norri 780), and are listed in pharmaceutical texts as one of the four major

cold seeds. Furthermore, some chymical medicines were prepared with distilled water of melon seeds or other cold seeds.

67 "Bebida que se hace de pepitas de melón y calabaza, con algunas almendras, todo machacado y exprimido con agua, y sazonado con azúcar. Dixose assi quasi Hordeata, porque las más veces se hace con agua de cebada" (*Dicc. Aut.* 177,1).

68 To clarify this connection, the *Diccionario de Autoridades* establishes a similarity between glovers and perfumers: given that gloves were scented, both engaged in distributing scents and fragrances.

69 "Poma: A little small box full of holes to carry perfumes in to smell to" (Stevens 312).

70 "Aviendo visto la relación de todos los votos y la declaración que ace dicho maestro boticario de todos ellos, somos de parecer que aunque los más, según la declaración de dicho maestro sean útiles en la medicina para fines medicinales y saludables, pero mirado el conjunto, y la persona en que se allaron, y los que declara dicho maestro ignorar su utilidad y fin para que sean, y principalmente los dos, en que se allaron escapias y el yerro, los otros en que se allaron plumas, la piedra yman y el antimonio, dicho conjunto es sospechoso vehementemente de ser apresado para maleficios y echiços, y otras obras supersticiosas. Así lo sentimos en este monasterio de la Victoria de Madrid"; AHN, INQ, 96, exp. 3, fol. 68v.

71 "Pedazos de vidrio blanco con unas peluças dentro juntas con vascosidad de muy mal olor y muy frío del tamaño de un real de a ocho"; AHN, INQ, 96, exp. 3, fol. 90v.

72 ARCHV, EJECUTORIAS, C. 3146,19.

WORKS CITED

Arredondo, Martin. *Verdadero examen de cirugia: recopilado de diversos autores: teorica y practica de toda la cirugia y anotomia con consultas muy utiles para medicos y cirujanos*. Madrid, por Iosep Fernandez de Buendia, 1674.

Boix y Moliner, Miguel Marcelino. *Hippocrates Aclarado*. Blas de Villanueva, 1716.

Boyle, Margaret E. *Unruly Women: Performance, Penitence and Punishment in Early Modern Spain*. U of Toronto P, 2014.

Broomhall, Susan. *Women's Medical Work in Early Modern France*. Manchester UP, 2004.

Cabré, Montserrat, and Teresa Ortiz-Gómez. "Mujeres y salud: Prácticas y saberes. Presentación." *Dynamis*, vol. 19, 1999, pp. 17–24.

– editors. *Sanadoras, matronas y médicas en Europa. Siglos XII–XX*. Icaria Editorial, 2001.

Cohen, Elizabeth S. "She Said, He Said: Situated Oralities in Judicial Records from Early Modern Rome." *Journal of Early Modern History* vol. 16, no. 4–5, 2012, pp. 403–30.

Cruz, Anne, and Rosalie Hernández, editors. *Women's Literacy in Early Modern Spain and the New World*. Ashgate, 2011.

Davis, James C., and Isabel Burdiel. *El otro, el mismo: Biografía y autobiografía en Europa (siglos XVII–XX)*. Universitat de Valéncia, 2005.

Evans, Jennifer, and Sara Read. *Maladies and Medicine: Exploring Health and Healing, 1540–1740*. Pen & Sword History, 2017.

Fissell, Mary. "Introduction: Women, Health, and Healing in Early Modern Europe." *Bulletin of the History of Medicine*, vol. 82, no. 1, Spring 2008, pp. 1–17.

Fragoso, Juan. *Cirugía universal*. Alcalá de Henares, en casa de viuda de Juan Gracián, 1608.

Guardia Herrero, Carmen de la. "La Sala de Alcaldes de Casa y Corte: Un estudio social." *Investigaciones Históricas: Época Moderna y Contemporánea*, vol. 14, 1994, pp. 35–64.

Harkness, Deborah. "A View from the Streets: Women and Medical Work in Elizabethan London." *Bulletin of the History of Medicine*, vol. 82, no. 1, Spring 2008, pp. 52–8.

Kinzelbach, Annemarie. "Women and Healthcare in Early Modern German Towns." *Renaissance Studies*, vol. 28, no. 4, 2014, pp. 619–38.

Klein, Ursula, and Emma C. Spary, editors. *Materials and Expertise in Early Modern Europe: Between Market and Laboratory*. U of Chicago P, 2009.

Klein, Ursula, and Wolfgang Lefèvre. *Materials in Eighteenth-Century Science: A Historical Ontology*. MIT P, 2007.

Laguna, Andrés. *Pedacio Dioscorides Anazarbeo*. Domingo Fernández de Arrojo, 1733.

Lanza, Janine M. "Women and Work." *The Ashgate Research Companion to Women and Gender in Early Modern Europe*, edited by Allyson Poska et al., Routledge, 2013, pp. 279–96.

Leong, Elaine. "'Herbals She Peruseth': Reading Medicine in Early Modern England." *Renaissance Studies*, vol. 28, no. 4, 2014, pp. 556–78.

– "Making Medicines in the Early Modern Household." *Bulletin of the History of Medicine*, vol. 82, no. 1, Spring 2008, pp. 145–68.

– *Recipes and Everyday Knowledge: Medicine, Science and the Household in Early Modern England*. U of Chicago P, 2018.

Leong, Elaine, and Sarah Pennell. "Recipe Collections and the Currency of Medical Knowledge in the Early Modern 'Medical Marketplace.'" *Medicine and the Market in England and its Colonies, 1450–1850*, edited by Mark Jenner and Patrick Wallis, Palgrave, 2007, pp. 133–52.

Lindemann, Mary. *Medicine and Society in Early Modern Europe*. 2nd ed., Cambridge UP, 2010.

López Barahona, Victoria. "La caza de vagabundas: Trabajo y reclusión en Madrid durante la Edad Moderna." *La prisión y las instituciones punitivas en la investigación histórica*, edited by Pedro Oliver Olmo and Jesús Carlos Urda Lozano. Ediciones de la Universidad de Castilla-La Mancha, 2014, pp. 31–48.

– *Las trabajadoras en la sociedad madrileña del siglo XVIII*. Madrid, ACCI ediciones, 2017.

López Terrada, María Luz, and Carolin Schmitz. "Licencias sociales para sanar: La construcción como expertos de salud de curanderas y curanderos en la Castilla del Barroco." *Studia Historica: Historia Moderna*, vol. 40, no. 2, 2018, pp. 143–75.

Martínez Galindo, Gema. *Galerianas, corrigendas y presas: nacimiento y consolidación de las cárceles de mujeres en España, 1608–1913*. Madrid, Ed. Edisofer, 2002.

Martínez Vidal, Àlvar, and José Pardo Tomás. "Un siglo de controversias. La medicina Española de los novatores a la Ilustración." *La ilustración y las ciencias. Para una historia de la objetividad*, edited by J.L. Barona et al., Universitat de València, 2003, pp. 107–35.

Mercado, Luis. *Libri duo de communi et peculiari praesidiorum artis medicae*. Valladolid, Diego Fernández de Córdoba, 1574.

Minuzzi, Sabrina. "'Quick to say Quack': Medicinal Secrets from the Household to the Apothecary's Shop in Eighteenth-Century Venice." *Social History of Medicine*, vol. 32, no. 1, February 2019, pp. 1–13.

Newman, William R., and Lawrence M. Principe. "Alchemy vs Chemistry: The Etymological Origins of a Historiographic Mistake." *Early Science and Medicine*, vol. 3, no. 1, 1998, pp. 32–65.

Norri, Juhani. *Dictionary of Medical Vocabulary in English, 1375–1550: Body Parts, Sicknesses, Instruments, and Medicinal Preparations*. Routledge, 2018.

Nummedal, Tara. "Alchemical Reproduction and the Career of Anna Maria Zieglerin." *Ambix*, vol. 48, no. 2, 2001, 56–68.

Ortiz, Teresa. "From Hegemony to Subordination: Midwives in Early Modern Spain." *The Art of Midwifery: Early Modern Midwives in Europe*, edited by Hilary Marland, Routledge, 1994, pp. 95–114.

Pablo Gafas, José Luis de. *Justicia, gobierno y policía en la Corte de Madrid: La Sala de Alcaldes de Casa y Corte (1583–1834)*. Universidad Autónoma de Madrid, 2000.

Pardo Tomás, José. *El médico en la Palestra. Diego Mateo Zapata (1664–1745) y la ciencia moderna en España*. Junta de Castilla y León, 2004.

Pardo Tomás, José, and Àlvar Martínez Vidal. "Medicine and the Spanish Novator Movement: Ancients vs. Moderns, and Beyond." *Más allá de la Leyenda Negra: España y la Revolución Científica. Beyond the Black Legend: Spain and the Scientific Revolution*, edited by Victor Navarro Bortóns and William Eamon, Universidad de Valéncia, 2007, pp. 323–44.

– "Stories of Disease Written by Patients and Lay Mediators in the Spanish Republic of Letters (1680–1720)." *Journal of Medieval and Early Modern Studies*, vol. 38, no. 3, 2008, pp. 467–91.

Pelling, Margaret, editor. *The Common Lot: Sickness, Medical Occupations and the Urban Poor in Early Modern England*. Longman, 1998.

– *Medical Conflicts in Early Modern London: Patronage, Physicians, and Irregular Practitioners 1550–1640*. Clarendon Press, 2003.

– "Older Women and the Medical Role." *Women, Science and Medicine, 1500–1700: Mothers and Sisters of the Royal Society*, edited by Lynette Hunter and Sarah Hutton, Sutton Publishing, 1997, pp. 63–88.

Rankin, Alisha. *Panaceia's Daughters: Noblewomen as Healers in Early Modern Germany*. U of Chicago P, 2013.

Ray, Meredith. *Daughters of Alchemy, Women and Scientific Culture in Early Modern Italy*. Harvard UP, 2015.

Roche, Daniel, editor. *Journal de ma vie: Jacques-Louis Ménétra, compagnon vitrier au 18e siècle*. Montalba, 1982.

Sarti, Raffaella. *Vida en familia: Casa, comida y vestido en la Europa moderna*. Crítica, 2003.

Sgobbi, Antonio de. *Universale theatro farmaceutico*. Presso Paolo Baglioni, 1682.

Society of Gentlemen in Scotland: *Encyclopædia Britannica; Or a Dictionary of Arts and Sciences, compiled upon a new plan*. Vol. 3, Bell and Macfarquhar, 1771.

Stevens, John. *A New Spanish and English Dictionary: Collected from the Best Spanish Authors, both Ancient and Modern*. London, Printed for George Sawbridge, 1706.

Stolberg, Michael. "Learning from the Common Folks: Academic Physicians and Medical Lay Culture in the Sixteenth Century." *Social History of Medicine*, vol. 27, no. 4, 2014, pp. 649–67.

Storey, Tessa. "Face Waters, Oils, Love Magic and Poison: Making and Selling Secrets in Early Modern Rome." *Secrets and Knowledge in Medicine and Science, 1500–1800*, edited by Elaine Leong and Alisha Ranking, Ashgate, 2011, pp. 143–63.

Strocchia, Sharon T. "Introduction. Women and Health Care in Early Modern Europe." *Renaissance Studies*, vol. 28, no. 4, 2014, 496–514.

Tausiet, María. *Ponzoña en los ojos: Brujería y superstición en Aragón en el siglo xvi*, Turner, 2004.

Terreros y Pando, Esteban de. *Diccionario castellano con las voces de ciencias y artes y sus correspondientes en las tres lenguas francesa, Latina e italiana* [...]. Viuda de Ibarra, 1786.

van Gijsen, Annelies. "Isaac Hollandus Revisited." *Chymia: Science and Nature in Medieval and Early Modern Europe*, edited by Miguel López-Pérez et al., Cambridge Scholars Publishing, 2010, pp. 310–30.

Villa, Esteban de. *Examen de boticarios*. Burgos, por Pedro de Huydobro, 1632.
Diccionario de autoridades. Real Academia Española, 1737.
Whaley, Leigh. *Women and the Practice of Medical Care in Early Modern Europe, 1400–1800*. Palgrave Macmillan, 2011.
Zapata, Diego Mateo. *Crisis médica sobre el antimonio*. Madrid: s.n., 1701.
Zemon Davis, Natalie. *Mujeres de los márgenes: Tres vidas del siglo XVII*. Cátedra, 1999.
– "Women in Crafts in Sixteenth-Century Lyon." *Feminist Studies*, vol. 8, no. 1, 1982, pp. 47–80.

Chapter Two

Killer Skin Care: Gender and Venereal Disease Experiences in Colonial Lima

KATHLEEN M. KOLE DE PERALTA

In April 1537, angry red sores and blisters covered Diego Almagro's skin. *Bubas*, a disease that manifested itself with these physical markers, imperilled Almagro's health and military strategy. En route to Cuzco via Vilcas, "allí [Diego Almagro] se cayó enfermo y estuvo a punto de muerte de bubas y dolores, y estuvo allí veinte o veinte cuatro dias" ("there he [Diego Almagro] fell ill and almost died from *bubas* and pain. He stayed there twenty or twenty-four days").[1] It is possible that Almagro's health ailments can be connected to his hesitation in attacking his rivals, the Pizarristas, supporters of the Pizarro brothers (Espinar 206; Stewart 412). Within a year, Almago was dead, but not because he carried *bubas*. He met a violent end, garroted by the Pizarristas.

Diego Almagro was a key player in the Spanish Conquest of Peru, yet most historical narratives gloss over his sexually transmitted infection and the *bubas* outbreak across the Pacific coast and Cuzco in 1530–1 (Tanteleán Arbulú 1171). Yet, sex is a sidebar for the Spanish conquistador. The same cannot be said for "La Malinche" (aka Marina or Malintzin), maligned for betraying Mexico's indigenous peoples by allying with Hernando Cortés and bearing his child (Townsend 6). Both Almagro and Malinche feature prominently in conquest narratives, but we remember them quite differently. Whether a colonial chronicle or quotidian account, gender informs both colonial experience as well as how we remember the past.

This essay posits that local healing practices matter within the larger field of medical history. Medical, municipal, and bureaucratic records from sixteenth-century Lima, Peru, reveal gendered and racialized responses to certain medical practices. Iberian men ran Lima's principal health-care institutions. They regulated Lima's medical trades through the office of the Royal Protomedicato, overseeing hospitals and pharmacies and Lima's university medical curriculum.[2] I argue that local responses to venereal disease demonstrate that Iberian men leveraged their race, gender, and education to assert a medical authority over women and peoples of African and indigenous descent. My argument builds on a discussion of the historiography, the history of early modern *bubas*, common medical therapies, the racialized and gendered reactions to lethal drug use, and hospital care for *bubas*. In short, we cannot understand health in the early modern Iberian world without examining the intersection between gender, medicine, and power.

Historiography

Medical histories on venereal disease increased in the late twentieth century. During the 1990s, disease historians, inspired by the similarities between the epidemic stages in syphilis and AIDS, dedicated more research to syphilis. Both are sexually transmitted infections, spread quickly, and were perceived "as a foreign disease which was contracted by (the promiscuous, drug users, and homosexuals) ... labeled as outsiders" (Petrie 4).

Within the medical history corpus, most authors stop short of integrating colonial Latin America. Despite syphilis's global reach in the early modern era, the majority of the secondary scholarship focuses on the European experience, especially England, Austria, and Germany (Petrie; Quétel; Stein; Siena; Jütte; and McGough). There are surprisingly fewer studies on early modern Spain and Latin America (Berco, Tello, and Ternaux-Compans). While several medical histories of Peru discuss *bubas*, only two provide extensive detail (Valdizán and Maldonado; Instituto de Estudios Histórico-Marítimos del Peru; Barrionuevo; Sociedad Peruana de Historia de Medicina). The first is an 1829 pamphlet on Arequipa that discusses mercury's healing properties (Ternaux-Compans). The second, a medical thesis, examines the linguistic history of syphilis in the indigenous Quechua and Aymara languages and its role in religious beliefs, practices, and superstitions (Tello).

This chapter aligns with more recent medical histories that contend disease is best understood in a local context. For example, Pablo Gómez's *The Experiential Caribbean* argues that black ritual healers in the Caribbean developed evidence-based medicine using sensorial experience rather than dogma. Following the work of Gómez and others, this essay uses hospital and town council records to examine colonial Lima. Here, endemic disease provides a pathway to examine local disease experiences.

Muddled Origins and Misinterpretations

At the end of the fifteenth century, a strange and dangerous disease known as "the pox" spread across Europe, from Italy to Austria. Its origins baffled physicians, who named multiple culprits including Christopher Columbus's recently returned crew from Hispaniola and Italian prostitutes interloping with French mercenaries during the Italian Wars (1494–1530) (Hayton 82; Petrie 2). While its origins remain inconclusive, undoubtedly the movement of merchants, soldiers, and sailors around Europe and the Americas during this period facilitated the infection's spread. Depending on the population, the disease went by a variety of names, including, "the French disease," "the great pox," "the Neapolitan sickness," "the Spanish illness," the *pudendagra* in Spain, or *bubas* in Peru (Quétel 20; Tarlach).

Treating venereal disease relied on a two-pronged approach addressing body and soul. Tending to the body, licensed physicians emigrated from Spain to Lima throughout the sixteenth century. The University of San Marcos opened in 1551 but lacked the funding for medical chairs until 1568 (Delgado Matallana 18). Without them, the university could not award medical degrees (Newson 28). Whether educated in Spain or Lima, local physicians were trained in Galenic medicine.[3] As treatment progressed, physicians might prescribe more intensive therapies that expelled fluids and thereby warmed and dried the humours.

Within this medical world view, different personalities experienced diseases differently, which also created problems diagnosing *bubas*. Physicians identifying and describing the disease noted that pustules could vary in size, shape, smell, and colour, and they explained these discrepancies by reasoning that the same illness could look different depending on whether or not an individual were sanguine, choleric, melancholic, or phlegmatic. For example, the 1500 treatise by Spanish writer Torella noted that some pustules were small and yellowish (an excess of yellow bile), others large and white (an excess of phlegm), and some were black (Stein 634).

Healing necessitated physical and spiritual interventions. Like Renaissance counterparts in Spain and Italy, Lima's hospitals all contained a chapel and many exhibited cruciform architecture (Henderson). Hospitals staffed priests who visited patients, heard confessions, and assisted with wills, testaments, and the last rites. Many early modern medical and theological writers assumed the disease was divine punishment for sins such as sex with prostitutes, sex out of wedlock, and sodomy (Berco 31). Repentance paved the road to recovery. Physicians and priests instructed syphilitics to turn away from lustful behaviour.

And when "cured" patients relapsed, physicians often blamed a moral lapse, rather than ineffective medicine (Berco 49). An Inquisition record about a prisoner with *bubas* wrote that the man got sicker until he was transferred to a hospital. There he confessed his sins and cured the disease (Medina, 235). As these experiences convey, disease causation could be a moving target.

Labelling specific diseases proved imprecise as well. Colonial authors and medical manuals incorrectly applied the word *bubas* to a range of medical symptoms. These observations often conflated, confused, and mislabelled diseases (Berco 22; McGough 10). For example, physicians might diagnose *bubas* due to a burning sensation while urinating when it was actually gonorrhoea (Petrie 5).[4] And while the medical term "syphilis" first appeared in 1530, it was not widely adopted for several centuries (McGough 10; Jütte 97). Furthermore, without archaeological corroboration, it is only possible to know how individuals labelled an illness. Therefore, this essay does not investigate syphilis or gonorrhoea specifically. Instead, it examines how women processed venereal disease's social and biological consequences.

Killer Skin Care

Before analysing women's navigation of venereal disease, it's important to take stock of the "treatments" inflicted on patients in colonial Latin America. Indeed, many medical treatments for *bubas* were lethal in the end. Common therapies included sweating, coca leaf, mercury, sarsaparilla root, and guaiacum. Sweating required the patient to cover up with many layers of clothing, and blankets to expel the "corrupt matter" (Grigsby 158). Sometimes patients would sit in a small room with a fire, and place medicinal plants or mercury over the flames. Other texts describe a warm room, blankets as cover, and a drink of the water of sarsaparilla root (see figures 3 and 4). Sweating out venereal and other diseases represented a long-standing medical tradition inherited from Europe. By contrast, coca leaf's medicinal properties were new to European physicians. An eighteenth-century medical student reported on the use of coca leaf powders mixed with sarsaparilla root water to treat "el morbo venero" (Unanue 258). Patients consumed the mixture and used it to wash their sores. They also mixed coca water into an unguent and applied it to the skin (Unanue 258).

Mercury, one of the most popular treatments, literally poisoned the patient. Mercury treatment came in the form of vapours, ointments, unction, and pastes. Because physicians classified the pox as an imbalance of wet and cold humours, mercury offered an antidote by

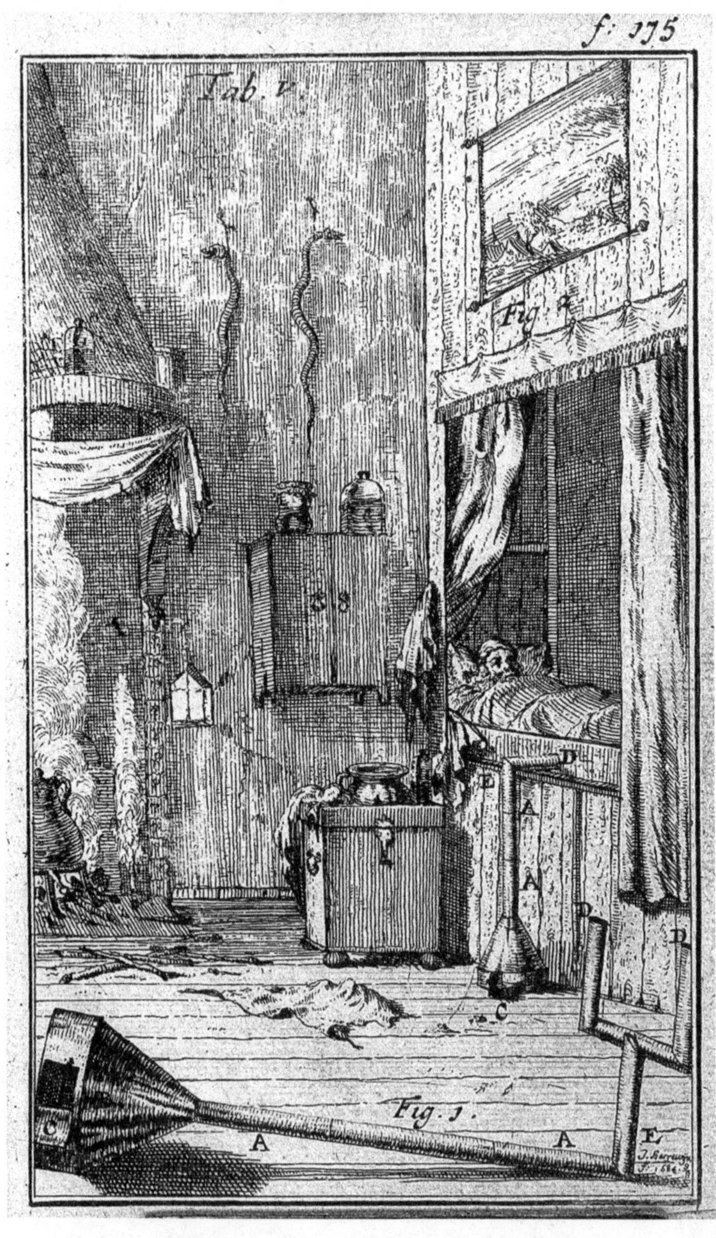

Figure 3. Sweating treatment for syphilis, first method: patient in bed over a hot pipe. Drawing by J. Harrewijns. Wellcome Collection.

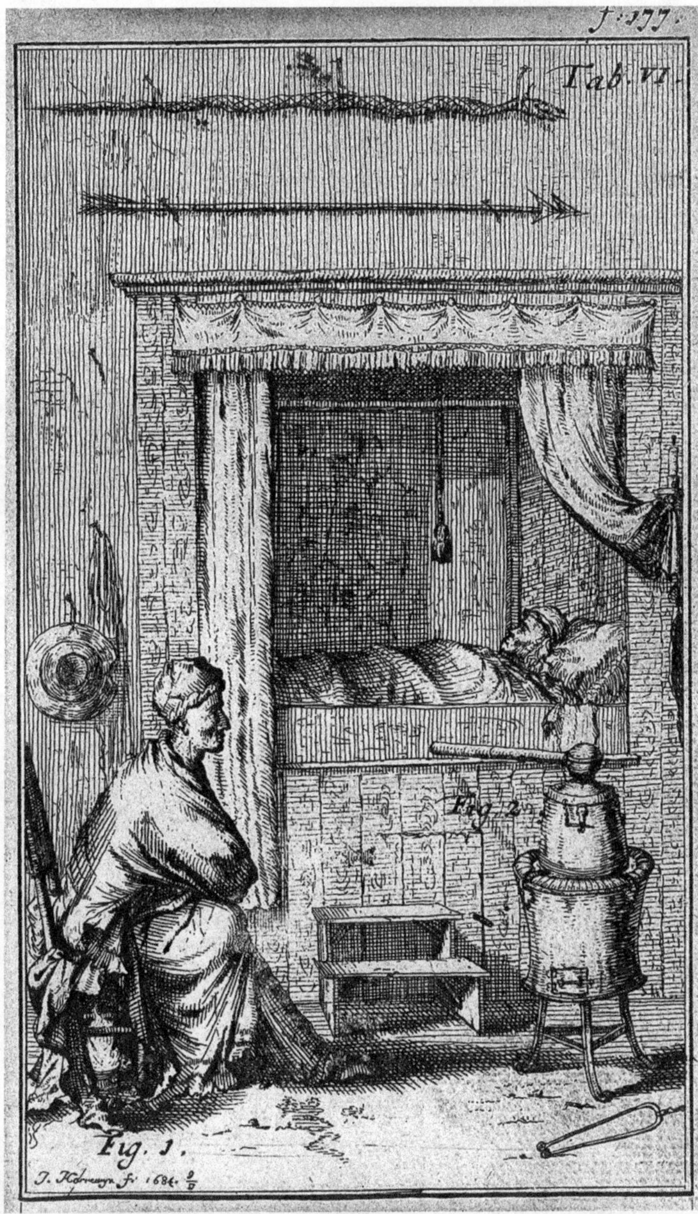

Figure 4. Sweating treatment for syphilis, second method: patient wrapped in sheet and blanket sits on a chair beneath which is a flaming spirit stove (Fig. 1), then gets into bed (Fig. 2). Drawing by J. Harrewijns. Wellcome Collection.

warming and drying the body. In any form it induced sweating, vomiting, and diarrhoea. With continued doses, patients might experience itchiness, incontinence, haemorrhoids, fever, insomnia, and black teeth. As Mary Lindemann writes, "Mercury corroded the membranes of the mouth, loosened teeth in their sockets, and even ate away jawbones, often turning the mouth and throat into one large stinking ulcer" (70). These outcomes were unpleasant, but in humoral terms they served their purpose: expelling bad humours.

Guaiacum and sarsaparilla root, found in the Americas, were lethal in the sense that they did not actually cure the disease. To prepare guaiacum, nurses mixed the greenish-brown resin from the guaiacum tree, also called holywood, into potions that patients drank in copious amounts (Jütte 108). The tea made from its bark also induced the sweating needed to satisfy medicinal practices based on humoral theory (Berco 101). Physicians believed the concoction thinned the humours, making them easier to expel, and that it alleviated secondary symptoms (Stein 632; Berco 102). Sarsaparilla was prepared as a drink and as an infusion and applied to skin lesions and ulcers. It is a mild antimicrobial and eases joint pain. Other uses called for placing sarsaparilla on a brazier and asking patients to inhale the fumes (Berco 102). If patients could afford it, they combined multiple therapies. But because they were unable to actually cure venereal disease, patients ultimately died from the disease, the treatment, or other causes.

Anyone with the disease might face a painful and ugly death. Without proper treatment, patients typically experienced four stages of decline, each with distinct physical markers. In the first stage, a single sore usually appeared around the site of infection (the genitals, anus, or mouth). During the second stage (two to eight weeks later), a rash appeared accompanied by spots on the soles of the feet and palms of the hands. Other symptoms included fever, headaches, fatigue, muscle ache, loss of appetite, sore throat, enlarged lymph nodes, and wart-like patches. During the third stage (two to six weeks), the symptoms subsided and the disease went dormant. When this happened, patients believed they were cured. But the absence of physical signs only belied the onset of a furious decline. In its final stage (ten to thirty years after the initial infection), the disease wreaked havoc on the skin, organs, bones, and nervous system. The infection eroded the cranium and tibia, causing limping or other paralysis. Facial cartilage disintegrated, collapsing the nose. Skin erupted into blisters and pustules. Chunks of hair fell out in patches. In fact, nicknames such as *el pelon* and *la pelona* (the bald man or bald woman) described those suffering from *bubas* (Berco 31).

Gender and Venereal Disease in Lima

Men and women experienced their illness within a larger Iberian context that combined medical knowledge, sin, and gendered notions of honour (Harrison 59–60). The miasma theory and the theory of four humours held that daily environmental interactions determined well-being, and that different sexes had different needs (Myers 483; Paster 8–9). Female body functions and emissions including menstruation, lactation, sweat, tears, and internal heat distinguished their bodies from men (Feerick 21 and 62). When compared to men, women possessed less heat, which theoretically made them weaker and more emotional, and fed into cultural constructions of inequality (Harvey 27; Howard 65; Socolow 75; Presta 47–9).

Early modern Christian medical knowledge travelled with Iberians to Peru, meaning that diseases were often associated with immoral/sinful behaviour (Johnson 108). Moreover, these diseases provided clues about their root cause. For example, venereal diseases like syphilis left sores around the genitals. In Peru, an old saying captured in a twentieth-century medical review declares "Males bubas te de dios" ("God gave you the *bubas* plight"; Sociedad Peruana de Historia de la Medicina 103). This combined with cultural constructions of honour meant that venereal disease undermined individual (especially female) and familial honour. Honour often refers to "reputation," which comprised status, virtue, and sexual restraint. While the term was used to qualify a person's character, the term must be used with caution. Its application was never absolute, and could be negotiated (Twinam 33).

Gender permeated Lima's health-care system. Venereal disease socially stigmatized women from diverse racial and economic backgrounds and cast aspersions on their virtue. Iberian honour encompassed a number of ideas such as sexual purity, discretion, and public behaviour (Socolow 84). Yet few women, on either side of the Atlantic, adhered ubiquitously to a sexual hegemony (Poska 40). Allyson Poska shows that class and ethnicity were more likely to shape expectations for women's behaviour, writing that whereas "aristocratic women were expected to remain chaste (although they often did not), lower class women could maintain their honor through hard work, honesty, and self-reliance, their chastity notwithstanding" (40). Like other colonial Latin American towns, Lima's women "may have understood and strategically employed the rhetoric of honor, but their lives did not conform to its ideals" (40).

Infected women and caregivers were prohibited from working with food because of the misconception that disease could be transmitted through physical contact with the ill themselves, their clothing, utensils, etc. On 9 January 1551, Sebastián Sánchez de Merlo, a municipal *procurador*, denounced Antonio Ramos's wife because she worked both as a baker and a health-care provider. In fact, town council records indicate several women found themselves in this position: "tantas españolas como negras, que tenían el negocio de hacer pasteles y pan cocido se descuidaban con la hygiene y los amasaban al tiempo que se ocupaban del cuidado de los enfermos de bubas" ("so many Spanish women, just like black women, bake bread and pastries but lack basic hygiene because they knead dough at the same time they cared for *bubas* patients"; Pons 26). Fears over cross-contamination shaped public health policies that restricted women from moving between medical and non-medical occupations.

Women with knowledge of mercury's medical and cosmetic properties undermined a social fabric that normalized everyday racism and misogyny. In 1551, town council records made an unusual comment, noting that local apothecaries were selling powerful drugs such as mercury and red arsenic of sulphate without a prescription. The entry revealed that "algunas mugeres y esclavas han tomado solimán y muertose con ello lo qual por ventura se oviera escusado sino se vendiese tan comúnmente el dicho solimán y otras cosas mortiferas para hevitar los dichos males y ynconvenientes" ("some women and female slaves have taken mercuric chloride and died, which might have been overlooked if it were not for the widespread sales of mercury and other fatal [medicines] used to avoid illness and inconveniences").[5] The death of several women was certainly a problem, but the targeted language about race, gender, and pharmaceutical sales suggests something else was at play, too. The town council's response intimates a colonial hierarchy that favoured elite white Iberian men.

Women with medical knowledge of mercury endangered Lima's racial hierarchy and authority of male medical practitioners. Its use highlights racial tensions especially between Lima's black female population and white Iberians. For one, mercury lightened the skin (Berco 31 and 81). While it could not dramatically change one's skin tone, the possibility threatened racial categories. Furthermore, the town council doubted black and indigenous could even handle dangerous drugs. After this incident, Lima's town council banned *mestizo* and African pharmacy assistants from preparing prescriptions and prohibited over-the-counter sales of mercuric chloride, red sulphate arsenic, or any other lethal drug.[6] Only men, women, and slaves, at least fifteen years old and with a prescription in hand, could purchase these medicines. Twenty years later in April 1572, the town council reiterated a similar version of this policy when it forbade black and indigenous peoples from purchasing mercury in a pharmacy, working in one, or even stepping foot inside.[7] Town councilmen reasoned that "la arte de boticarios require mucha ciencia e habilidad e fidelidad lo cual no puede haberse en los dichos negros ni indios" ("the art of pharmacy requires a lot of science, aptitude, and responsibility, which cannot be found in blacks or indigenous peoples").[8] Social conventions relegated control over mercury's proper use to a small group of educated, white medical professionals (Snook 32).

The town council record provides one more clue about female disease experiences in Lima. Allegedly, the victims were treating "inconveniences."[9] Venereal diseases were about as socially damning as any disease could be. If, by chance, these women experienced an illness deemed not to be linked with gender or sexuality, it is likely the town council would have identified the problem with a precise term like *peste* (pestilence). Their records, after all, are full of references to specific illnesses. "Inconvenience" erases the medical vocabulary and replaces it with a social problem. Furthermore, the women circumvented traditional medical channels by making purchases without a prescription. It is unclear if they did this because they possessed sufficient medical knowledge of mercury or because cultural norms dictated clandestine actions.

Bubas in Hospitals

Hospitals upheld the medical authority of Iberian men and preserved the honour of female patients. They institutionalized *bubas* care and the primacy of Iberian scholastic medicine. Hospitals employed Iberian medical professionals like physicians, barbers, and surgeons. They in turn relied on a staff comprising nurses, assistants, and chefs. Women facing economic uncertainty or changes in social or health status relied on hospitals to weather difficult times (Lindemann 178). Lima's first hospitals accepted people from all backgrounds, but over time the addition of new facilities allowed each institution to become more specialized (see table 1). Founded in 1559 and erected in 1596, Hospital San Cosme y San Damián de la Hermandad de Santa María became the first hospital dedicated to the care of women and orphans. (It was later renamed Hospital de la Caridad.) Social and physical welfare coalesced in these institutions.

Hospital de la Caridad provided medical and social services to Lima's women and orphans. In Hospital de la Caridad "se curan por año mucho numero de mujeres honradas, pobres, y honestas porque no hay

Table 1. Hospital Foundations in Lima, 1538–1669 (Kole de Peralta)

Hospital	Founded	Clientele	Additional details
Nuestra Señora de la Concepción	1538		Merged with Hospital Santa Ana in 1549
San Andrés	1549	Spanish men	
Santa Ana	1549	Indigenous men and women	
La Caridad	1559	Spanish and mestiza women	Also a place for divorcees and widows
San Lázaro	1563	Lepers	
Espíritu Santo	1575	Sailors	Physician on staff visited mariners' wives and children at home
San Toribio	1589	Indigenous men and women	Opened in response to a smallpox epidemic
San Juan de Dios (Hospital San Pedro)	1594	Clergymen	Used as a depository for prisoners
San Diego	1598	Convalescing men	
Santa Cruz	1603	Orphans	
San Bartolomé	1646	Slaves and free blacks	Used by slaveowners as a depository for free black men and women who could no longer work
Santa Cruz de Atocha	1649	Female orphans/ abandoned children	
Santo Refugio de Incurables	1669	Invalids, the chronically ill, and the elderly	

otro hospital dónde se puedan curar mujeres en esta ciudad y dan cría y se crían muchos niños a que no se les conocen" (they cure a large number of honourable, poor, and honest women annually. And those women care for and raise children who they do not know).[10] This facility also housed divorced and abandoned women (van Deusen 66).

Like facilities in Toledo, Spain, and Mexico City, Lima's hospitals also treated *bubas* patients (Socolow 132; Berco 23 and 72). *Bubas* care appealed to urban men and women from different economic and ethnic backgrounds. In 1591, Hospital San Andrés' founder and administrator, Francisco de Molina, reported that there were twenty patients ill with *bubas* in the unction infirmary.[11] Hospital La Caridad had among its staff a specialist for the disease and someone to "administer plasters and ointments" (Warren 46). And Hospital Santa Ana's staff treated *bubas* with both mercury unction and sarsaparilla.[12] Records from the seventeenth century reveal that Hospital San Andrés's and Santa Ana's *mayordomo* stocked mercuric oxide for its *bubas* patients.[13] Medical historian Linda Newson found that *solimán* (mercuric chloride) could be purchased from local shops and was "quite widely employed in the form of unctions to treat syphilis, which in the Hospital of Santa Ana were applied by African slaves" (181).

Hospital Nuestra Señora de Atocha's discretion aided post-partum women to maintain privacy and their reputation, concepts that wove into local understandings of female honour. Hospital Atocha received orphans and abandoned children anonymously.[14] In 1649, Atocha's founder, Luis Pescador, installed a turnstile door for that purpose. This way, mothers would be less likely to abandon the child out in the open. According to witnesses, before the hospital existed, people dumped babies in trash heaps, into irrigation canals, or onto the doorways of religious institutions. Unfortunately, exposed infants were sometimes eaten by stray dogs and pigs if found by them first.[15] The pattern of women abandoning babies suggests serious circumstances for unmarried, pregnant women.

Hospital architecture further separated men and women into gendered spaces, each designed to cater to the specific and distinct needs of men and women. In Europe and Latin America, builders designed hospitals to improve patient health and establish social relations via the physical environment (Howe 63). Gender divisions became more common in Europe by the fifteenth century and were rooted in the theories of urban planners such as Leon Battista Alberti and Antonio Averlino. For example, Alberti's *On the Art of Building in Ten Books* advocates the division of patients according to illness and gender.

Physical separation safeguarded women physically and socially (Socolow 118). Before Hospital San Andrés's completion, Lima's archbishop called for hospitals to rigorously separate male and female spaces.[16] In 1549, a royal order underwrote construction with the understanding that there would be at least "[t]wo rooms, one for men and another for women, with a central patio in the entranceway, and large chambers for the reception of patients."[17] Eventually, these guidelines even encouraged women to cook their own food in their "cocina propia y separada para guisar la comida de las enfermas, de acuerdo con sus gustos y necesidades (muy bien aderezada), ya que las mujeres se acomodan mejor para hacer las viandas" ("own separate kitchen where the female patients can cook according to their tastes and needs [very well-seasoned], since they are better suited to make the food").[18]

San Andrés's layout catered to the gendered body by separating the women's infirmary, patio, and garden. Barring movement between male and female spaces preserved the reputation of the hospital and its patients. Hospital inspectors insisted that "Los enfermeros no pueden tener acceso alguno a la sala de mujeres, que cuenta para su servicio con una enfermera y sirvientes encargadas" (Male nurses will not have any access to the female ward, which is accounted for by the nurse and the servants in charge).[19] Only female nurses and slaves tended to female patients and cleaned their living quarters. For example, black women cleaned the bathroom and dispensed patient medications.[20] Similar rules governed Hospital Santa Ana, which had a separate women's infirmary, to be overseen by a Spanish woman, who was at least fourteen years old, prudent, careful, and able to manage the ward with the same discipline as the hospital's head nurse and wardrobe attendant.[21] According to the hospital's constitution, the space remained enclosed and guarded with a locked door ensuring that no man, regardless of ethnicity, nor indigenous women enter the infirmary without a licence from the physician or barber-surgeon.[22] These rules reinforced social norms regarding male and female interaction and safeguarded women's reputations.

Conclusion

In sixteenth-century Lima, Iberian men controlled the major medical channels: the Royal Protromedicato, hospitals, pharmacies, and University San Marcos. Yet, they were by no means the only ones with medical savvy. Women, indigenous people, and people of African descent possessed medical knowledge too. Hospitals presented less contentious spaces where hierarchies remained clear and orderly. Support staff like nurses, cooks, cleaners, and assistants deferred to Iberian medical practitioners. Within this infrastructure, physicians could properly oversee *bubas* treatments and prescribe therapies.

By contrast, *bubas* treatment outside of hospitals became subversive in the eyes of university-trained physicians. When non-licensed individuals handled lethal drugs like mercury and arsenic it threatened their medical authority. At stake was the question of who had the right to practise all levels of medicine. In the interest of preserving patriarchal and racial barriers to medical power, town councilmen restricted women, and black and indigenous peoples, from accessing lethal drugs and exercising coveted medical knowledge. This led to policies that blocked women and black and indigenous peoples from purchasing lethal medicines without a prescription and questioned their intellectual capacity to practice medicine.

NOTES

1 Manuel de Espinar, "Battle of Las Salinas" (15 June 1539) in Cabildo de Lima, *Libros de Cabildos de Lima* 1:206.

2 The Spanish crown depended on the Protomedicato to regulate, monitor, and adjudicate medical practice in Iberia and Latin America. The position held the power to resolve medical disputes, approve licences, and inspect pharmacies. Lima's first Protomedicato, Hernando Sepúlbeda, arrived in 1537.

3 See the introduction to this volume along with Mujica for an extended discussion of Galenic theory and practice.

4 For example, gonorrhoea's symptoms (burning urination, pain, pus, and swelling) were frequently labelled as "pox."

5 Cabildo de Lima, *Libros de Cabildos de Lima,* 4:416 (24 July 1551).

6 Ibid.

7 2 April 15 in *Libros de Cabildos* 7:270.

8 Ibid.

9 Ibid.

10 Here I translated *calidad* as "social status." AGI, Lima, 211, N.10, ff. 3r. "Información sobre la hospital de la Caridad" (15 February 1596).

11 Francisco de Molina, "Información y averiguaciones hechas del oficio en esta real audiencia de los reyes de la necesidad que tienen el hospital de los Españoles," in AGI Lima, 131, N. 1, f. 8r. (2 April 1591).

12 ABPL 9806 ff. 104–105 "Visita de Santa Ana sin fecha" [1588] cited in Newson and Minchin 247.

13 IRA, Maldonado, A-III-227 (1611–1612) and IRA, Maldonado, A-III-306, ff. 87r–109r.

14 AGI, Lima, 216, N. 11, "Informaciones: Hospital Nuestra Señora de Atocha de Lima" (1604).

15 Ibid.

16 "Real Cédula" (29 May 1559) in ibid., 32.

17 "En principio edificaron dos salas, una para hombres y otra para mujeres, con un patio principal de entrada, así como aposentos grandes para la recepción de los enfermos." "Las primeras ordenanzas" (1549), in Miguel Rabi-Chara, *Del Hospital de Santa Ana,* 41.

18 "Real Cédula," 3 July 1587 in Miguel Rabi-Chara, *Del Hospital de Santa Ana*, 72.

19 "Los enfermos no pueden tener acceso alguno a la sala de mujeres, que cuenta para su servicio con una enfermera y sirvientes encargadas." Ibid., 73.

20 "Reglas de funcionamiento," in ibid., 72.

21 Hosptial Real de Santa Ana, "Constituciones y ordenanzas del Hopsital Real de Santa Ana de Lima," s.f. in *Lima: Reimpresas, por decreteo de 29 Febrero 1778*, housed at the U.S. National Library of Medicine.

22 In ibid, s.f.

WORKS CITED

Berco, Cristian. *From Body to Community: Venereal Disease and Society in Baroque Spain*. U of Toronto P, 2015.

Cabildo de Lima. *Libros de Cabildos de Lima*.

Comisión para Escribir la Historia Marítima del Perú. *Historia marítima del Perú*. Instituto de Estudios Histórico-Marítimos del Perú, 1977.

Delgado Matallana, Gustavo. *Evolución de la Facultad de Medicina de San Fernando, Universidad Nacional Mayor de San Marcos*. Universidad de San Marcos, Facultad de Medicina, 2006.

Duthurburu, J.A. del Busto. *Historia marítima del Peru*, vo. 3. Lima: Editorial Ausonis, 1972.

Espinar, Manuel de. "Battle of Las Salinas (15 June 1539)." Cabildo de Lima, *Libros de Cabildos de Lima* 1:206, cited from Betram T. Lee and Juan Bromley, eds., *Libros de cabildos de Lima*, 23 vols., Concejo Provincial de Lima, 1935–62.

Feerick, Jean E. *Strangers in Blood: Relocating Race in the Renaissance*. U of Toronto P, 2010.

Grigsby, Bryon Lee. *Pestilence in Medieval and Early Modern English Literature*. Routledge, 2004.

Gómez, Pablo. *The Experiential Caribbean: Creating Knowledge and Healing in the Early Modern Atlantic*. U of North Carolina P, 2017.

Harrison, Regina. *Sin and Confession in Colonial Peru: Spanish-Quechua Penitential Texts, 1560–1650*. U of Texas P, 2014.

Harvey, Tamara. *Figuring Modesty in Feminist Discourse across the Americas*. Ashgate Publishing Limited, 2008

Hayton, Darin. "Joseph Grünpek's Astrological explanation of the French Disease." *Sins of the Flesh: Responding to Sexual Disease in Early Modern Europe*, U of Toronto P, 2005, pp. 81–108.

Henderson, John. *The Renaissance Hospital: Healing the Body and Healing the Soul*. Yale UP, 2006.

Htun, Mala. *Sex and the State: Abortion, Divorce, and the Family under Latin American Dictatorships and Democracies*. Cambridge UP, 2003.

Howard, Skiles. *The Politics of Courtly Dancing in Early Modern England*. U of Massachusetts P, 1998.

Howe, Eunice D. "The Architecture of Institutionalism: Women's Space in Renaissance Hospitals." *Architecture and the Politics of Gender in Early Modern*

Europe: Women and Gender in the Early Modern World, edited by Helen Hills, Ashgate Publishing Limited, 2003, pp. 63–82.

Johnson, Holly. "A Fifteenth-Century Sermon Enacts the Seven Deadly Sins." *Sin in Medieval and Early Modern Culture: The Tradition of the Seven Deadly Sins*, edited by Richard G. Newhauser and Susan J. Ridyard, York Medieval P, 2012, pp. 107–31.

Jütte, Robert. "Syphilis and Confinement Hospitals in Early Modern Germany." *Institutions of Confinement: Hospitals, Asylums, and Prisons in Western Europe and North America, 1500–1950*, edited by Norbert Finzsh and Robert Jütte, Cambridge UP, 1996, pp. 97–116.

Kent, Susan Kingsley. *Gender and Power in Britain, 1640–1990.* New York: Routledge, 1999.

Lastres, Juan. *Médicos y cirujanos de Pizarro y Almagro.* Universidad San Marcos, 1958.

Lindeman, Mary. *Medicine and Society in Early Modern Europe.* Cambridge UP, 2010.

McGough, Laura. *Gender, Sexuality, and Syphilis in Early Modern Venice: The Disease That Came to Stay.* Palgrave MacMillan, 2011.

Medina, José Toribio. *Historia del Tribunal del Santo oficio de la Inquisicion de Lima (1569–1820).* Imprenta Gutenberg, 1887.

Myers, Kathleen. "The Mystic Triad in Colonial Mexican Nuns' Discourse: Divine Author, Visionary Scribe and Clerical Mediator." *Colonial Latin American Historical Review*, vol. 6, no. 4, 1997, pp. 479–524.

Newson, Linda. *Making Medicines in Colonial Lima, Peru: Apothecaries, Science, and Society.* Brill, 2017.

Newson, Linda, and Susie Minchin. *From Capture to Sale: The Portuguese Slave Trade to Spanish South America.* Brill, 2007.

Paster, Gail Kern. *The Body Embarrassed: Drama and the Disciplines of Shame in Early Modern England.* Cornell UP, 1993.

Petrie, Hugh. *The French Pox: Concepts and Cures for Syphilis and Gonorrhea in the 16th and 17th century.* Stuart Press, 1999.

Pons, Frank Moya. *Lima El Cabildo y la vida local en el siglo XVI (1535–1553).* Editoria Coripio, 1985.

Poska, Allyson. "An Ocean Apart: Reframing Gender in the Spanish Empire." *Women of the Iberian Atlantic*, Louisiana State UP, 2012, pp. 37–56.

Presta, Ana María, "Doña Isabel Sisa, A Sixteenth-Century Indian Woman Resisting Inequalities." *The Human Tradition in Colonial Latin America*, edited by Kenneth J. Adrien, Rowman & Littlefield Publishers, Inc., 2013, pp. 47–62.

Quétel, Claude. *History of Syphilis.* Polity Press, 1990.

Schleiner, Winifried. "Moral Attitudes toward Syphilis and Its Prevention in the Renaissance." *Bulletin of the History of Medicine*, vol. 68, no. 3, 1994, pp. 389–410.

Scorr, Joan. "Gender: A Useful Category of Historical Analysis." *The American Historical Review*, vol. 91, no. 5, 1986, pp. 1043–75.

Siena, Kevin P. "Pollution, Promiscuity, and the Pox: English Venereology and the Early Modern Medical Discourse on Social and Sexual Danger." *Journal of the History of Sexuality*, vol. 8, no. 4, 1998, pp. 553–74.

Snook, Edit. *Women, Beauty and Power in Early Modern England: A Feminist Literary History*. Palgrave MacMillan, 2011.

Sociedad Peruana de Historia de la Medicina. *Anales de la Sociedad de Historia de la Medicina*, v. 6. Sociedad Peruana de Historia de la Medicina, 1944.

Socolow, Susan Migden. *The Women of Colonial Latin America*. Cambridge UP, 2000.

Stein, Claudia L'Engle. "The Meaning of Signs: Diagnosing the French Pox in Early Modern Augsburg." *Bulletin of the History of Medicine*, vol. 4, 2006, pp. 617–48.

Stewart, Paul. "The Battle of Las Salinas, Peru, and Its Historians." *The Sixteenth Century Journal*, vol. 19, no. 3, 1988, pp. 407–34.

Tantaleán Arbulú. *Pirú: La irrupción hispana y transición hacia el orden colonial (1532–1572)*. Vol. 3, Fondo Editorial del Congreso del Perú, 2002.

Tarlach, Gemma. "First Ancient Syphilis Genomes Reveal New History of the Disease," *Discover Magazine*, vol. 21, June 2018, http://blogs.discovermagazine.com/deadthings/2018/06/21/ancient-syphilis/#.W05G4VMvyRs.

Tello, Juan C. "Antigüedad de la sífilis en el Perú." B.A. thesis, Universidad Nacional de San Marcos, Lima, Peru, 1909.

Ternaux-Compans, Henri. *Influjo del clima y de la policia sobre el escsito de varias enferemedades reynantes en Arequipa*. Imprenta del Gobierno: administrada por Pedro Benavides, 1829.

Townsend, Camila. *Malintzin's Choices: An Indian Woman in the Conquest of Mexico*. U of Albuquerque P, 2006.

Twinam, Ann. *Public Lives, Private Secrets: Gender, Honor, Sexuality, and Illegitimacy in Colonial Spanish America*. Stanford UP, 1999.

Unanue, Joseph Hipolito. *Disertación sobre el aspecto, cultivo, comercio y virtudes de la famosa planta del Perú nombrada coca*. Imprenta Real de los Niños Huérfanos, 1794.

Valdizán, Hermillo y Angel Maldonado. *La medicina popular peruana*, v. 3. Torres Aguirre, 1922.

van Deusen, Nancy E. *Between the Sacred and the Worldly: The Institutional and Cultural Practice of "Recogimiento" in Colonial Lima*. Stanford UP, 2001.

Warren, Adam. *Medicine and Politics in Colonial Peru: Population Growth and the Bourbon Reforms*. U of Pittsburg P, 2010.

Chapter Three

Convent Medicine, Healing, and Hierarchy in Arequipa, Peru

SARAH E. OWENS

It is clear that Peruvian nuns spent considerable sums of money on drugs, medicines, and herbal remedies. They purchased simple syrups made of sugar and violets to treat diarrhoea; ointments composed of animal fats, wax, and resins to treat burns and skin infections; and purgatives made of rhubarb imported from China to induce vomiting. Nuns who were cloistered behind convent walls and separated from men are an interesting population to study because they actively sought out health care for their members. They relied on hybrid medical forms, including Galenic medicine and indigenous practices. Behind their convent walls lived a broad cultural milieu of society. From a servant class of indigenous and African descent to the black-veiled nuns of white European descent, this diverse group of women shared close quarters. Nuns across the Spanish Empire cultivated healing herbs in their convent gardens and bought ointments, powders, minerals, and pills to stock their medicine cabinets. Skilled nurses cared for sick nuns in convent infirmaries. They ground herbs using pestle and mortar, boiled roots in large vats, and steeped rosebuds, thistle, and orange blossoms into curative waters. They often turned to indigenous and African women who resided in the convent to help care for sick nuns and novices. When they could not obtain ingredients from their own gardens and orchards, they used convent funds to buy *materia medica* from local pharmacies and distributors. Abbesses, treasurers, and nurses kept meticulous records of all convent expenditures, including doctor visits, bloodletting from barber-surgeons, and money spent on food and medicines. Earthquakes, hurricanes, fires, and wartime upheaval destroyed countless documents and others were lost during the closing of many convents at the end of the nineteenth century, but there still remain a surprising number of convent ledgers, letters, and other documents in archives across Latin America and Spain. What the written records often leave blank, however, is the role of indigenous healing and ingredients used in treating religious women. To what extent did these women participate in convent healing and what types of local ingredients did they employ? Only from the interstices and vague references to home remedies within those documents can we surmise the usage of native plants and recipes in convent infirmaries (see figure 5).

This essay focuses on the infirmary ledgers and healing practices of three convents in Arequipa, Peru, during the late eighteenth century as a microcosm of convent health care and healing in colonial Latin America. Based on archival research surrounding the communities of Santa Catalina, Santa Rosa, and Santa Teresa, this essay explores how Peruvian nuns adopted pharmaceutical traditions from Europe (very few of the convent ledgers mention medicines from the Atlantic World), while at the same time it analyses how the nuns adapted to the strict reforms enacted by the Bourbon Crown of Spain during the latter half of the eighteenth century. Combined with an analysis of convent ledgers detailing medicines, ingredients, and prices recorded for each convent's medicine cabinet (*botica*), this essay also probes first-person letters written by one abbess between 1792 and 1801 about the ailments and requests of nuns and their servants whose movements were severely restricted by communal life and a bishop's strong desire to control their movement. The abbess's repeated requests to the bishop to allow for more visits from physicians and other types of healers hint at the agency of these women, especially in the context of their own medical care. This series of about seventeen letters also allows us to see firmly entrenched hierarchies that were not erased by Bourbon reforms. Wealthy nuns still employed servants, and when one got sick, they often petitioned the bishop for a replacement. These convent ledgers and letters provide us a glimpse into health and healing in Peruvian convents through the lens of gender, class, and race. Through these letters we can find vestiges of indigenous healing absent in the convent ledgers. We see that the abbess used the written word to fight for better medical care for all members of her convent at the same time that she sought to maintain the class distinctions and racial norms within her community.

Any tourist who has travelled to Arequipa, Peru, surely has visited the convent museum of Santa Catalina de Sena. Founded in 1579 by Dominican nuns, one can appreciate the size of this large convent from the period of the Viceroyalty of Peru. During this time period *conventos grandes* (large convents) could house hundreds of women from diverse social classes.[1] Black-veiled nuns of white Spanish descent ruled the convents followed by a hierarchy of women from white-veiled nuns, often mestizas of mixed Spanish and indigenous descent, to a cadre of servants and slaves of indigenous and African descent. Shadowed by the towering

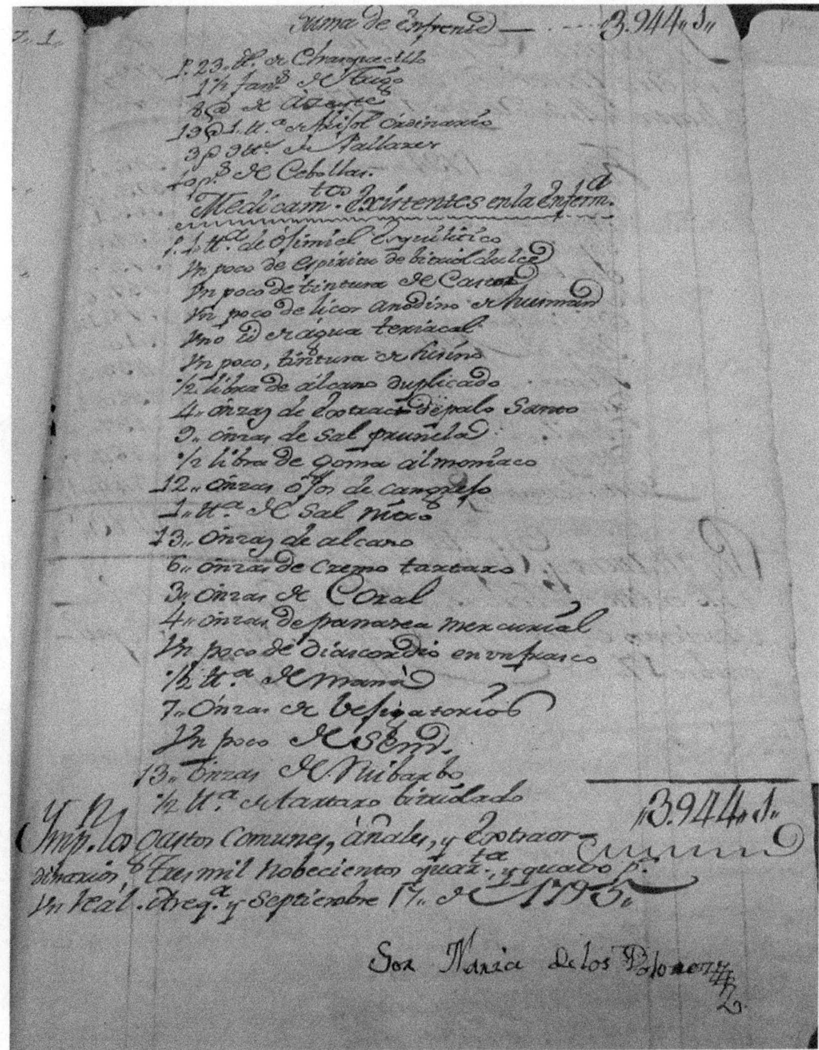

Suma de Enfermería — . . . 3.944 ps

[illegible]
1½ fan.s de Trigo
8 @ de Azúcar
13 @ 1 lb. de [illegible] ordinario
3 p 3 lb. de [illegible]
[illegible] de Cebollas.

Medicam.tos Existentes en la Enferm.ria

1 lb. de [illegible]
Un poco de Espíritu de [illegible] dulce
Un poco de tintura de Castor
Un poco de licor anodino de Hoffman
Uno de agua teriacal
Un poco tintura de [illegible]
½ libra de alcanfor duplicado
4 onzas de extracto de palo Santo
3 onzas de Sal prunela
½ libra de goma almoniaco
12 onzas ojos de cangrejo
1 lb. de Sal nitro
13 onzas de alcanfor
6 onzas de crémor tártaro
3 onzas de Coral
4 onzas de panacea mercurial
Un poco de diacordio en un frasco
½ lb. de maná
7 onzas de vejigatorio
Un poco de Sen
13 onzas de Ruibarbo
½ lb. de tártaro vitriolado

Importan los gastos comunes, anuales, y extraordinarios, tres mil novecientos cuarenta y cuatro p.s un real. Areq.a y Septiembre 17 de 1795. — 3.944 ps 1 r.

Sor María de los Dolores

Figure 5. Convent ledger from Santa Rosa, 1795. Photo by author.

snow-covered volcano of El Misti, this convent was built in the heart of colonial Arequipa. To this day, a small group of cloistered nuns still lives in a section of the convent closed off to the public, but tourists have access to the museum grounds covering several city blocks. One can visit the original nuns' "cells" or apartments with their own kitchens, *estrados* or sitting rooms, bedrooms, and servants' quarters. Some apartments had terraces, chicken coups, and oratories. Before the emphasis on *vida*

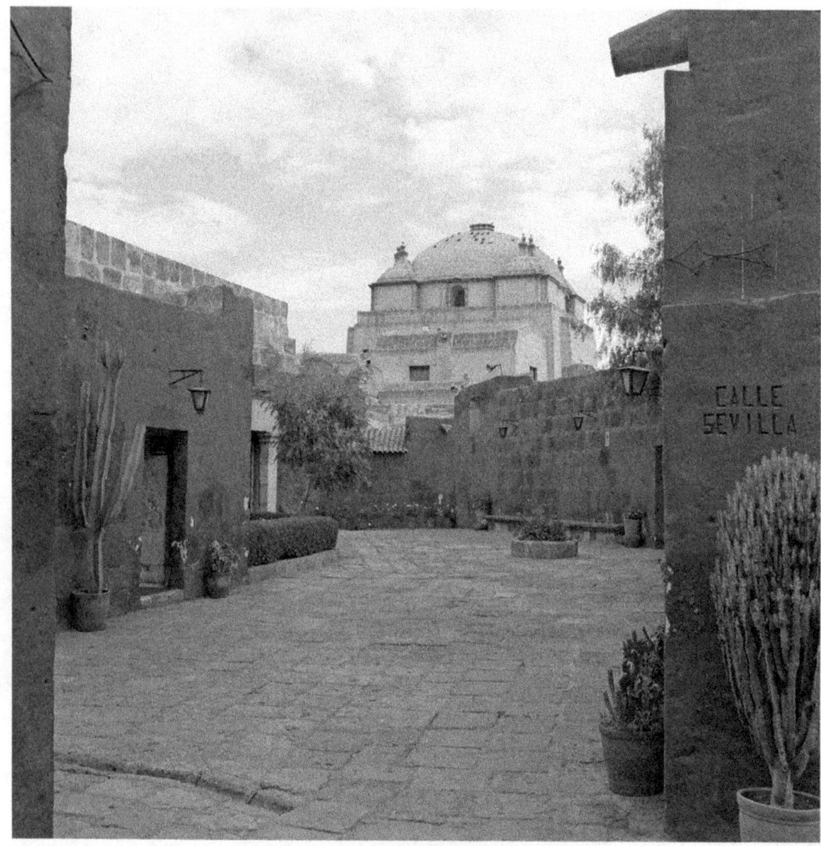

Figure 6. Convent of Santa Catalina. Photo by author.

común, or communal life, of the 1780s, young women who wanted to profess as black-veiled nuns brought with them large dowries. Mostly teenagers from the highest echelons of society, they had the purchasing power to buy the finest china, linens, and furniture to decorate their own private living quarters. Servants and slaves accompanied the young women into the convent, and they brought with them some of their local customs and cuisines. Servants kept *cuy*, or guinea pigs, in pens near the warm kitchen stoves, and the nuns dined on this delicacy typical of the Andean region. They used large quantities of *ají*, or hot peppers, to season food. They soaked *chuño* (freeze-dried potatoes), reconstituting it for thick stews, and they produced vats of *chicha*, an alcoholic beverage from fermented corn and sugar (see figures 6 and 7).

While in Arequipa, a tourist can also visit the Museo de Arte Virreinal de Santa Teresa. Similar to Santa Catalina, this convent museum still has a part of the convent closed off for cloistered nuns. One can buy sweets and embroidered cloth at the *torno*, a type of revolving door, but you cannot physically see the nuns without special permission. This Carmelite convent built in the early 1700s is not as large as Santa Catalina, but it still has impressive artwork, gardens, and a small display of items used in the convent infirmary, including various jars, pots, vases, small presses, mortar and pestle, weights and measures, and a balance. Visitors are greeted by the convent mascot, "Misti," a hairless Peruvian dog who roams the grounds without restriction. Renowned for the healing properties of its warm skin, this type of dog is similar to the hairless Mexican variety, Xoloitzcuintli. The latter is still used in Mexico to treat aches and pains in the elderly like a living "hot-water bottle" (*National Geographic*).

In the 1740s, Dominican nuns from Santa Catalina went on to found the convent of Santa Rosa, but of the three convents analysed in this essay, it is not open to the public. The cloistered nuns of these three communities are very private and rarely grant access to their convent archives. Instead, this study focuses on the archival holdings of the Archivo Arzobispal of Arequipa. That archive has rich sources, including convent ledgers and letters written by the nuns from the late 1700s. As mentioned earlier, these documents correspond to the period of the Bourbon reforms from the Spanish Crown that tried to control the movement of nuns by requiring them to follow the *vida común*. These reforms also obligated the abbesses to request permission from their bishop for anyone to enter or leave the convent such as servants, physicians, and priests. Prior to the *vida común*, wealthy nuns could hire their own doctors and surgeons, but during this time period they could do so only with special permission, otherwise they were obligated to use the official convent physician.

Before delving into the world of health care in colonial Peru, it is important to take stock of convent medicine in Europe and Spain during the early modern period. As Sharon Strocchia has demonstrated in her research on Renaissance Italy, nuns have long cultivated a culture of convent pharmacies. In the sixteenth century, nuns from Florence, Italy, sought out exotic ingredients such as manna and violets to produce extracts, unguents, oils, tinctures, and tonics. They bought large quantities of sugar to sweeten bitter ingredients into palatable essences, syrups, and medicinal waters. They sold their own fruit conserves and other sugar concoctions that according to Galen had healing properties (633). This convent culture of producing medicines and healing extended throughout the early modern Catholic world. Although nuns in Mexico and Peru did not sell their wares to the extent of the Italian nuns, we do know that they did produce small quantities of specific items such as tonics for the general public. In Mexico City, for example, nuns from the convent of Regina Coeli sold to the public a purgative powder that they fabricated from their own secret formula. They also provided free of charge a liquid to treat eye problems (Muriel 76).[2]

Returning to colonial Peru, Linda Newson's study *Making Medicines in Early Colonial Lima, Peru* (2017) provides solid research on *materia medica* found in Lima's hospitals and pharmacies during the latter half of the 1500s and the early 1600s. She concludes that only a handful of these ingredients were native in origin. As the introduction to this volume has made clear, physicians, surgeons, and pharmacists still relied heavily on a Galenic framework that prioritized humoral theory. According to Newson, pharmacists in Lima stocked many plant-based materials thought to be effective in correcting these imbalances, mainly used for purgatives and emetics. In general, apothecaries viewed native plants and minerals with scepticism and relied heavily on Old World botanicals.[3] Her study notes, however, that some plants gathered in Latin America could have been mislabelled with Old World names and that we might underestimate the use of native plants (158–85).

During the colonial period, the Spanish Crown attempted to regulate pharmacies and standardize pharmacopoeia sold to the general public through the institution of the Protomedicato in the first half of the sixteenth century in New Spain and Peru.[4] But these first attempts at regulating medicine, hygiene, public health, and apothecary shops were slow and ineffective. It was not until the universities in Mexico City in 1621, and in Lima in 1634, began to award medical degrees that the Spanish Crown slowly began to exert more control in these large cities (Lanning 327–8). As John Tate Lanning and Newson have shown, however, the hinterlands of Latin America received much less oversight. Although Spain tried to regulate medicines sold to the general public, it was not until the end of the eighteenth century that it took a real interest in classifying the diverse flora of its territories. Before that time, Spain relied heavily on medicinal imports and often did not value the tremendous biodiversity of its own empire.[5]

Although it is difficult to ascertain if some of the botanicals discovered on these expeditions made their way into the medicine cabinets of Arequipa's convents, we certainly can see some new items such as *ojos de cangrejo*, or crab's eye (*Abrus precatorius*), found in the ledgers of Santa Rosa, but absent from the inventories of Newson's study (1550s–1618). To be sure, some items consistent with late eighteenth- and nineteenth-century medicine such as *esperma*, or sperm whale oil, was documented in the Peruvian convent ledgers, but the majority of the items were not new, and they did not necessarily reflect any drastic changes from previous centuries.

What we can note, however, is the long arm of the Protomedicato and a standardization of pharmacopoeia used in religious communities at the end of the eighteenth century. For example, Norma Balderas Sánchez's research on the medicine cabinet of the Colegio de Vizcaínas in Mexico City from 1775 to 1780 provides an excellent point of comparison with the products used by the Arequipan nuns. Despite the vast distances separating Arequipa and Mexico City, these religious women stocked many of the exact same items in their medicine cabinets.[6] It is important to note, also, that Spanish women and *criollas* (women of Spanish descent born in the Americas) dominated these communities and that they would opt to buy remedies prescribed by physicians from their same social class. The Colegio de Vizcaínas was not a convent but was established as an educational residence for widows and poor women of Basque and Navarren descent. Similar to a religious community, the residents lived enclosed and were served by a convent doctor, a surgeon, and a phlebotomist. The Vizcaínas used a specific pharmacist to stock its medicine cabinet. This pharmacist also kept a yearly log of prescriptions and medicines, all in Latin, but never mentioned the actual ailments. Compared to the medicine cabinet in the convent of Santa Rosa, we can find many of the same products including sperm oil, castor oil, coral, crab's eye, licorice, and chicory. Moreover, as noted by Balderas Sánchez, the majority of the herbs and plants are originally of European and Asiatic origin like roses and wormwood, and very few are from indigenous plants native to the Americas.

Although the *materia medica* from the three convents in Arequipa is from the late 1700s, it appears that the nuns still relied heavily on medicine based on humoral practices. The accounting ledgers from the Convent of Santa Rosa provide the best snapshot of the types of materials used by the nuns for the medicines in the convent infirmary. We also learn a lot from these ledgers about the basic make-up of the community and how the budget was allocated. For example, on 27 October 1788, the prioress Sor María Ignacia de Santa Teresa notes that the community was composed of thirty-three black-veiled nuns, five white-veiled nuns, one *donada* (part of the servant class), and a large contingent of approximately thirty servants assigned to the kitchen, laundry, and infirmary. She also explains that there were several more servants who could not work due to poor health, but had grown old during their service to the community. In addition, there were eight female *mandaderas*, or messengers, who lived outside the cloistered walls, but who also received rations and clothing. According to Sor María Ignacia, in order to support these women and care for their illnesses, she gave each of them a ration of sugar and herbs, which amounted to two *reales* a piece, totalling 2,737.4 pesos a year. To put these numbers in perspective, between 1788 and 1795, the community spent on average around 8,500 pesos a year.

Of that total budget the convent paid its own convent administrator 600 pesos, its chaplain 400 pesos, its physician 180 pesos, and a phlebotomist 25 pesos. Much of the rest of the budget went towards other convent personnel (sacristan, lawyer, gardener), expenditures on wax for candles, clothing, shoes, fuel, meats and vegetables, and supplies for the infirmary (AAA, Santa Rosa, 1762–99, leg. 1).

It is difficult to ascertain from the convent ledgers if the nuns were using native plants and remedies in their infirmaries, some of which they may have grown themselves, but they do clearly reveal the importance of native foods and ingredients in their diets. Nuns did buy considerable quantities of quinoa, chocolate, *ají*, and *chuño*. Most likely the indigenous women who served as cooks for the convent brought with them their traditional recipes that combined local ingredients altered to satisfy European tastes. The large quantity of sugar allocated to the servants and nuns alike indicates their addiction to sweets. The nuns bought extra honey and milk to prepare *mazamorras* (purple corn pudding); sugar, cherries, cinnamon, and snow to make ice cream; almonds, peanuts, pepper, cloves, cinnamon, anise, and cloves to make *alfajores* (a traditional cookie) served to celebrate nuns' vows of profession; and they set aside special funds to purchase sweets during feast days and religious holidays such as *dulce de almíbar* (candied fruit), "rosquetes de pan con manteca" (ringed-pastries made with lard), *turrón*, chocolate (for drinks), and coffee.[7] It is not hard to imagine that the consequences of this diet would have produced a propensity towards diabetes in some women, if not, at the very least, a lot of rotten teeth. Surprisingly, the ledgers only document money spent to extract teeth on a handful occasions. At the end of the same year for the sweets listed above, the convent of Santa Teresa paid one peso to the surgeon to extract a single molar.

The nuns of Arequipa also consumed a lot of meat. Several pages of the convent ledgers are dedicated to the purchase of meat, but it should also be noted that the records only indicate money spent on animals of European origin. The nuns also ate animals from the Andean region such as *cuy* (guinea pig), which were raised in the convent kitchens by indigenous servants. In the month of June 1797, for example, the nuns of Santa Rosa purchased seventy *carneros* (rams), three *arrobas* (pounds) of *carne de vaca* (beef), two *cecinas* (cured meat), and one *torillo* (small bull) for a total of 52.45 pesos.[8] Although that appears to be a large amount of meat, the nuns of Santa Rosa spent 79.5 pesos in bread for that same month. Again, to put these numbers in perspective, the nuns spent considerable sums of money on food items in comparison to medicinal herbs, pills, and other *material medica*. As indicated in the table below, for that same month of June they only spent a total of 1.4 pesos in supplies for the medical cabinet (see table 2).

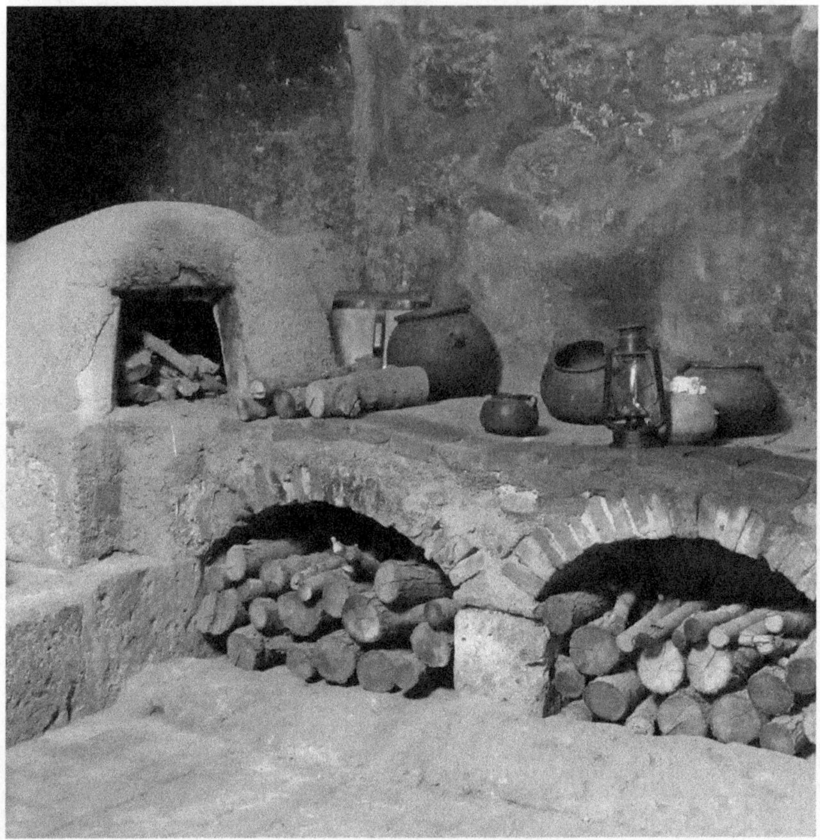

Figure 7. A kitchen in the Convent of Santa Catalina. Photo by author.

The convent ledgers provide information about ingredients, quantities, and prices of medicinal supplies purchased by the convents, but they rarely mention the actual diseases or circumstance that the nuns and their servants faced during this time period. For that, we can turn to a fascinating set of about seventeen letters written between 1792 and 1801, by the prioress of Santa Catalina, Sor Paula Francisca del Tránsito y Barreda, to the bishop of Arequipa, don Pedro José Chávez de la Rosa. Bishop Chávez de la Rosa was a strong advocate of communal life imposed on the nuns by his predecessor, Bishop Miguel de Pamplona, in 1784 (Santner 92).[9] He was especially concerned with the movement in and out of the enclosed convent and obligated the abbess to petition him every time unauthorized personnel entered the community. Santa Catalina was not the only convent to experience the Bourbon reforms

Table 2. Expenses from Santa Rosa Infirmary, June 1797

Junio de 1797 Enfermería [Santa Rosa]	
Día 3 por 2 reales gastados en ajenjos	0.2 [pesos]
Día 15 por 4 reales que costó media onza de diascordio	0.4
Día 17 por 1 ½ real que se gastó en cebada y chicoria	0.15
Día 19 por 1 real gastado en un jarabe	0.1
Día 27 por 4 ½ reales gastados en leche y cuajo	0.45
En dicho por 1 real gastado en piedra alumbre	0.1
Sor María de la Asensión	**1.4**
Expenses from Santa Rosa Infirmary, June 1797	
Day 3 for 2 *reales* spent on absinthe	0.2 [pesos]
Day 15 for 4 *reales* that cost half an ounce of astringent	0.4
Day 17 for 1 ½ *real* spent on barley and chicory	0.15
Day 19 for 1 *real* spent on a syrup	0.1
Day 27 for 4 ½ *reales* spent on milk and whey	0.45
On the same [day] 1 *real* spent on Alum stone	0.1
Sor María de la Asensión	**1.4**

Source: AAA, Santa Rosa, 1762–1799, leg. 1.

of the *vida común*. Ecclesiastical authorities across Latin America subjected calced convents to a strict regimen of shared dormitories, dining, and overall communal living. At times nuns fought back against these austere reforms. In Puebla, Mexico, for example, nuns embarked on a letter-writing campaign to lessen the stringent rules. Abbesses and supporting nuns complained that they did not profess under those rules and it was unfair for them to give up their apartments and servants.[10] At times these rules divided convents, pitting nuns from different factions against one another.[11]

In the case of Arequipa, Sor Paula's letters provide valuable insight into how the nuns of Santa Catalina dealt with these reforms. Interestingly, the majority of Sor Paula's requests revolve around illness and health care. Even before the reforms, Santa Catalina, like many convents, paid an annual salary to its own physician and barber-surgeon, but some of the wealthy nuns often secured their own specialists for certain ailments. Not only do Sor Paula's letters reveal how many of these same women still demanded the option to contract physicians outside the convent, but they also shed light on the fact that many wanted to maintain their same lifestyle, one that included a servant class. For example, "Sor Melchora del Costado de Cristo y Pérez suplica a Vuestra Señoría Ilustrísima se digne darle licencia para entrar otra criada nombrada María Josefa Llamosas, huérfana de Camaná aunque tiene dos criadas, la una no le sirve porque está imposibilitada" ("Sor Melchora del Costado de Cristo y Pérez begs Your Lord Grace to deign licence for another servant named María Josefa Llamosas, an orphan from Camaná, to enter the convent. Although she already has two servants, one of them cannot serve because she is incapacitated"; Sor Paula to Bishop Chávez, 10 January 1801, AAA, Santa Catalina, leg. 2). In a similar case, the abbess requested permission for an orphan to enter the convent as a servant to Sor Josefa de la Mercedes y Loaisa [*sic*]. Her current servant, a white-veiled nun, was "malísima de ético, ha mandado el médico que le administren los sacramentos y la Extremaunción" ("very ill with tuberculosis and the doctor ordered she be given last rites and Extreme Unction"; Sor Paula to Bishop Chávez, 4 October 1792, AAA, Santa Catalina, leg. 2.).

We can see from these letters that the nuns wanted to maintain a class hierarchy, but they also shine a light on their concern for the health care of their servants. On 3 January 1792, Sor Paula wrote Bishop Chávez de la Rosa concerning María Soto Mayor: "una india anciana está malísima e hidrópica [*sic*]" ("an elderly Indian is very ill and dropsical"; Sor Paula to Bishop Chávez, 3 January 1792, AAA, Santa Catalina, leg. 2). María worked for the nuns as a *mandadera* who lived in one of the small rooms outside the enclosed portion of the convent, but within the closed walls of the garden. The abbess requested special permission "para que puedan las muchachas enfermeras allí fuera al cuarto a hacerle los medicamentos y ponerle las ayudas estando huerta cerrada porque allí no hay quien se los haga" ("for the young nurses to be able to go outside [the convent walls] to her room so they can give her medicines and treatments since the garden is closed and there is no one on the outside who can do it"; Sor Paula to Bishop Chávez, 3 January 1792, AAA, Santa Catalina, leg. 2). This example also speaks to the nuances of enclosure. It was quite common for convents to provide rooms to servants and even priests on the periphery of their nunneries. Most likely, in this case before the strict Bourbon reforms, the nuns could have treated the servant without permission.

In another curious case, we hear echoes of the rare voice of a *donada*. *Donadas*, mostly of indigenous or African descent, were "donated" to the convent by their parents or committed by themselves. They took lesser vows in exchange for their servitude, but because of their race and lack of a dowry, they never could aspire to become nuns. In some cases, however, their extreme piety could lead to adoration by others and the formation of spiritual cults.[12] On 3 December 1792, the abbess wrote the bishop requesting the services of a *partera* (midwife), not because the *donada* was pregnant, but because "se le ha descompuesto la madre [la matriz] de una fuerza que se hizo en el ejercicio de la cocina" ("her uterus was damaged from an exertion while working in the kitchen"; Sor Paula to Bishop Chávez, 3 December 1792, AAA, Santa Catalina, leg. 2). She elaborates, explaining how the servant was embarrassed to be examined by the convent physician and would much prefer a *partera*. In a subsequent letter on 17 January 1792, the bishop denied her request, and the abbess had the convent doctor examine the *donada*.

Why did the *donada* really want a *partera*? Can we take her justification at face value that she felt embarrassed being examined by a male physician? There may be some truth in her request; even today many women opt for female gynecologists and obstetricians. It is also possible that she preferred the alternative remedies of a midwife of indigenous or African descent. Maybe she knew someone in particular that had been recommended to her. Even during the late colonial period, in the Andes and Mesoamerica, traditional healers and indigenous midwives were still valued by many communities. Although the Protomedicato of these regions tried to eliminate their influence, they could not always control these unlicensed healers, especially midwives, who were highly valued for their "comprehensive approach" (Birn 247). According to Adam Warren, however, the Bourbon reforms in Lima of the late 1700s took a harsh stance against midwives and wet nurses, and in some documents accused them of "inflicting harm on mother and child, increasing their chances of death" (*Medicine* 60).[13] For an excellent study on the tensions between indigenous medical knowledge and Western medicine we can turn to Martha Few's *For All of Humanity: Mesoamerican and Colonial Medicine in Enlightenment Guatemala.* I agree with Few's position when she notes that we must be careful with gender and racial stereotypes and try to find a more nuanced view of the diverse milieu that participated in colonial medicine. She writes, "conflicts surrounding medicine in colonial settings cannot be seen as exclusively categorizable along racial and ethnic lines in a narrative pitting modernizing Western medicine against indigenous medicine, or as only divided along gendered lines between university-trained male medical professional and female midwives" (20).

The more we examine the context of the letters between the abbess and the bishop, the more we find the complex interplay between gender dynamics, racial tensions, power struggles, and the backdrop of the Bourbon reforms. Although Bishop Chávez often says no, as in the case of the midwife, this does not stop the abbess from listening to the nuns and their servants. And yet, there is no denying the racial and class hierarchy that permeates convent life. While *criolla* and Spanish women like the abbess reigned at the top, poor mestiza, *mulata*, black, and indigenous women worked as servants on the bottom rungs of the community.[14] In the same vein, sanctioned male medical doctors were more esteemed than female midwives, and the abbess was required to follow the bishop's orders.[15]

The following letter from 14 February 1792, from Sor Paula to Bishop Chávez, illustrates the class structure, while at the same time it reveals the abbess's concern for the unnamed servant's physical and spiritual well-being:

> Mi Señor, después de ponerme a los pies de V.S. Ilustrísima se me hace preciso darle noticia como una negrita de Sor Margarita de la Asunción y Tornalvo ha amanecido hecha un tronco, ya la han visto los médicos él del convento y Trujillo como que está entrando a Sor Ana le han hecho varios remedios, volvió un poquito y apenas se empezó a confesar y se volvió a quedar sin acabar la confesión y está así no más. Y estando actualmente con el Mayordomo quien me trajo recaudo de V.S.IL. para que no entre otro médico fuera del convento, a ese tiempo me mandó recado la dicha Sor Margarita pidiéndome licencia para que entre el Dr. Revollar y le he respondido que ocurra a V.S. Ill. a pedirla la licencia; la suplico a V.S. me conceda licencia para que si se puede se le administre los sacramentos y si muriese se le haga su entierro porque está de riesgo.[16]
>
> Febrero 14 de 1792
>
> Sor Paula Francisca del Tránsito, priora
>
> My Lord, after prostrating myself at the feet of Your Lord Grace, I find it necessary to tell you about the *negrita* of Sor Margarita de Asunción y Tornalvo, who has woken up like a tree trunk. The doctors, the one from the convent and Trujillo, have already visited her when they came to see Sor Ana. They gave her some remedies, which helped revive her a bit, but as soon as she started her confession she relapsed before she finished it and has stayed like that ever since. At the same time I was with the [convent] administrator who gave me the message from Your Lord Grace that no outside doctors should enter the convent, I received a message from the aforementioned Sor Margarita, asking me for permission so that Dr. Revollar could enter. I responded to her that it was Your Lord Grace's decision to grant the licence. I beg Your Lord to grant the licence so that

> she can be administered the sacraments and if she should die, to have her burial because she is at grave risk.
>
> February 14 of 1792
>
> Sor Paula Francisca del Tránsito, prioress

This letter puts into clear view the juxtaposition of the abbess's concern for the physical and spiritual well-being of the black servant, with her clipped description of her as a nameless woman on her deathbed. Without ever mentioning the actual name of the ill woman – the abbess only refers to her as the *negrita*, or little black woman, of Sor Margarita – she goes on to use terse language to describe her illness: "who has woken up like a tree trunk," a colloquial phrase indicating that she experienced a paralyzing stroke. This letter, like many others in the series, brings to the fore the complex fabric of class, race, and gender enmeshed in the microcosm of a colonial convent. On the one hand the nuns cared for their servants by providing them with doctors' "remedies," for example, but on the other, they were also concerned about their own well-being and replacing a dying or incapacitated servant with a new one.

Even though the abbess often petitions the bishop to allow additional doctors to enter the convent, she also alludes to the toxic effects of their prescriptions. In a letter from 18 May 1792 she writes: "Sor Tomasa de San Pedro y Portu, está muy mala, desahuciada de todos los médicos, han recetado sacramentos, olios, y todos los auxilios, V.S.Ill me conceda licencia para todo lo que se ofreciere y para que entre con más frecuencia su confesor; la ha visto Revollar, Trujillo, y le han recetado cáusticos y temo que en el puesto se quede" ("Sor Tomasa de San Pedro y Portu is very ill, declared terminal by the doctors. They have prescribed the sacraments, oils, and all remedies. I ask Your Lord Grace to grant me licence for whatever she might need and so that her confessor can visit her more frequently. [Doctors] Revollar and Trujillo have seen her and they have prescribed caustics. I fear that she will die in this condition"; Sor Paula to Bishop Chávez, AAA, 18 May 1792, Santa Catalina, leg. 2).

In the abbess's opinion, Sor Tomasa now needed spiritual care from her confessor, not caustic medicines, which appear to have been a last resort. Caustics or corrosive substances such as arsenic were sometimes mixed into a paste to treat diseases such as breast cancer. A surgeon, for example, would smear the caustic paste on the breast to corrode the infected tissue so that it could be cut off on a daily basis (Owens 326). Other toxic ingredients were formulated as strong purgatives, mixing toxic ingredients such as potassium nitrate, arsenic, mercury, and sometimes lead into spirits (Newson 180).[17] Unfortunately, this letter does not give us any more clues as to Sor Tomasa's ailment. We can assume, however, that the doctor's use of caustic remedies exacerbated her terminal illness. Without hope of a physical cure, the abbess pleads with the bishop to allow more spiritual care. Just as this letter emphasizes the role of prayer and spiritual healing in the care of sick nuns, it also points to the continued control of the bishop who limited the confessor's visits – a solace that could have deeply affected some women who had developed close bonds with their spiritual advisors (Bilinkoff 90–2).

Obviously, the bishop tried to control the power of the nuns by severely restricting the movement in and out of the convent. He used his authority and that of the strict Bourbon reforms by micromanaging doctors' visits, meetings with confessors, and even funeral services. Yet, as revealed by these letters and ledgers from the convents of Arequipa, we can also conclude that behind the thick walls of the cloister, away from the sharp eyes of ecclesiastical authorities, the nurses cared for their patients much as they did before the imposition of *vida común.* To be sure, the hierarchies of race and class persisted without much change, but the nurses also treated their charges with companionship and prayer, a diet rich in protein, and remedies prepared from their own medicine cabinet. This essay demonstrates that medical treatment in the Arequipan convents primarily relied on European medicine, but that there is some indication of indigenous influence, especially with the incorporation of indigenous foods.

Convent ledgers provide important insight into the purchasing habits and types of ingredients used to stock medicine cabinets. But the ledgers tell only half the story. It is the combination of the ledgers with nuns' concerns and requests documented in their letters that reveals a deeper understanding of health and healing among colonial Latin American nuns.

NOTES

1 For more on "conventos grandes" of colonial Peru, see Kathryn Burns (3) and Luis Martín (174–92).

2 For a detailed overview of convent infirmaries in Madrid, see María Elena del Río Hijas (325–421).

3 For a discussion of *materia medica* in the Ancient Mediterranean, see Paula De Vos (283–7).

4 For a fuller introduction to the position, see chapter 2 of this volume authored by Kathleen M. Kole de Peralta. Spain appointed its first *protomédicos*

in New Spain and Peru in 1527 and 1537, respectively, but the first royal *protomédicos* were not appointed until the second half of the sixteenth century. See John Lanning (58–62), Abraham Zavala Batlle (n.p.), Linda Newson (7).

5 Between 1770 and 1816, Spain financed the Royal Botanical Expeditions to the Caribbean, Latin America, and the Philippines. There exist approximately twelve thousand illustrations from those exhibitions in the archives of the Royal Botanical Garden of Madrid, many of which can be perused in their digitized collection. See the Real Jardín Botánico de Madrid: http://www.rjb.csic.es/jardinbotanico/jardin/index.php?Cab=114&len=es. For excellent commentary and select images, see Daniela Bleichmar's *Visual Empire: Botanical Expeditions & Visual Culture in the Hispanic Enlightenment*.

6 See also a book on convent inventories from Queretaro by María Concepción de la Vega Macías (225–67).

7 All of these ingredients and others are listed for the expenses of June through September 1794 in the Convent of Santa Teresa. AAA, Santa Teresa, 1745–1898, leg 2.

8 The price of one ram was approximately half a peso as compared to six pesos for one small bull and two pesos, two *reales* for three pounds of beef, and four pesos for two cecinas. These tables come from a section of the Santa Rosa documents titled "Cuaderno de cuentas de este año de 1797 en que son porteras sor Fernandina de la Presentación y sor María de la Asensión y se cuenta desde el día 26 de mayo de 97 hasta igual día de 98." AAA, Santa Rosa, 1762–1799, leg. 1.

9 I want to extend a special thanks to Kathryn Santner, who first alerted me to the documents in Arequipa. Her dissertation, "Art and Devotion at the Convent of Santa Catalina de Sena, Arequipa, Peru, 17th–19th Centuries," also provided me with excellent background information on convent life in Arequipa.

10 For example, see Nuria Salazar Simarro's *La vida común en los conventos de monjas de la cuidad de Puebla.*

11 As demonstrated throughout Margaret Chowning's *Rebellious Nuns*.

12 For one such example in Peru, see van Deusen's *The Souls of Purgatory*. See also Lavrin (32–3).

13 In general, the Bourbon crown vilified informal healers, and midwives' presumed incompetence was fuelled by colonial writers such as Lima's Juan Antonio de Olavarrieta in his journal, *Semanario Crítico*. For more on Olavarrieta and critiques from other later colonial writers, see Adam Warren's "Between the Foreign and the Local" (182–8). On the backlash of Olavarrieta's harsh words against indigenous and African wet nurses, see Bianca Premo (169–75).

14 Exceptions did exist to this hierarchy. For example, there are cases of poor and sometimes illegitimate Spaniards working as servants in convents.

15 For the role of female healers in Mexico City's convents, see Salazar and Owens ("Cloistered Women in Health Care").
16 Sor Paula to Bishop Chávez, AAA, 14 February 1792, Santa Catalina, leg. 2.
17 Many of these same ingredients can be found in the medicine cabinet of Santa Rosa.

WORKS CITED

Archival Sources

Archivo Arzobispal de Arequipa (AAA). Sección: Curia Diocesana. Serie: Monasterios Santa Catalina, 1784–1853, legajo 2.

Archivo Arzobispal de Arequipa (AAA). Sección: Curia Diocesana; Serie: Monasterios Santa Rosa, 1762–1799, legajo 1.

Archivo Arzobispal de Arequipa (AAA). Sección: Curia Diocesana. Serie: Conventos, Santa Teresa, 1745–1898, legajo 2.

Print Sources

Balderas Sánchez, Norma. "La herbolaria en la Nueva España y su empleo en la botica del Colegio de Vizcaínas 1775–1780." *Multidisciplina*, no. 11, 2012, pp. 47–59.

Birn, Anne-Emanuelle. "Public Health and Medicine in Latin America." *The Oxford Handbook of the History of Medicine*, edited by Mark Jackson, Oxford UP, 2011, pp. 243–65.

Bilinkoff, Jodi. *Related Lives: Confessors and Their Female Penitents, 1450–1750*. Cornell UP, 2005.

Bleichmar, Daniela. *Visual Empire: Botanical Expeditions and Visual Culture in the Hispanic Enlightenment*. U of Chicago P, 2012.

Burns, Kathryn. *Colonial Habits: Convents and the Spiritual Economy of Cuzco, Peru*. Duke UP, 1999.

Chowning, Margaret. *Rebellious Nuns: The Troubled History of a Mexican Convent, 1752–1863*. Oxford UP, 2006.

de la Vega Macías, María Concepción. *Fragmentos de la vida cotidiana: Cinco inventarios del Real Convento de Santa Clara de Jesús Santiago de Querétaro (siglos XVIII–XIX)*. Consejo del IV Centenario de la Fundación de Convento de Santa Clara de Jesús, 2007.

De Vos, Paula. "Apothecaries, Artists, and Artisans: Early Industrial Material Culture in the Biological Old Regime." *Journal of Interdisciplinary History*, vol. XLV, no. 3, Winter 2015, pp. 277–336.

Few, Martha. *For All of Humanity: Mesoamerican and Colonial Medicine in Enlightenment Guatemala*. U of Arizona P, 2015.

Lanning, John Tate. *The Royal Protomedicato: The Regulation of the Medical Professions in the Spanish Empire*. Edited by John Jay TePaske, Duke UP, 1985.

Lavrin, Asuncion. *Brides of Christ: Conventual Life in Colonial Mexico*. Stanford UP, 2008.

Martín, Luis. *Daughters of the Conquistadors: Women of the Viceroyalty of Peru*. U of New Mexico P, 1983.

Muriel, Josefina. *Conventos de monjas en la Nueva España*. Editorial Jus, 1995.

National Geographic. https://news.nationalgeographic.com/2017/11/hairless-dog-mexico-xolo-xoloitzcuintli-Aztec/.

Newson, Linda A. *Making Medicines in Early Colonial Lima: Apothecaries, Science and Society*. Brill, 2017.

Owens, Sarah E. "The Cloister as Therapeutic Space: Breast Cancer Narratives in the Early Modern World." *Literature and Medicine*, vol. 30, no. 2, Fall 2012, pp. 295–314.

Premo, Bianca. *Children of the Father King: Youth, Authority, and Legal Minority in Colonial Lima*. U of North Carolina P, 2005.

Río Hijas, María Elena del. "El desarrollo de las enfermerías en las órdenes religiosas en Madrid capital, durante los siglos XVII, XVIII y XIX." *Archivo Ibero-Americano*, vol. 53, no. 209/212, Feb. 1993, pp. 325–421.

Salazar Simarro, Nuria, and Sarah E. Owens. "Cloistered Women in Health Care: The Convent of Jesús, María, Mexico City." *Women of the Iberian Atlantic*, edited by Sarah E. Owens and Jane E. Mangan, Louisiana State UP, 2012, pp. 128–47.

Salazar Simarro, Nuria. *La vida común en los conventos de monjas de la cuidad de Puebla*. Gobierno del Estado de Puebla, 1990.

Santner, Kathryn. "Art and Devotion at the Convent of Santa Catalina de Sena, Arequipa, Peru, 17th–19th Centuries." PhD Diss, University of Cambridge, 2015.

Strocchia, Sharon T. "The Nun Apothecaries of Renaissance Florence: Marketing Medicines in the Convent." *Renaissance Studies*, vol. 25, no. 5, 2011, pp. 627–47.

van Deusen, Nancy. *The Souls of Purgatory: The Spiritual Diary of a Seventeenth-Century Afro-Peruvian Mystic, Ursula de Jesús*. U of New Mexico P, 2004

Warren, Adam. "Between the Foreign and the Local: French Midwifery, Traditional Practitioners, and Vernacular Medical Knowledge about Childbirth in Lima, Peru." *História Ciências Saúde-Manguinhos*, vol. 22, no. 1, Jan.–March 2015, pp. 179–200.

– *Medicine and Politics in Colonial Peru: Population Growth and the Bourbon Reforms*. U of Pittsburgh P, 2010.

Zavala Batlle, Abraham. Acta méd. peruana v.27 n.2 Lima abr./jun. 2010. Online version ISSN 1728–5917: http://www.scielo.org.pe/scielo.php?script=sci_arttext&pid=S1728-59172010000200013.

Chapter Four

Leche and *lagartijas*: Injecting the Local into Eighteenth-Century Spanish American Medical Discourse[1]

KAREN STOLLEY

The eighteenth-century Hispanic world stands at the intersection of coloniality and modernity, and perhaps in no area is this more provocatively reflected than in writings about late colonial medical practices. Jorge Cañizares-Esguerra shows in *How to Write the History of the New World* that colonial intellectuals in the eighteenth-century Americas were not merely passive recipients of metropolitan knowledge but rather creators, observers, and disseminators of knowledge who participated in a lively transatlantic epistemological exchange. Taking up Cañizares-Esguerra's invitation that we rewrite the Eurocentric history of the New World to recognize the agency of indigenous and *criollo* thinkers and practitioners, this essay explores the ways in which a wide range of medical cultures that came into contact in Spain's sixteenth- and seventeenth-century global empire continued their interactions well into the late colonial period in Spanish America.[2] In what follows I will argue that eighteenth-century medical beliefs and practices in Spanish territories in the Americas were informed by an ongoing negotiation of the local and the global, a negotiation in which categories of difference, including gender and race, played a key role. How does this negotiation play out? I've organized my argument around two examples: *leche* (criollo anxieties about the prevalence of indigenous or mixed-race wet nurses) and *lagartijas* (debates about the medicinal uses of New World lizards), using textual evidence from letters and essays published in the emerging periodical press by enlightened scientists and practitioners in the viceregal capitals of New Spain (now Mexico) and Peru.[3]

These examples, which involve introducing a carefully calibrated amount of New World substance – breast milk or lizard meat – into a transplanted or newly colonized imperial body, suggest parallels with much-celebrated advances in inoculation taking place at the same time.[4] As is commonly known, inoculation – the introduction of a disease agent into an organism with the intention of producing well-being through immunity – was revolutionized by Edward Jenner's 1796 use of cowpox to promote immunity against smallpox. Less widely appreciated is the enthusiastic appropriation of Jenner's cowpox vaccine by Spanish and Spanish American physicians and its employment in imperial vaccination campaigns as part of a larger program of enlightened Bourbon reforms related to public health. This oversight is characteristic of the way the Hispanic world has figured – or not – in the history of science and medicine.[5] Notwithstanding the tendency to overlook the role played by science in Spain's global empire, John Slater, Maríaluz López-Terrada, and José Pardo-Tomás note in their introduction to *Medical Cultures of the Early Modern Spanish Empire*: "In the early modern world of the Hapsburg empire, medical cultures proved powerful tools for imaging the spaces of the body politic and for extending the ideologies of the Spanish state" (2).[6] The same can be said for medical cultures during the Bourbon Empire, which reflect continuity and rupture with those of early modern Spain. In the examples I will study, breastfeeding and the so-called "lizard cure" function as much-debated methods for inoculating the body politic that carry with them risk and reward for individuals and the imperial state. By focusing on how medical cultures and practices were negotiated on the ground in eighteenth-century Spanish America, we can better understand a distinctive Hispanic Enlightenment in its transatlantic dimensions and in a context that was at the same time global and local, ideologically informed by enlightened ideas and deeply pragmatic.

Eighteenth-century Spanish American medical cultures were predicated upon a body politic inscribed in power relationships defined by gender and other categories of difference such as *casta* (race or ethnicity) and *calidad* (status or social class).[7] Gender as a category of analysis has traditionally been a neglected topic in studies of the Hispanic Enlightenment (itself another often overlooked field of study), with the notable exception of historian Mónica Bolufer Peruga's *Mujeres e Ilustración*.[8] Yet, as Catherine M. Jaffe and Elizabeth Franklin Lewis argue in their introduction to *Eve's Enlightenment* any assessment of the Hispanic Enlightenment must take into account gendered experiences: "Given the empirical orientation of the Enlightenment, experience was integral to its epistemology" (4). Rebecca Haidt, who has studied the importance of the body and embodied knowledge in eighteenth-century enlightened writers such as Benito Jerónimo Feijoo (1676–1764) and Gaspar Melchor de Jovellanos (1744–1811), proposes a working definition of the construction of gender as "the education and training of persons to inhabit bodies in such a way as to evidence their alignment within such categories as 'masculine' and 'feminine,' 'active' and 'passive' ... effected through the contingent operation of a number of institutions, proscriptions and practices such as schools, churches, marriage laws and bodily deportment" (9). The work of Haidt, Jaffe, and Lewis provides a necessary foundation for my reading of the embodied knowledges implicit in eighteenth-century Spanish American medical discourses on *leche* and *lagartijas*, as access to first-hand experience and empirical observation privileged criollos in enlightened debates with armchair philosophers about the nature of the New World. Recent scholarly work that has begun to take into account the role of indigenous peoples, women, and slaves in the creation and dissemination of knowledge about plants and healing practices in the Americas is also fundamental to my reading.[9]

Leche

In the early modern European world, breast milk was understood to be part of the body's humoral system, almost a kind of blood whose benefits were both biological and moral.[10] For example, Spanish theologian Fray Luis de León offered counsel in *La perfecta casada* about the importance of breastfeeding. As Alison Krögel explains, Fray Luis felt that "a mother's milk provided not only the perfect nutritional sustenance for her child, but also served as a liquid conduit for the transfer of maternal values and morality into the body and soul of her offspring" (237). Breast milk, according to Fray Luis, "se bebe y convierte en substancia, y como en naturaleza, todo lo bueno y lo malo que hay en aquella de quien se recibe; porque el cuerpo ternecico de un niño, y que salió como comenzando del vientre, la teta le acaba de hacer y formar" ("is drunk and converts into substance, and as in nature, all the good and evil that exists in the one from whom it is received; because the tender body of a child, begun and sprung from the womb, is completed and formed by the breast"; trans. mine; 170; quoted by Krögel). Arguments against using wet nurses were traditionally articulated on moral grounds – the unnaturalness of a mother choosing not to breastfeed her baby – or religious grounds – the threat of heresy being transmitted through polluted breast milk.[11] These debates about wet nursing reflected anxieties not only about childrearing practices but also larger issues of social and religious hygiene that continued to resonate.

As Claudia Rosas Lauro has observed, enlightened debates about breastfeeding, which Bolufer Peruga called "the metaphor of maternity," reflect long-standing ideas about the role of women as exemplary figures of domestic instruction. These debates, employing medical and philosophical discourse, blur the boundaries of public and private space, elite and popular agency (Rosas Lauro 313). Women were encouraged to care for themselves and their children as part of their patriotic and civic responsibilities. The anti-wet nurse rhetoric that appeared in Spanish American eighteenth-century medical literature incorporated new approaches to childrearing, but it also reflected increasing criollo anxieties about miscegenation and its implications for public health. Mixed-race wet nurses were seen as a particularly pernicious threat to social order, and in the viceregal centres of Lima and Mexico this argument was made vociferously on hygienic, epidemiological, philosophical, and patriotic grounds, often in the nascent periodical press.

A couple of examples will serve to illustrate these anxieties. The first is an article that appeared in the *Mercurio Peruano,* which was published in Lima from 1790 to 1795, entitled "Amas de Leche (Segunda carta de Filómates sobre la educación)" ("Wet Nurses [Second letter from Philomates on education]"). The anonymous author had previously addressed the question of childrearing in criollo families, lamenting the excessive reliance on slaves and the resulting lack of formality in familial relations. In this letter, addressed to "Gentlemen who love their country," he turns to the detrimental influence of wet nurses of colour. His focus is on wet nurses of African descent, although other letters published around the same time reflect similar anxieties regarding indigenous or mestiza wet nurses. While indigenous women served as wet nurses during the early years of the colonial period, by the eighteenth century women of African descent and *mulatas* primarily performed this function, as evidenced by job ads in the periodical press. Acknowledging the "amor casi materno" ("almost maternal love") that his own daughter's wet nurse María has demonstrated, Filómates complains that she carries the child everywhere: "María viste a la muchachita, la lleva a la cocina, al lavadero, a la calle, a la pulpería y adonde quiere" ("María dresses the little girl, she takes her to the kitchen, to the laundry, out in the street, to the 'pulpería' and wherever she wants"; Clément 44). And he concludes with a warning: "esta libertad de las amas suele ser fatal a la inocencia de los niños, que éstos, rosándose sólo con la gente de esta ralea, se familiarizan con sus modales groseras, y que aprenden y adoptan todas las llanezas que entre sí practican los esclavos" ("This freedom on the part of wet nurses tends to be fatal for children's innocence, as when they only have contact with this sort of person, they become familiarized with vulgar manners and learn and adopt all the informalities that are practised among slaves"; Clément 44). In other words, the child ventures out with her wet nurse into an increasingly diverse terrain of private and public spaces, housing demographically diverse crowds of dubious customs. The danger only increases as the little girl becomes a young woman, susceptible to greater threats to her honour, while at the same time the wet nurse comes to expect special favours from the family in exchange for her devotion. In Filómates's complaints, the practice of wet nursing seems to open a door to social and moral contagion and to the breakdown of the social, moral, and hygienic hierarchies that are essential to the preservation of viceregal order.

In her work on the *Mercurio Peruano* in *Deviant and Useful Citizens: The Cultural Production of the Female Body in Eighteenth-Century Peru* (2011), Mariselle Meléndez has analysed these letters in the context of a larger argument about the cultural production of the female body in late colonial Peru. She notes that male contributors to the periodical pursued a discussion of "the social preoccupations that the white Creole elite thought were fundamental for the good social order and progress of society ... [and] central to the production of healthy citizens and to social progress" (128).[12] The bodies of mixed-race women, in need of constant monitoring and moral and physical containment, were seen as especially disruptive to these goals. In this instance, the behaviour of María, the African-descendant criolla wet nurse in question, and that of others like her reveals the fragility of rules governing the behaviour of wet nurses (Meléndez 165); she threatens social and familial order because other members of the household saw her as a figure of authority (166). Meléndez emphasizes that these complaints are as much about power as breastfeeding practices; the writer is not saying that wet nurses shouldn't be used, but rather that husbands and fathers need to control their engagement and access. The tension between the ideal and the real permeates every line of the letter. Meléndez concludes by quoting José Ignacio Lequanda, who argued in an article published in the *Mercurio Peruano* in 1794 that the disease of indolence and social disorder requires the intervention of "un doctor diestro que no solo aplique el *antidoto,* sino que sepa aplicarlo lentamente y con cordura" ("a skilful doctor who not only is able to apply the *antidote* but knows how to apply it slowly and with reason"; Clément 171; emphasis mine). I am intrigued by the employment of medical vocabulary in Lequanda's assessment. The rampant use – even abuse – of mixed-race wet nurses is presented in pathological terms, and the prescribed response is described as an "antidote."

Alison Krögel explores another example of anti-wet nurse rhetoric, published under a pseudonym in the satirical "Ordenanzas del Baratillo de México" (1734), in which the author focuses on the lax childrearing practices of a criollo elite surrounded by an increasingly disorderly and diverse urban population. The author worries that the common practice of mothers abdicating their maternal role to wet nurses leads to weak, whiny, and dishonest offspring who will not grow up to be responsible citizens worthy of self-rule. The author of the "Ordenanzas" even includes a shocking case of a wet nurse who has taught the toddlers in her care to smoke cigars and prostitute themselves (242–3). The mention of cigars is particularly striking, since tobacco was a New World plant that even in the eighteenth century still occupied an uncertain space between uncivilized indigenous customs and commercialized adoption by Europeans, between poison and cure. Like chocolate, tobacco is a local product in the process of becoming a global commodity; excessive consumption risked upsetting the balance of indigenous and European customs.[13]

Krögel notes that "colonial Spanish-American satire often served as a 'diagnostic tool' for identifying societal ills with the ultimate goal of affecting real sociopolitical change" (245).[14] While this is no doubt true, these particular examples of satire repeat, rather than challenge, the entrenched racial hierarchies implicit in eighteenth-century taxonomies. The condemnation of breastfeeding by *castas* is seen as a necessary check on a pernicious cultural mediation that brought the offspring of the criollo elite into close proximity with the unhealthy customs of the urban underclass, exposing them to the risk of uncontrollable cultural contagion.

Enlightened medical discourse increasingly highlighted the figure of the male doctor who practised his profession on the basis of science and experience, unlike the superstitious midwives who had traditionally cared for women during pregnancy and childbirth – a racialized and misogynist stereotype, to be sure. The fear of contagion reflected in critiques of mixed-race wet nurses informs related concerns about infant mortality, the prevalence of popular customs like not washing babies immediately after birth, or the use of herbal remedies for female maladies. Such concerns ultimately led to attempts to limit the involvement of midwives in childbirth. As the Protomedicato redoubled its critique of the lack of professionalization in medicine in the eighteenth century, midwives were an easy target (Rosas Laura 332). One means of controlling their participation in medical practice was a new requirement that they be officially examined on questions of female anatomy (Zegarra 371). But these concerns also reflected deeper worries about paternity: to whom would the children of Spain's territories in the Americas belong, and who would claim responsibility for them?[15]

Gendered racial and social hierarchies intersected with politics and the Bourbon reform agenda against a background of profound changes in the teaching and practice of medicine that were widely discussed in the emergent periodical press.[16] Medical care in colonial Spanish America had long been racially and socially stratified; however, neither members of the criollo elite nor the *casta* population were averse to consulting a range of practitioners. Although folk healers were officially seen as a threat to public health, they were often used in combination with medical techniques of Peninsular origin (Jouve Martín 17), and the medical practices of the educated criollo elite incorporated New World elements such as plant remedies and the lizard cure, to which I now turn.

Lagartijas

There is, of course, a long tradition of integrating New World nature into the systemic knowledge of the Old World, rewriting Plinian natural history on the basis of American experience. This tradition includes early chronicles like Gonzalo Fernández de Oviedo's *Historia general y natural de las Indias* (1535) and his *Sumario* (1526), José de Acosta's *Historia natural y moral de las Indias* (1590), Francisco Ximénez's Spanish translation of Francisco Hernández de Toledo's *De la naturaleza, y virtudes de las plantas, y animales que estan receuidos en el vso de medicina en la Nueua España* (1615), as well as the lesser-known *Códice de la Cruz Badiano* (1552) – all of which incorporate discussion of medicinal uses in their depiction through text and image of American nature.[17] The interest in the therapeutic application of American fauna and flora led to the exploration of autochthonous resources and indigenous traditions carried out by Europeans with curiosity and, on occasion, trepidation. These explorations were guided by the principles of Galenic medicine; humoralism provided the foundation for European understandings of bodily differences that informed their encounters with indigenous peoples in the sixteenth and seventeenth centuries and well into the eighteenth century, even as new medical discoveries about the circulation of blood or the role of germs in the spread of disease gained currency. We see the traces of humoral thinking in ideas about hot and cold or wet and dry elements in folk medicine, for example.

In the eighteenth century, criollo intellectuals turned to local knowledge to engage in enlightened debates that took place in the viceroyal capitals of Mexico City and Lima and also crossed the Atlantic. Instead of the display of curiosities and the power of possession represented by the *Wunderkammer* tradition, they focused on the scientific opportunities of studying flora and fauna alive and in situ.[18] Moving beyond the *enumeratio caotica* (that is, the enumeration of a series of diverse items) that characterized Pliny and earlier chroniclers, their enlightened descendants in the eighteenth century used their American experiences to put received cultural and scientific authority to an orderly test.

Miruna Achim discusses one example of these debates in *Lagartijas medicinales*.[19] The debate about "medicinal lizards" was sparked by the publication in 1781 of a brief pamphlet titled "Específico nuevamente descubierto en el Reyno de Guatemala, para la curación radical del horrible mal de cancro y otros más frecuentes" ("A medicine newly discovered in the Kingdom of Guatemala, for the radical cure of the horrible affliction of cancer, and other more frequent ones"). Authored by José Felipe Flores, who held a Chair in Medicine at the Royal University of Guatemala, the pamphlet offered a cure for cancer, based on indigenous practices that had been "newly discovered."[20] The cure involved lizards, and Flores provided detailed instructions:

> Toman una Lagartija, y con diestra ligereza le cortan la cabeza, y cola. Inmediatemente les extraen los Intestinos, y de un tirón le arrancan la pielezilla. En este estado, cruda, la carne aun caliente, y en toda la vitalidad posible, la mascan, y tragan con gran serenidad. De este modo se tragan una Lagartija cada dia. Dicen que suele bastar una, y si no, toman hasta tres: asegurando que por este medio han sanado siempre de las llagas, y las bubas, enfermedad endémica de aquel Pueblo.

> They take a Lizard, and with quick skillfulness they cut off its head, and tail. Immediately they remove the Intestines, and all at once tear off the little skin. In this state, raw, the flesh still warm and with all possible vitality, they chew it and swallow it with great serenity. In this manner they swallow one Lizard every day. They say that one is usually enough, and if not, they digest up to three: assuring that by these means they have always cured themselves of ulcers and inflammations endemic in that people. (trans. mine; Achim 232)

For the squeamish (or *melindrosos*), Flores provided the option of dicing the lizard meat and forming it into a little pill to be ingested.

Following the publication of Flores's pamphlet, experts and laymen weighed in on the kinds of lizards that should be used, the reliability of the experiments that had been conducted, and the advisability of official sanctions of the newly discovered radical cure.[21] One of the first and most significant of these interventions was a document published in 1782 by the distinguished criollo scholar Antonio de León y Gama, "Instrucción sobre el remedio de las lagartijas" ("Instruction on the lizard cure"). In addition to including first-hand accounts of the therapeutic experiments he had conducted with various patients, the author drew on his extensive knowledge of indigenous culture, Nahua language, and New World botany to urge caution with the lizard cure, recommending instead further study of indigenous plant remedies:

> Ojalá, y como se ha propagado este descubrimiento de los Indios, resucitara en esta Nueva España la medicina herbaria de ellos! Con ella se tomaría un perfecto conocimiento de todas sus plantas: se aprovecharían los trabajos del Doctor Hernández, de que se ha hecho tanto aprecio en los países extrangeros, donde solo se han contentado con las noticias de sus descubrimientos; sin poder aprovecharse de las yervas de que carecen: se caminaría, con toda seguridad, en el uso de ellas, sin los escollos en que tropieza la Antigua Medicina tantas veces dañosa a la salud.
>
> I hope, and just as this discovery by the Indians has been propagated, that their herbal medicine might resuscitate here in New Spain! With that, one would have perfect knowledge of all their plants: one would be able to take advantage of the work of Doctor Hernández, who is much appreciated in foreign lands, where they have had to be content only with the news of his discoveries, without being able to take advantage of the herbs themselves, which they do not have; one would advance with all certainty in their use, without the mistakes which Ancient Medicine has made, so often a danger to good health. (trans. mine; Achim 263)

The "lagartijas" question reflects the heightened sense of intellectual engagement among members of the enlightened criollo elite around the issue of traditional versus modern knowledge, clearly visible in the quote from León y Gama. His lament that foreigners had given greater credence than Spaniards to the work of naturalists such as Francisco Hernández is counterbalanced by his reminder that only those living in the Americas had access to the plants themselves. This intense local debate reflects the negotiation of local and global knowledge that informed discussions of New World nature, most notably studied by Antonello Gerbi in *The Dispute of the New World*. Lance Thurner, moreover, relates the medical community's fascination with the lizard cure as a therapeutic equivalent of Francisco Javier Clavijero's *Storia antica di Messico* (1780–1) – an attempt to appropriate and deploy ancient indigenous wisdom as a counterbalance to the perceived view of the Americas as degenerate and in decline.

The lizard cure was part of a transatlantic pharmacopeia that included New World flora and fauna and combined indigenous, African-descendant and early modern European medical practices. Londa Schiebinger has explored this phenomenon in two important books, *Plants and Empire: Colonial Bioprospecting int the Atlantic World* (2004) and *Secret Cures of Slaves: People, Plants and Medicine in the Eighteenth-Century Atlantic World* (2017). One of the most fascinating examples she studies pertains to the circulation of knowledge about exotic abortifacients, including the *flos pavonis*, or peacock flower. Schiebinger argues that botanical knowledge was applied in the service of empire in ways that were deeply inflected by notions of race and gender. These debates point to the importance of scientific experimentation as a means of creating and transmitting knowledge, and to the potential benefits of the commercialized dissemination of that knowledge.[22] Given the high stakes, there was frequently a tension between the desire to disseminate knowledge and a sense that the knowledge was a valuable secret to be jealously guarded. The registry for the Real Gabinete de Historia Natural de Madrid includes a 1782 entry acknowledging receipt of Flores's "Específico nuevamente descubierto," noting as well his intention to send six lizards to accompany the report. We know that Flores's pamphlet circulated widely in Europe, although it's not clear if the lizards ever arrived (Achim 173–4).

I argue that lizards occupy a special place in these discussions by virtue of their very strangeness. As in European accounts of indigenous practices related to tobacco and smoking practices that were both ritualistic and therapeutic, lizards represent something that is at the same time noxious and compellingly attractive. Lizards are a kind of "local hero" that functions as a *pharmakon*, that is, remedy, poison, and scapegoat; the lizard cure – during which small amounts of raw flesh are ingested by the patient – is presented almost as an experiment in inoculation, one that must be carried out in accord with a deep understanding of the cultural context from which it had emerged if it is to be successful. Yet the very process of understanding – the integration of European medical knowledge, products, and practices with those of the indigenous inhabitants, flora, and fauna of the Americas – carries with it a certain degree of risk.[23]

This is one of the takeaways from decades of smallpox inoculation campaigns carried out in the eighteenth century by the Protomedicato and viceroyal authorities, as Martha Few has studied in *For All of Humanity: Mesoamerican and Colonial Medicine in Enlightenment Guatemala* (2015). Plans for the prevention and containment of the disease included a combination of quarantine, inoculation, and civilian and military oversight; colonial administrators recognized that these measures were more successful when they involved collaboration with local indigenous leaders and *curanderos* and an appreciation of indigenous medical practices.[24] Negotiations between local and imperial infrastructures and belief systems had to be carefully carried out in order to successfully combat the ravages of the disease; in the process, the boundaries between the two became blurred. This is not unlike what had happened in the scientific sphere. As Few explains, "In late eighteenth and early nineteenth-century colonial Latin America, the word "inoculación" ("inoculation") could refer to both the use with human-derived smallpox matter and to vaccination with cowpox after the development of the Jenner vaccine in 1796 (203).[25] The linguistic interchangeability reflects the scientific advance represented by Jenner's cowpox vaccine; however, it also underscores the complexities of introducing a foreign substance into the body in order to provoke a therapeutic development while recognizing the risk that the foreign element might prove too powerful or noxious. Perhaps not coincidentally, José Flores, the physician whose pamphlet had touched off the "lizard cure" controversy, was the designer and chief advocate for an ambitious smallpox vaccination campaign, authorized by Carlos IV and the Council of the Indies and intended for the entire Spanish Empire (Few 3).[26] In all these instances, a willingness to inject the local into imperial considerations of public health proved to be a strategic and enlightened contribution to colonial medicine, operating in a broad humanitarian context in which individual patients and their gendered, racialized bodies were understood to form part of a larger body politic. As Few notes, "'colonial medicine' absorbed and responded to indigenous, gendered, and local medical cultures even as it may have presented itself as the autonomous project of peninsular and creole elites connected to European metropoles" (16).

The examples I've discussed in this essay remind us that medical cultures are as much about context and process as they are about outcomes. They challenge us to study the eighteenth century not through the retrospective lens of independence or belated modernity but rather alive and *in situ,* following the model of the enlightened scholar-practitioners I've highlighted here. Debates about breastfeeding and the lizard cure represent a negotiation of European and indigenous medical practices and home-grown or scientific remedies that attempt to weigh the risks and benefits of introducing the "new" world into the "old." These are questions that continue to resonate. Londa Schiebinger notes that in the eighteenth century, "funding priorities, global strategies, national policies, the structures of scientific institutions, trade patterns, and gender politics all pushed investigation toward certain parts of nature and away from others" (*Plants and Empire* 226). Schiebinger makes a larger argument that reproductive control worked against imperial and, later, national projects involving expansion of population and wealth. She discusses colonial efforts to enlist midwives as agents of the state (*Plants and Empire* 237) and links Alexander von Humboldt's resistance to knowledge about abortifacients and abortion practices to his embrace of mercantilist emphasis on population growth (239). In the realm of fiction, Julia Alvarez's 2006 novel *Saving the World* tells the alternating stories of two women, a Latina novelist suffering from writer's block, and Isabel Sendales y Gómez, the smallpox survivor and orphanage director who accompanied the orphan boys who served as human carriers on the Balmis Expedition. The novel, albeit flawed, reflects the importance of bringing to the fore the forgotten protagonism of women in early modern and colonial science. As these stories demonstrate, eighteenth-century medical discourses and practices in Spanish America "injected the local" in ways that continue to inform us today.

NOTES

1 I presented an early version of this essay at the International Conference on Medicine, Literature and Culture in the Early Modern Hispanic World (St. Andrews University, July 2017); my deepest thanks to co-organizers Ted Bergman and María Luisa Lobato and to the distinguished keynote presenters and panelists whose comments are reflected in this revised version.

2 See John Slater, Maríaluz López-Terrada, and José Pardo-Tomás, "Introduction" in *Medical Cultures of the Early Modern Spanish Empire* (2).

3 In addition to demonstrating how the eighteenth-century negotiation of the local and the global expands our thinking about medical cultures in general, I am also interested in disseminating recent work on eighteenth-century Spanish America that may not be familiar to scholars of other periods.

4 Martha Few has studied inoculation campaigns in viceregal Spanish America in *For All of Humanity*.

5 See Antonio Barrera-Osorio's *Experiencing Nature*. Although Barrera-Osorio focuses on the sixteenth century, his observation that "historians of science tend to overlook the program for researching nature in the Atlantic world" holds for later periods as well (3). See also Daniela Bleichmar et al., eds., *Science in the Spanish and Portuguese Empires, 1500–1800* (2009).

6 They understand medicine as "on the one hand, a varied form of cultural practice and production, and on the other, a significant matrix for the

intersection of a wide range of cultural phenomena (political, literary, religious, or otherwise)" (2). This understanding is my point of departure for the analysis that follows.

7 Mariselle Meléndez notes that "it was in the eighteenth century that factors such as race and social class came to play a major role when defining what was to be considered a useful citizen" (138); she cites Ruth Hill's seminal discussion of "intersecting principles of hierarchy in colonial Spanish America" (*Hierarchy, Commerce, and Fraud*, 215).

8 An English translation of Bolufer's groundbreaking study is forthcoming. See Arcos Herrera.

9 See Londa Schiebinger, and Pablo F. Gómez. Schiebinger identifies barriers to the circulation of knowledge about medicine and healing in the Atlantic world: the extermination of the indigenous population during the colonial period, enslavement, secrecy, prejudice, and the linguistic differences that reflected and shaped different world views. Nevertheless, she concludes that "the flow of knowledge in the Atlantic World medical complex was promiscuous and multidirectional" (*Secret Cures of Slaves* 147).

10 See the next essay in this volume by Emily Colbert Cairns for a detailed study of the depiction of breast milk in early modern art and literature.

11 Alison Krögel notes that "throughout medieval Europe, papal and royal decrees sought to prevent wet nurses from suckling infants of a different faith"; the *Siete partidas* addressed this concern, and later José de Acosta worried that indigenous mothers might pass religious heresy on to their mestizo offspring (234–5). There is an extensive bibliography on breastfeeding in colonial Spanish America that includes Bianca Premo's "'Misunderstood Love': Children and Wet Nurses, Creoles and Kings in Lima's Enlightenment" (2005) and Claudia Rosas Lauro's "La visión ilustrada de las amas de leche negras y mulatas en el ámbito familiar, Lima, siglo XVIII" (2005)."

12 Meléndez notes that these articles frequently focused on cases of monstrous births that built on long-standing associations of the female with the monstrous and suggested larger threats of "disorder, ambiguity, deviance and anomaly" (130).

13 Marcy Norton discusses the Atlantic World history of tobacco and chocolate as cultural commodities in *Sacred Gifts, Profane Pleasures*, focusing on the seventeenth century. She concludes, "The imagery of enchantment that surrounded tobacco and chocolate, both because of their American origins and because of Europe's Eucharistic culture, did not disappear. Rather, it was displaced; the images of chocolate as divine elixir and tobacco as a diabolical, but ever-useful substance flourished in the pretend-world of art and literature" (265). In her conclusion, however, she makes short shrift of the eighteenth century.

14 Krögel is drawing here on Julie Greer Johnson's work on colonial satire in *Satire in Colonial Spanish America: Turning the New World Upside Down*.

15 See Premo, "Misunderstood Love" and *Children of the Father King*.

16 Beyond questions of gender, efforts to professionalize medicine also bring to the fore questions about how to categorize – legally, racially, socially – individuals of African descent in colonial society and about the relationship between race and knowledge, as José Jouve Martín explores in *The Black Doctors of Colonial Lima. Science, Race and Writing in Colonial and Early Republican Peru* (2014).

17 The second part of Fernández de Oviedo's *Historia general y natural*, unfinished at the time of the author's death, was not published until 1852. The *Códice de la Cruz-Badiano* refers to the Spanish translation, completed by Juan Badiano, of a Latin manuscript, *Libellus de medicinalibus indorum herbis*, written by Martín de la Cruz.

18 The "cabinet of curiosities" emerged in the sixteenth century as a way of exhibiting strange and exotic objects, often collected by travellers to the Americas.

19 Achim's volume includes lengthy appendices with the primary documents she mentions.

20 José Felipe Flores (1751–1824) is considered one of the pioneers of medicine and medical education in Guatemala. He studied medicine at the University of San Carlos, played a leading role in official inoculation campaigns during the 1780 smallpox epidemic, and served as Protomedicato of Guatemala (1794–6). Achim discusses Flores's pamphlet at length in her introduction (11–18) and returns to it in the context of eighteenth-century rediscoveries of indigenous "materia médica" (75). Few discusses Flores's contributions (8); see also José Aznar López, *El doctor Don José Felipe Flores* (1960).

21 Europeans had long been fascinated by "New World" lizards, large and small. Gonzalo Fernández de Oviedo recounts in an addendum to his chapter on iguanas in the *Historia general y natural de las Indias* (1548) that he sent an iguana to Venetian scholar Giovanni Battista Ramusio, recommending it as a delicious delicacy when seasoned with bacon and kale (*berzas*); it "tastes like chicken," he claimed. Unfortunately, the iguana did not survive its transatlantic crossing, perishing of hunger because its Spanish captors didn't fully appreciate that it was herbivorous and sent it on its translantic crossing trapped in a barrel of mud with nothing else to eat (Paden 203). Oviedo's concern in the *Sumario* and the *Historial general y natural de las Indias* – beyond the gastronomic possibilities – has to do with the nature of the animal itself.

22 For a discussion of the commercialization of cincona bark, see Matthew Crawford, *The Andean Wonder Drug: Cinchona Bark and Imperial Science in the Spanish Atlantic, 1630–1800* (2016); Christophe Strosetzki also addressed this topic in his keynote address at the International Conference "Medicine, Literature and Culture in the Early Modern Hispanic World." For additional context, see too Schiebinger, *Plants and Empire*, and *Secret Cures of Slaves*.

23 As Jacques Derrida argued in "Plato's Pharmacy," "This pharmakon, this 'medicine,' this philter, which acts as both remedy and poison, already introduces itself into the body of the discourse with all its ambivalence ... Operating through seduction, the pharmakon makes one stray from one's general, natural, habitual paths and laws" (429).

24 "for antiepidemic campaigns to succeed in colonial Central America and elsewhere in the Americas, indigenous cultures, practices, and responses had to be taken into account" (Few 18).

25 Few continues, "This can also be translated into English as variolation and variolization. 'Vacuna' (vaccine, vaccination; from the Latin 'vaca' [cow]) referred specifically to the use of the cowpox virus to confer immunity to smallpox" (203).

26 Eighteenth-century poets joined the chorus celebrating Jenner's discovery and its imperial implementation by Flores and Don Francisco Balmis, who organized the Real Expedición Filantrópica de la Vacuna (1803–6). Manuel José Quintana's "A la expedición española para propagar la vacuna en América bajo la dirección de Don Francisco Balmis" (1806) is a lengthy poem whose title seems more appropriate for a medical report than an ode. Quintana highlights the pain and suffering caused by smallpox among the innocent peoples of America before going on to acclaim the role played by Jenner in inventing the vaccine and Balmis in disseminating it (both surnames are always written in capital letters in the text). Andrés Bello also penned an "Oda a la vacuna" praising Jenner and Balmis (1804). For a consideration of political and epidemiological discourse in both poems, see Pereiro-Otero's essay "Conquistas Vi(r)olentas y Vacunas Independentistas."

WORKS CITED

Achim, Miruna. *Lagartijas medicinales: Remedios americanos y debates científicos en la Ilustración*. Universidad Autónoma Metropolitana-Cuajimalpa/ Consejo Nacional para la Cultura y las Artes, 2008.

Alvarez, Julia. *Saving the World*. Algonquin Books, 2006.

Arcos Herrera, Carol. "Sujetos de controversia: Aportes para una bibliografía sobre las mujeres en el siglo XVIII y la Ilustración." *Revista de Crítica Literaria Latinoamericana*, vol. 34, no. 67, 2008, pp. 111–22.

Aznar López, José. *El doctor Don José Felipe Flores. Una vida al servicio de la ciencia*. Editorial Universitaria, 1960.

Balaguer Perigüell, Emilio y Rosa Ballester Añon. *En el nombre de los Niños. Real Expedición Filantrópica de la Vacuna, 1803–1806*. Monografías de la AEP, 2003.

Barrera-Osorio, Antonio. *Experiencing Nature: The Spanish American Empire and the Early Scientific Revolution*. U of Texas Press, 2006.

Bello, Andrés. *A la Vacuna*. http://www.cervantesvirtual.com/obra-visor/poesias--35/html/.

Bentancor, Orlando. *The Matter of Empire: Hispanic Metaphysics and Mining in Colonial Peru, 1520–1640*. U of Pittsburgh P, 2017.

Bleichmar, Daniela, et al., editors. *Science in the Spanish and Portuguese Empires, 1500–1800*. Stanford UP, 2009.

Bolufer Peruga, Mónica. *Mujeres e Ilustración. La construcción de la feminidad en la España del siglo XVIII*. Institució Alfons El Magnanim y Diputació de Valéncia, 1998.

Cañizares-Esguerra, Jorge. *How to Write the History of the New World: Histories, Epistemologies, and Identities in the Eighteenth-Century Atlantic World*. Stanford UP, 2001.

Casalino Sen, Carlota. "Hipólito Unanue y la ciencia ilustrada en el Perú." *Passeurs, mediadores culturales y agentes de la primera globalización en el Mundo Ibérico, siglos XVI–XIX*, edited by Scarlett O'Phelan and Solange Alberro, Pontificia Universidad Católica del Perú/Instituto Riva-Agüero/Instituto Francés de Estudios Andinos, 2005, pp. 605–28.

Clément, Jean-Pierre, editor. *El Mercurio Peruano, 1790–1795. Vol. II: Antología*. Iberoamericana Vervuert, 1998.

Crawford, Matthew James. *The Andean Wonder Drug: Cinchona Bark and Imperial Science in the Spanish Atlantic, 1630–1800*. U of Pittsburgh P, 2016.

Derrida, Jacques. "Plato's Pharmacy." *Dissemination*, translated by Barbara Johnson, U of Chicago P, 1981, pp. 63–171.

Earle, Rebecca. *The Body of the Conquistador: Food, Race and the Colonial Experience in Spanish America, 1492–1700*. Cambridge UP, 2012.

Few, Martha. *For All of Humanity: Mesoamerican and Colonial Medicine in Enlightenment Guatemala*. U of Arizona P, 2015.

Foucault, Michel. *The Birth of the Clinic: An Archaeology of Medical Perception*. 1963; translated 1973, Vintage, 1994.

Gerbi, Antonello. *The Dispute of the New World: The History of a Polemic, 1750–1900*. Translated by Jeremly Moyle, 1955; U of Pittsburgh P, 1973.

Gómez, Pablo F. *The Experiential Caribbean: Creating Knowledge and Healing in the Early Modern Atlantic*. U of North Carolina P, 2017.

Haidt, Rebecca. *Embodying Enlightenment: Knowing the Body in Eighteenth-Century Spanish Literature and Culture*. St. Martin's Press, 1998.

Hernández, Francisco. *De la naturaleza, y virtudes de las plantas, y animales que estan receuidos en el vso de medicina en la Nueua España, y la methodo, y correccion*. En casa de la viuda de Diego Lopez Davalos, 1615.

Hill, Ruth. *Hierarchy, Commerce and Fraud in Bourbon Spanish America: A Postal Inspector's Exposé*. Vanderbilt UP, 2005.

Jaffary, Nora E. *Reproduction and Its Discontents in Mexico: Childbirth and Contraception from 1750 to 1905*. U of North Carolina P, 2016.

Jaffe, Catherine M., and Elizabeth Franklin Lewis, editors. *Eve's Enlightenment: Women's Experience in Spain and Spanish America, 1726–1839*. Louisiana State UP, 2009.

Johnson, Julie Greer. *Satire in Colonial Spanish America: Turning the New World Upside Down*. U of Texas P, 1993.

Jouve Martín, José R. *The Black Doctors of Colonial Lima: Science, Race and Writing in Colonial and Early Republican Peru*. McGill-Queen's UP, 2014.

Krögel, Alison. "Mercenary Milk, Pernicious Nursemaids, Heedless Mothers: Anti-Wet Nurse Rhetoric in the Satirical *Ordenanzas del Baratillo de México* (1734)." *Dieciocho*, vol. 37, no. 2, Fall 2014, pp. 233–48.

Lafuente, Antonio, and Nuria Valverde. "Linnaean Botany and Spanish Imperial Biopolitics." *Colonial Botany. Science, Commerce, and Politics in the Early Modern World*, edited by Londa Schiebinger and Claudia Swan, U of Pennsylvania P, 2005, pp. 134–47.

León y Gama, Antonio de. *Instrucción sobre el remedio de las lagartijas nuevamente descubierto para la curación del cancro, y otras enfermedades*. Felipe de Zúñiga y Ontiveros, 1782.

León, Fray Luis de. *La perfecta casada* [1583]. Edited by Joaquín Antonio Peñalosa. Editorial Porrúa, 1999.

Meléndez, Mariselle. *Deviant and Useful Citizens: The Cultural Production of the Female Body in Eighteenth-Century Peru*. Vanderbilt UP, 2011.

Norton, Marcy. *Sacred Gifts, Profane Pleasures: A History of Tobacco and Chocolate in the Atlantic World*. Cornell UP, 2008.

O'Phelan, Scarlett, and Solange Alberro, editors. *Passeurs, mediadores culturales y agentes de la primera globalización en el Mundo Ibérico, siglos XVI–XIX*. Pontificia Universidad Católica del Perú/Instituto Riva-Agüero/Instituto Francés de Estudios Andinos, 2005.

Paden, Jeremy. "The Iguana and the Barrel of Mud: Memory, Natural History, and Hermeneutics in Oviedo's *Sumario de la natural historia de las Indias*." *Colonial Latin American Review*, vol. 16, no. 2, 2007, pp. 203–26.

Pereiro-Otero, José Manuel. "Conquistas Vi(r)olentas y Vacunas Independentistas: Andrés Bello y Manuel José Quintana ante la Enfermedad de la Colonia." *Hispanic Review*, vol. 76, no. 2, 2008, pp. 109–33. *JSTOR*, www.jstor.org/stable/27668833.

Premo, Bianca. *Children of the Father King: Youth, Authority, and Legal Minority in Colonial Lima*. U of North Carolina P, 2009.

– "'Misunderstood Love': Children and Wet Nurses, Creoles and Kings in Lima's Enlightenment." *Colonial Latin American Review*, vol. 14, no. 2, 2005, pp. 231–6.

– Quintana, Manuel José. "A la expedición española para propagar la vacuna en América bajo la dirección de Don Francisco Balmis." *Poesía del siglo XVIII*, edited by John H.R. Polt, 3rd ed., Castalia, 1987, pp. 376–80.

Reyes-Foster, Beatriz, and Shannon K. Carter. "Suspect Bodies, Suspect Milk: Milk Sharing, Wetnursing, and the Specter of Syphilis in the 21st Century." Author's draft.

Rosas Lauro, Claudia. "La visión ilustrada de las amas de leche negras y mulatas en el ámbito familiar (Lima, siglo XVIII)." *Passeurs, mediadores culturales y agentes de la primera globalización en el Mundo Ibérico, siglos XVI–XIX*, edited by Scarlett O'Phelan and Solange Alberro, Pontificia Universidad Católica del Perú/Instituto Riva-Agüero/Instituto Francés de Estudios Andinos, 2005, pp. 311–43.

Schiebinger, Londa. *Plants and Empire: Colonial Bioprospecting in the Atlantic World*. Harvard UP, 2004.

– *Secret Cures of Slaves: People, Plants, and Medicine in the Eighteenth-Century Atlantic World*. Stanford UP, 2017.

Schiebinger, Londa, and Claudia Swan, editors. *Colonial Botany: Science, Commerce, and Politics in the Early Modern World*. U of Pennsylvania P, 2005.

Slater, John, et al., editors. *Medical Cultures of the Early Modern Spanish Empire*. Ashgate, 2014.

Thurner, Lance. "Lizards and the Idea of Mexico." https://nursingclio.org/2018/04/12/lizards-and-the-idea-of-mexico/.

Tuells, José. "Francisco Xavier Balmis y las Juntas de Vacuna, un ejemplo pionero para implementar la vacunación." *Salud pública de México*, vol. 53, no. 2 (marzo-abril 2011), pp. 172–7.

Unanue, Hipólito. "Decadencia y Restauración del Perú. Oración inaugural que, para la estrena y abertura [*sic*] del Anfiteatro anatómico, dijo en la Real Universidad de San Marcos el día 21 de noviembre de 1792." *El Mercurio Peruano, 1790–1795. Vol. II: Antología*, edited by Jean-Pierre Clément, Iberoamericana Vervuert, 1998, pp. 213–31.

– *El Clima de Lima y su influencia en los seres organizados, en especial el hombre*. Imprenta de los Huérfanos, 1812.

Warren, Adam. *Medicine and Politics in Colonial Peru. Population Growth and the Bourbon Reforms*. U of Pittsburgh P, 2010.

Zegarra, Margarita. "Olavarrieta, la familia ilustrada, y la lactancia maternal." *Passeurs, mediadores culturales y agentes de la primera globalización en el Mundo Ibérico, siglos XVI–XIX*, edited by Scarlett O'Phelan and Solange Alberro, Pontificia Universidad Católica del Perú/Instituto Riva-Agüero/Instituto Francés de Estudios Andinos, 2005, pp. 345–73.

PART TWO

Representing Health

Chapter Five

Breastfeeding in Public? Representations of Breastfeeding in Early Modern Spain

EMILY COLBERT CAIRNS

The oil painting by Bartolomé de Cardenas (aka Bartolomé Bermejo, 1440–1500) entitled *Virgen de la leche* (*Virgin of the Milk*, ca. 1465), portrays a seated Virgin Mary nursing her child. The Virgin is depicted in this work as a humble mother and a regal figure; looking at her child, her gaze is cast down and she is sumptuously dressed in pearls and a lush velvet dress of deep reds and blues. The chubby child appears full of health and is playing with the rosary beads that belong to his mother. Her left breast is exposed and is spraying milk abundantly, and the baby is wearing a transparent diaper but is otherwise naked. The Virgin's one bare breast is removed from a slit in her clothing that is typical in other paintings of the *virgo lactans*. Crucially, this peaceful image of the Virgin's exposed breast and naked Christ Child would be banned for viewing in the Counter-Reformation (1545–63). Although the divinity celebrates the Holy Mother, her female status became increasingly problematic in the male-dominated patriarchal social order of the early modern world.[1] Despite the scene's serenity, the politics of church and state that surround this painting urge us to consider a tension between the centrality of the Virgin's figure within the Iberian Empire and the regulation of lactation, the female body, the infant in relationship to mothers, and by extension the Christian nation.

Two discourses, one of Catholic identity building and the other seeking to enforce ideal mothering habits, dialogue with each other throughout the medieval and early modern periods. On the one hand, paintings such as Bermejo's *Virgen de la leche* exist within a high-concept battle for empire, one proposing a pure Catholic state equated with a pure body. Presenting embodied deities receiving milk within this context is deeply codified. Close to a century later, Juan Luis Vives, in *Instrucción de la mujer Cristiana* (*The Education of the Christian Woman*, 1523) writes "con la leche se toma lo bueno o lo malo" ("in milk one drinks the good or the bad") (10). This ongoing idea reinforces that a child is born unfinished and finished at the breast as shown by Charlene Villaseñor Black ("The Moralized Breast" 194). Simultaneously, early modern writers were interested in normalizing and enforcing motherly habits. As the Cult of Mary was growing in Spain, she represented a female body for model behaviour. While women became the carriers of difference, well-known early modern authors including Fray Luis de León (1527–91) and Antonio de Guevara (ca. 1481–1545) wrote about women's roles as mothers and everyday practices including breastfeeding and childrearing.[2] In this essay, I also consider a less commented work, Pedro de Luján's *Coloquios matrimoniales* (*Colloquies on Marriage*, 1571), to understand the advice that shaped the early modern Spanish woman's world view regarding her own body and breastfeeding.

As the visual works depicting the *virgo lactans* are limited due to Counter-Reformation mandates, advice manuals about lactation grows in the same period. In fact, the female body in this period is particularly open to public debate, and the regulation of milk both maintains and ensures the survival of the family. In order to access how the breast appeared in both written and visual culture in the early modern period, in this essay I discuss the first Castilian medical treatise by Mallorcan physician Damian Carbón, *Libro del arte de las comadres o madrinas, del Regimiento de las preñadas y paridas y de los niños* (*Book of the Art of Midwifery and the Treatment of Pregnancy, Birth and Children*, 1541) and the behaviour manual *Coloquios matrimoniales* by Pedro de Luján.[3] I analyse these texts alongside three visual works including the thirteenth-century Cantiga 48 from the *Cantigas de Santa María* (*Canticles of Holy Mary*), *La virgen de la leche* (1465) by Bermejo, and *Virgen con el Niño* (*Virgin with Child*) (ca.1500) by Pedro Berruguete. These works help understand how breast milk and breastfeeding was understood as both a social and health practice by different audiences within Spanish society. In focusing on the late medieval period (thirteenth century) through the early modern period (sixteenth century), the representation of the female body and breast milk underscores the tensions surrounding a newly reframed Christian Spain. I begin to explore the feminization of impurity in an early modern Spanish context.[4]

In order to fully appreciate the context of the *virgo lactans* in early modern Spain, it is useful to study one of the earliest representations of this figure, the illustrated manuscript that depicts the Virgin in Cantiga 48.[5] Written in Gallego-Portuguese, this late medieval text recounts numerous Marian miracles. Accompanying each miracle is a highly detailed illustration in six progressive panels. Cantiga 48 depicts a breastfeeding Virgin Mary and the conversion politics associated with her milk that leads a Muslim woman to become Christian. The religious background of this Muslim family and policies of conversion would later have ramifications with the Spanish Reconquista.[6] The *Cantigas* is a foundational work that helped establish a literary base of texts promoting conversion to Catholicism, a policy that became increasingly pervasive within Reconquista Spain. According to Pamela A. Patton, "the illustrated codices have much more to disclose about the process by which Spanish Christians began to reframe the Jewish-Christian [and Muslim-Christian] relationship after the reconquest had peaked" (135). Patton argues that "both the newness and the foreignness" of different ethnic groups in the *Cantigas* allowed for a reshaping and a reframing of identity within Spanish Christendom (145).

The images in Cantiga 48 dialogue with Bermejo's *Virgen de la leche* and Berruguete's *Virgen con el Niño* (see figures 8 and 9). Maternal milk highlights the complicated religious identities of Spanish subjects. The miracle presented in this painting is the breast coming to life and spraying milk in order to convince Muslim subjects to convert to Catholicism. As Charlene Villaseñor Black states, "paintings were preachers" ("Inquisitorial Practices" 184), and as this essay demonstrates, the two early modern Spanish painters Bermejo and Berruguete painted this sacred image to connect with a contemporary audience that had a deep interest in this critical practice of everyday life.[7]

The plentiful milk that the Virgin sprays in Bermejo and Berruguete's painting and in the *Cantigas* is full of meaning: it was simultaneously a practical health concern, a marker of religious and ethnic identity, and a means of controlling women. Both blood and breast milk were defined as contaminating agents that transmitted impurities by the mid-fifteenth-century purity of blood statutes, namely, Jewish and Muslim ethnic and racial difference. Since the Hellenic period, breast milk and breastfeeding were understood to be beneficial for infants.[8] Many early modern thinkers propose that mothers not only pass characteristics to their children in the womb, but that they also continue to develop their personalities through breast milk.[9]

In this discussion of breastfeeding, both maternal breastfeeding and the use of wet nurses are relevant and highly charged. The wet nurse amplifies many tensions; she both cares for the child of another using her body and in large part is responsible for the thriving of the child. At the same time her role is restricted, guided, and monitored.[10] The wet nurse is a complex figure that implies abundance and scarcity, power and powerlessness.[11] In extension of the metaphor of Mary as a mother to the whole Christian nation, another way of interpreting her figure is as a highly celebrated and revered wet nurse for all of Christendom.

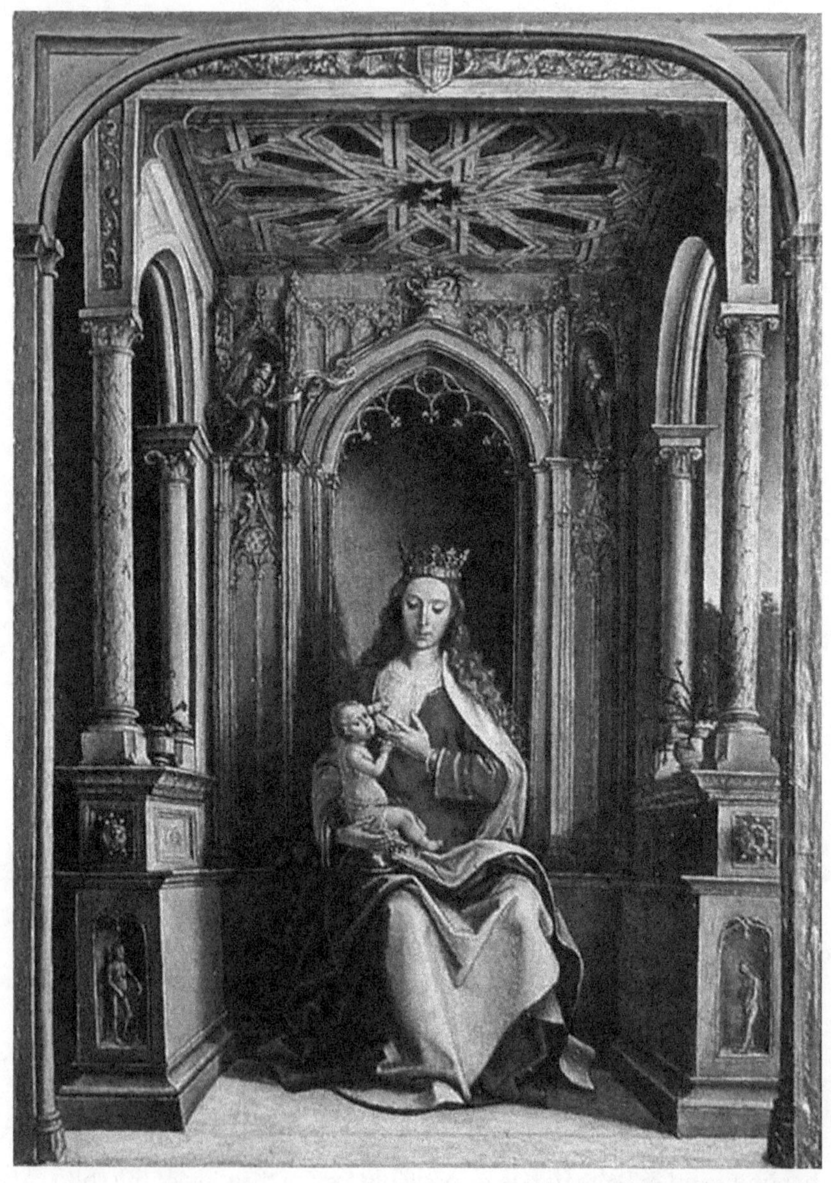

Figure 8. Pedro Berruguete, *Virgen con el Niño*, 1620. Oil on panel, 24" x 17.3". The Prado Museum, via Wikimedia Commons.

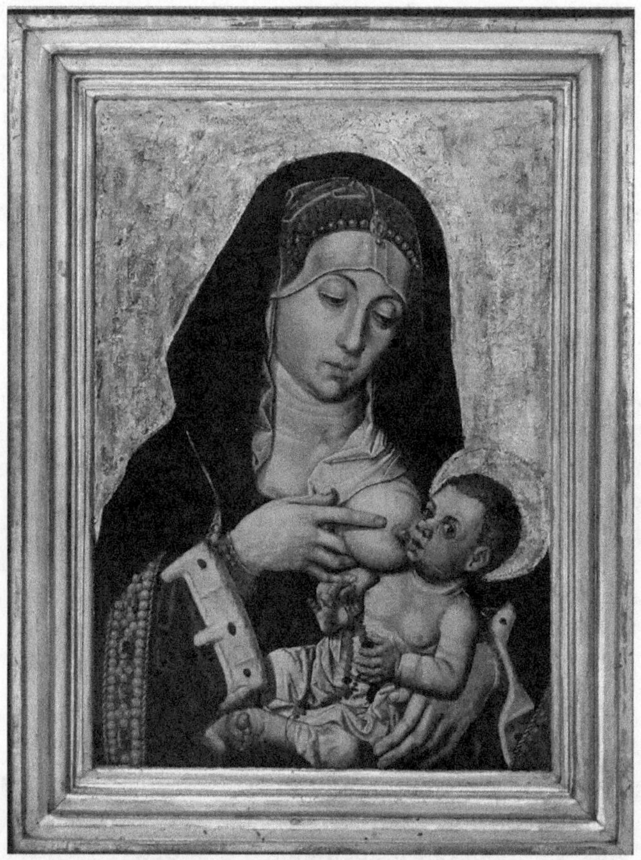

Figure 9. Bartolome Bermejo, *Virgin de la leche*, 1468. Oil on panel, 22.9" x 17". Convent of Santo Domingo in Valéncia, via Wikimedia Commons.

Bermejo and Berruguete's paintings present a Virgin who is breastfeeding in public for her public.[12] This type of feminization is important because it would end by the Counter-Reformation period, when prohibitions of nudity did not allow women's breasts to be exposed. Inquisitorial censorship and the Council of Trent (1545–63) would play a fundamental role in the transformation of the portrayal of the breast and the way that early modern society related to it. As Margaret R. Miles argues, it is in this period that the breast is secularized, and what was a religious image becomes eroticized and medicalized (*A Complex*

Delight: The Secularization of the Breast 1350–1750 1).[13] Curiously, as images of a relatable nursing Virgin decline, early modern authors in behaviour manuals increasingly write in favour of the mother's breast over that of the wet nurse; in fact, according to writers like Luján, mother's breast is best in early modern Spain. Although the nursing Virgin was no longer part of visual culture in daily life, the breast gained interest as a mechanism for social control. This resonates today, as many different people with varying interests attempt to regulate the visual aspects of a breastfeeding woman's public life.

Maternal Milk

Milk from the birth mother or from the breast of a paid wet nurse was the main option in the late medieval and early modern period to nourish a baby.[14] As an important commodity, milk became regulated in accordance with the politics of reconquest and conversion. Heath Dillard shows that the "1258 Cortes of Valladolid prohibited Christian women from becoming nurses to Jewish and Muslim children and at the same time barred minority women from nursing Christians, an order repeated by the same body at Jerez ten years later" (207). The topic of infant nutrition and breast milk has been well studied by scholars. Breast milk was associated with purity and the regulation of feeding practices was associated with race (Alexandre-Bidon 154). In this period, breast milk was considered to be a "purified form of menstrual blood that changed color as it passed between the breast and the womb" (Miller 4–5). These early modern thinkers drew upon Greek medical sources including the Galenic medical model of four humours that determined that breast milk was "blood twice cooked" (Martínez 48). Similarly, Avicenna and Aristotle determined that where blood manifested as sperm in men to create life, it manifested as breast milk in women to sustain life.[15] Galen advised that women abstain from sexual relations while nursing in order to maintain a superior quality of their breast milk (48). Conflating biology and cultural traits, the Greek medical sources determined that bodily fluids would impact the psychology of the child. Late medieval and early modern thinkers would draw upon these conclusions when writing their medical texts and guidebooks. Milk-as-blood was understood to transmit moral qualities from the mother and wet nurse (Alexandre-Bison 175), as women were seen "as sources of contamination" (Martínez 42). In this way, impurity was transmitted from a mother's body to the child. As Emilie Bergmann states, "the milk-as-blood model placed wet-nursing in a contested position" ("Language and Mother's Milk" 107). As impurity was feminized, regulation over the mother and the female body became increasingly important in controlling Spanish subjects.

Although wet nursing was a widespread practice among elite women and often a symbol of social status, in this period it became an oft-discussed topic for its role in managing epidemics of disease and famine.[16] In the *Cantigas de Santa María* the Virgin is juxtaposed with a Muslim woman, and significantly both are depicted breastfeeding their own children. Although the milk-as-blood model would argue that the Muslim woman's milk is contaminated, conversion allows her religious impurity to be corrected and made pure. It is keenly relevant how this physical impurity can be undone in a spiritual encounter; in fact, it reveals a type of shifting discourse that served to justify the monarchial powers of the Spanish Catholic royals that sought to create a homogeneous Christian nation centuries later. Further problematizing the milk supply, Jutta Gisela Sperling writes, "the promiscuity of milk exchange seems to provide a counter-discourse to the 'straight' and heavily policed line in which paternal blood was supposed to be passed down the generational ladder, [such that] the lactating virginal breast signified the utopian dimension of spiritual desire in Catholicism" (*Roman Charity* 339). Regulation of milk would be inconsistent and yet a fundamental necessity for the survival of a family and society as a whole; in fact, both Antonio de Guevara and Pedro de Luján consistently argue for the benefits of maternal breastfeeding for both the state and the family. This type of discourse that blended ideology and health practice flourished well into the early modern period in Spain.

The first Castilian medical treatise, entitled *Libro del arte de las comadres o madrinas, del Regimiento de las preñadas y paridas y de los niños* (*Book of the Art of Midwifery and the Treatment of Pregnancy, Birth, and Children*, 1541), reflects contemporary norms and popular culture surrounding breastfeeding. Authored by Mallorcan physician Damián Carbón, it is divided into two books and contains fifty-six chapters. This text was written in the vernacular to be accessible to midwives, unlike the majority of other early modern medical treatises, which were written in Latin (Gallego-Caminero et al. 603). Although Carbón himself had never attended a birth, he gathered the material that comprises his treatise in order to share knowledge with nurses and midwives (603). As he sets out in the introduction, he had a moral obligation to write this didactic text to further educate this network of female practictioners. He acknowledges the primary roles that midwives, or *parteras*, play in childbirth as they are consulted in preference to male physicians. Carbón says that he has written this book for these women: "Y porque tenemos hoy una platica que las mugeres preñadas y paridas, en sus necessidades y para las criaturas, a las comadres antes que a los médicos piden consejo. Y elas poco instruidas en su arte, no saben buenamente que hazer, y ansi caen en errors como vuestra merced tiene experimentado" ("Today we are saying that pregnant women and women who have recently given birth, because of their own and their babies' needs, request advice from their midwives before asking a doctor. But since they [midwives] have limited training, they don't really know what to do, and therefore, they make the mistakes that your excellency has experienced"; 11). Carbón recognizes that these midwives had a visible and valued role in their society.[17] Written to share "their art" with a broad audience (with some help from the medical establishment), two of the chapters of this treatise are dedicated to the topic of nursing.

In this book, the pregnant female body is open to public debate, a dynamic that continues until the present day. The unborn child is the responsibility of all society, and patriarchal society inexorably claims masculine dominion over it. Other discourses, including blood purity, are written into what is seemingly well-meant medical advice. The wholly conceptual imaginary of the "pure Christian body" is written into the nitty-gritty of the self-help "good mother" book. Carbón dedicates two chapters entirely to breastfeeding and the role of the wet nurse: chapter 33, "Del regimiento del mamar del niño" ("The regiment to nurse a child"), and chapter 34, "De la election de la ama" ("The election of a wet nurse"). He furthers the blood-as-milk conception and writes about the central role of breast milk: "Dizen que la leche de la propia madre es nodrimiento de la misma calidad del que tomava en el vientre porque la leche es del mismo sangre nutrimental de la madre: y mas que el niño con mayor delectancia lo toma por la semajaça y uniformidad y más que la leche maternal es maás conveniente que otra: y porque tiene conveniencia en la material" ("It is said that the mother's milk has the same quality as that which the baby drank in the womb because that milk comes from the same source as the mother's blood; moreover, the child prefers his mother's milk because of its similarity and uniformity and because it is more convenient than anything else: and in its substance it is beneficial"; 54). In arguing for the benefits of maternal breastfeeding in the former he describes the four conditions necessary for successful nursing for the mother, including her age, fitness level, and, crucially, her character. He also lists in chapter 34 seven conditions that the wet nurse should have. Her manner is of primary importance because Carbón describes that the baby takes on the traits of his wet nurse over those of his own parents; breast milk "trae más costumbres de ama que de madre y padre" ("the wet nurse passes down more characteristics than either mother or father"; 92).

Daniele Alexandre-Bidon explains that breastfeeding and maternal milk, like blood, was understood to transmit hereditarily both physical and moral qualities (170).

In addition to the medical treatises, early modern behaviour and conduct manuals, generally authored by men, gave women specific instructions regarding childrearing, how to best nurse a child and the arrangements that ought be made should the mother be ill and not able to breastfeed.[18] In Luján's fourth colloquy he outlines "las causas por mal parir" ("the causes of faulty births"; 119) including the mother going out too much, wearing tight clothes, attending banquets, entering into a garden with a lot of fruit whereupon she could overindulge, drinking wine, jumping, dancing and running, and any other acts that required physical exertion. The main characters of these colloquies include the recently married Marcelo and Eulalia, and the more experienced Dorotea. Basically, a pregnant woman is compared with a sick woman. Upon the birth of the child, Luján's *Coloquios* advise that (in order) the parents give thanks for a safe birth and thank God, and then nurse the child. Luján includes a list of items that are bad for breast milk including rosemary seeds, pepper, dry bread, cheese, and vinegar (142). Luján was not alone in the prescription of proper food for breast milk; earlier, for example, the Castilian legal text *Siete partidas* (*Seven Divisions*, ca. 1265) codified the specific foods that wet nurses should eat, and royal wet nurses had a special diet as shown by María del Carmen Simón Palmer in *Cocina de palacio* (*Royal Cookery*).

In no subtle tones, *Coloquios matrimoniales* shows preference for maternal nursing, as is standard in many early modern behaviour guides including Guevara's *Relox de los príncipes* (*The Dial of Princes*, 1529). In practice, however, many elite women and women of means sought the services of a wet nurse. For Luján, having another woman besides the birth mother feed the baby is described as a monstrous and uncaring act: "parece cosa muy monstruosa que haya ella parido la criatura de sus entrañas y que otra mujer extraña le dé sus tetas" ("it appears to be a very monstrous act that a woman should give birth to a baby from her own body and that a stranger would feed that baby from her breasts"; 133). Luján calls the birth mother that does not nurse a "half mother," and he calls upon the "naturaleza" ("nature") of a true mother in order to guilt women who do not breastfeed. He makes a case of maternal deficiency in his text: "una mujer ha de criar a su fijo ha de ser por madre entera, y no media madre, porque la mujer que solamente pare es media madre mas la que lo cría es madre entera" ("A mother who raises her child must do it as a complete mother, and not a half mother, because the woman who only gives birth is just a half mother, whereas she who nurses her child is a complete mother"; 134). Similarly, Guevara accuses women who do not nurse their own babies of being monstrous and cruel mothers.[19]

In comparatively analysing Fray Luis's *La perfecta casada* (*The Perfect Wife*), Guevara's *Relox de príncipes*, and Luján's *Coloquios Matrimoniales*, Carolyn Nadeau shows that Luján's text is a type of rewriting of Guevara's text as was common in the traditions of Renaissance imitation ("Authorizing the Wife/Mother" 32). The central difference is the more intimate tone of Luján's work, and wheareas the purpose of the *Relox* is to reconconcile the needs of the family and the state for the elite group of the nobility and royalty, Luján's text is dedictated to a wider audience of all upper-class families (22). For Nadeau, the *Coloquios* has a "social agenda" that is crucial to the reception of this work (22). *Coloquios* shares with the paintings of the *virgo lactans* after the fourteenth century the common value of accessibility and the goal of reaching a wide audience. Luján writes to connect with a broader audience than Guevara, and the paintings are meant to connect with a broader public that would be looking to connect with a humanized Virgin who was engaged in practices of daily life that women would face in their own lives. Both sets of works serve to make breastfeeding personal and intimate.

Luján argues that the baby is safer in the care of the birth mother: "la madre debría criar a su fijo por tenerlo más seguro ... cada día veemos más hijos se mueren en poder de amas que no valen" ("the mother should care for and nurse her child to keep him safe ... every day we see more children who die in the care of unfit nurses"; 136). The idea of well-being "tenerlo más seguro" – literally, "to keep him safe" – is both a directive regarding child safety and also directly relates to the assurance of healthy milk/blood and the pure background of the nursing mother. As stated, early modern politics of separation and contagion were linked to the female body. The female body as the creator and nurturer of life is also the transmitter of a community's honour and *limpieza* (religious and ethnic purity).[20] The female body has long been used as a space to fulfil patriarchal desires, and this text is no exception; the female body is a recipient that through control contains and maintains male honour.[21]

Although Luján calls wet nurses "muy descuidadas" ("very careless"), he does stipulate that their use is acceptable if the mother is sick or cannot produce enough milk. He carefully outlines which women make the best wet nurses: the best *ama* should "sea sana" ("be healthy"), "regalada en el comer" ("balanced in what they eat"), "no beba vino" ("not drink wine"), "que no esté preñada" ("not be pregnant"), and "bien acondicionadas" ("be in good shape"). Luján also racializes the task of finding the best nurse, saying, "Todos los medicos tienen que la leche de una mujer morena es mejor que la de la muy blanca" ("All the doctors understand that the milk from a dark woman is better than that of a white woman"; 138). In this way, he dialogues with the ethnically and racially produced politics of empire that associated darker women with being closer to nature and more prolific in their bodily abilities, including milk production. This argument is also economically driven, as darker women in this period generally occupied lower social standing and were part of a domestic service class. María Elena Martínez shows that the system of *limpieza de sangre* (purity of blood statues) directly influenced the creation of the system of *castas* (casts) in New Spain. The Viceroyalty of New Spain was part of the Iberian Empire and under Spanish colonial role (1535–1821). Divided into the Republic of Spaniards and the Republic of Indians, there were many hybrid identities as indigenous peoples lived and married alongside Spaniards and slaves from Africa. New identities born of mixed racial background were created and terms were employed to categorize and establish hierarchies; for example, *criollo* (a person born in the "New World" and of two Spanish parents), *mestizo* (a mixture of indigenous and Spanish), and *mulato* (a mixture of black and Spaniard). Study of Luján's *Coloquios* reveals how the politics of racial categorization would in turn shape the way that subjects conceived of their own ethno-religious identity (New or Old Christian).[22] The "mujer morena" here could be a woman of Andalusian background or of Muslim descent; she could have been enslaved or the child of enslaved parents, or a woman of mixed background from the colonial world.

Scholars of early modern Italy including James Bruce Ross, David Herlihy, and Christiane Klapisch-Zuber have detailed records of the number of wet nurses and their place of residence (either with the infant's family or in their own house); Spain, however, lacks exhaustive information to these ends (García Herrero, *Del nacer y el vivir* 80). García Herrero shows that both church and state established that a three-year period was the ideal time to nurse a child (81).[23] It was a deeply important, personal and difficult task. Ximena Illanes Zubieta confirms that in the fifteenth century, wet nurses would be paid less if the child was taken ill. Of the 424 cases of abandoned children in the hospital de la Santa Creu in Barcelona that she researched, many wet nurses came from the countryside, and slaves were also used in this function. In line with Carbón's stipulations, the primary concerns in hiring a wet nurse include the age of the woman, the quality of her milk, and whether she was nursing two children simultaneously (169). As discussed, contamination both regarding religious impurity and disease would directly influence early modern writers, usually male, who preferred maternal nursing above that of a wet nurse. Carolyn Nadeau shows that in the courts of 1258, midwives were examined because minority women were often associated with witchcraft and superstition. Although Jewish and Muslim wet nurses were officially banned from taking on Christian charges, in practice this directive was challenging to maintain. The regulating of the impurity in particular becomes difficult in the early modern period when religious others officially disappeared from Spain. In the case of Cantiga 48, the life-giving properties of the Muslim woman's milk overcome any stigma of impurity and make an argument that through conversion her "impure" milk (and blood) can be purified. Let us now discuss this foundational text in detail.

Cantiga 48 of the *Cantigas de Santa María*

Written in Gallego-Portuguese and during the reign of Alfonso el Sabio (Alfonso the Wise, reigned 1252–84), the thirteenth-century *Cantigas de Santa María* reflects the daily lives of Iberian subjects within the larger framework of reconquest. The *Cantigas* are compelling for the rich and varied representations of life in late medieval Spain. As Elisa Ruiz García and Laura Fernández Fernández state, they have a political and propagandistic purpose (109). As there are multiple original manuscripts of this text; this article focuses on the 1270 Códice Rico located in El Escorial.[24] Bound in leather, each of the 420 *cantigas* in this manuscript is accompanied by a musical score and panel of images. These manuscripts are well preserved because they were not intended for everyday use and instead housed in important libraries, such as the case with the Códice Rico. Each plate is divided into six panels with adorned borders and subtitles that indicate the action to the viewer. The written text is embellished in calligraphic letters and the illustrated panel is drawn using gold and silver pigments.

The number of cantigas dedicated to the miracle of breast milk shows the importance of this topic within the court of Alfonso (the Wise) as well as the everyday life of subjects. The Virgin Mary is the heroine of these songs, which narrate a series of miracles. In fact, many deal with various health practices related to women including childbirth, breastfeeding, and the relationship between the birth mother, mother, and the wet nurse she hires.[25] In addition to Cantiga 48, a number of other cantigas depict the miraculous powers of a lactating Virgin Mary; not only does her milk have the power to convert, it also heals, as in Cantiga 54: "All health comes from the Holy Queen, for She is our medicine" (Kulp-Hill 70).[26]

Other cantigas that treat the healing powers of the Virgin's milk include how she heals a monk in Cantiga 54 when she "sprinkled milk on the monk's mouth and face," cures leprosy in Cantiga 93, a cripple in Cantiga 77, and a priest in Cantiga 404.[27]

The thirteenth-century conversion Cantiga 48 under enquiry presents a portrait of the Virgin breastfeeding within the context of a Muslim household. The title of the Cantiga 48 reads: "Esta é como a omagen de Santa María, que un mouro guardava en sua casa onrradamente, deitou leite das tetas" ("This is how a statue of Holy Mary, which a Moor kept respectfully in his house, gave milk from its breasts"). Returning from the Crusades with loot, the Moor sells some of his bounty, but keeps a painting of the Virgin Mary and Child (panel 3). She is holding the Christ Child in her arms, and both are fully dressed. Upon returning to his home, he puts the painting on an Arabic-style alter. Crucially, this image is juxtaposed with his real-life wife, who is embracing their child (panel 4).

The fifth image in this panel is the most critical; the painting changes and the Virgin's breast comes to life, turning into flesh and squirting breast milk in two streams. Like the early modern paintings of Bermejo and Berruguete, it offers a realistic depiction of a nursing mother of a young child. This panel is not naturalistic and lifelike in the depiction of the faces and bodies of the subjects, but it does express a repeated dynamic in the early modern paintings of the *virgo lactans*. Although the conversion narrative is no longer required within Iberia, this visual representation in the Cantiga informs how the early modern mother and society would later view breastfeeding. In asking for proof as to the existence of God, we read in the text: "Apenas pudo acabar / el moro este discurso, / cuando vio en la imagen / un par de pechos / de carne que no de otra cosa, de los que empezó a mamar / y a salir / leche como si fuesen caños" ("The Moor had scarcely uttered this when he saw the statue's two breasts turn into living flesh and begin to flow with milk in gushing streams"; 68r). Unlike most imagery of the *virgo lactans*, both of her breasts are prominently visible to the viewer. Where other images present a breast that drips milk in careful drops, this image clearly squirts the milk in two constant streams. Although the transubstantiation of the painting is miraculous, the vigorous streams of lactations are depicted in a way that rings true to life to any recent mother. In this panel, the Moor's wife also nurses her child, and like the Virgin, her nipple is exposed. Where the gaze of Mary and the child are straight ahead, the mother looks ahead while the child looks at his mother.

In this visual representation, the Christ Child nursing at the Virgin's breast is juxtaposed with a Muslim woman breastfeeding her child. While the idea of godly conquest and conversion is patriarchal, here the mechanism denies and complicates patriarchal discourse. Here the Virgin is embodied and humanized (or made corporeal) through the act of breastfeeding, and this cantiga parallels the Muslim woman who feeds her child the same way that the Christ Child is fed.[28] The flowing of maternal milk connects these two mothers and calls into question various ideas of conquest, conversion, and background. The miracle of the spontaneous lactation in the portrait is the heroic act that ultimately achieves the family's conversion to Catholicism. In the conclusion of the cantiga, it reads: "Quand' esto viu, sen / mentir / começou muit' a chorar, / e un crérigo viir / fez, quo o foi baticar; / e pois desto, sen falir, / os séus crischaos tornar / fez, e ar / outres bees connoscudos" ("When he saw this, verily he began to weep and had a priest called in who baptised him. Afterward, without fail, he had all his followers become Christians as well as many of his other acquaintances"; 68r; Kulp-Hill 62). The final image of the panel celebrates the conversion and posits the centrality of this conversion narrative. Portrayed through the use of breast milk as a health practice and religious identity marker, Christianity is upheld through the connection of milk as blood.

In this panel, breastfeeding crosses lines of religious practice and underscores the human connection of all people regardless of their confessional identity. Part of the daily reality of many Iberian subjects, the illuminations portray the corrective nature of religious conversion for an emerging Catholic state in the late medieval period. According to Pamela Patton, "illustrations thus are best understood not as snapshots of their day, but as the inventive marriage between a new interest in the observable world and a respect for authoritative visual models that would retain their centrality to the image making for centuries to come" (138). This clear depiction of reconquest occurs within a Christian perspective. The Iberian landscape was populated with religious others including Muslim subjects "ready" for conversion to Christianity. In addition to religious instruction, this panel also provides instruction on nursing practices, depicting what is a key practice of everyday life – swollen breasts and strong milk production for recent mothers. In this way, the images that are found in the *Cantigas de Santa María* help explain the important role that nursing had in the court of Alfonso the Wise and the lives of the citizens under his rule.[29] As these examples make clear, the primary role of breast milk and the practices surrounding the breast and the baby would be oft discussed and even more at the forefront into the early modern period. At the same time, this panel underscores the tensions that existed surrounding breastfeeding and the identity politics that impact maternal milk production – a discussion that continues to exist in the present day. If breastfeeding is blood-as-milk, and was policed as such, then having the Virgin Mary share her breast, against legal practice, with religious others goes against the purity of blood statues. Mary's breast and her breastfeeding later become vanished by censorship as society implores mothers to nurse their own babies precisely to avoid blurring the lines from this cantiga. In this miracle of instantaneous conversion that involves neither a man nor the state, readers are confronted with the biological reality of miscegenation.

Bermejo's *Virgen de la leche* and Berruguete's *Virgen con el Niño*

This essay began with a brief analysis of Bermejo's *Virgen de la leche* (1465). Although in technique and style there are significant differences between Bermejo's painting and Cantiga 48, the topic of maternal lactation and the realistic spray of breast milk connect the two visual works. The depiction of the Virgin and nursing child was part of a movement (*devotio moderna)* to humanize the figures of Mary and Christ that began in late medieval Spain (Villaseñor Black 180).[30] This practice of *devotio moderna* shifted between the late medieval period and the early modern period, where stricter theological intepretations were replaced with more direct representations of the realities of everyday life including nursing.[31] In this way, the depiction of a realistic nipple spraying milk in Bermejo's painting marks it within the genre of naturalism.[32] The style is important because the painter connected to real women and men who would be viewing this image. They could see themselves, their children, their breast, and their everyday life in these images. The reception of this painting is also carefully monitored by the child's gaze, which is directed at the audience.

This painting reflects the artistic trends made popular internationally at Northern European schools, and at the same time demonstrates the topics that were important to everyday people at home in Spain. Judith Berg-Sobré reflects that the happy and chubby appearance and behaviour of the distracted child also designates the naturalistic style. It is a realistic scenario, for example, in which the baby plays with the rosary beads. The rosary signifies how Catholic practice is connected to material objects and serves to remind the viewer of an expectation of daily observance and faith. The golden background and halos including discrete floral designs are traditional elements of the Early Netherlandish school led by Rogier van der Weyden. Berg-Sobré explains how the "religioso local al combinar tema y forma tradicional con nueva tecnicá y composición extranjera" ("local religious character combines in its theme and traditional form with a new foreign technique and composition"; 40). From its Italian origins, to its Dutch influences, and the centrality of religious imagery like the rosary beads, this painting can be seen as both local and global. This painting illustrates that Spain was part of an international dialogue regarding the changing expectations for mothers. Whereas her physical role as central provider of nourishment is highlighted in these paintings, as the woman's body became more contested upon the expulsion of religious others from Spain, her naked breast also disappeared from public view.

Pedro Berruguete's *Virgen con el Niño* (ca. 1500) also presents a naked Christ Child gazing at the audience.[33] Again, one breast is exposed, highlighting the breast as the primary source of nourishment. Margaret Miles demonstrates that the paintings of the Renaissance *Maria lactans* are situated within the historical context of a malnourished Europe (*Complex Delight* 35). This realistic portrayal of the breast upholds the tradition that humanizes the *virgo lactans*. The Virgin holds her breast with a V-position of her fingers (a correct nipple hold for nursing mothers) and offers her nipple and milk to her child. The child faces his mother's breast and looks at the viewer.[34] The pensive Virgin in this image is seated on an altar and has downcast eyes and a dress of rich velvet brocade. She is depicted wearing a crown decorated with rubies.[35] The regal nature is highlighted for both painters; in Bermejo's, Mary is painted within a golden backdrop, and in Berruguete's, she is located on a throne.

In these images the audience encounters two serene and peaceful images of a mother that is calm and a baby that is well fed, happy, and serene. As Alexandre-Bidon explains, "la forma de 'dar' el pecho es cultural" ("the way that one nurses is cultural"; 155). These images are clearly instructing their audience that the mother is the best nurse for her baby, and this beautiful exchange is natural and relaxing. Some scholars argue that the nursing Virgin was a didactic strategy to instruct mothers to breastfeed (Sperling, *Roman Charity* 323). In these seemingly peaceful images, a palpable apprehension is related within the larger social and historical context. As Miles discusses, what these paintings present is the fantasy of the good mother. These visuals could very well be anxiety producing for a struggling new mother who does not have a throne to nurse her baby upon, let alone clean clothing to wear.

Although the Counter-Reformation limited Iberian proliferation of the *virgo lactans* images, these paintings stand as excellent examples of the power that this image had for an early modern audience.[36] They also stand as an Iberian counterpart to the pan-European interest in this topic as both painters had influences from Italy and the Netherlands. Whereas the origins of Bermejo's painting are unknown, Berruguete's painting was commissioned by the church. These images had a specific relationship with contemporary Flemish artistic trends. Whereas Berruguete is considered by Pilar Silvia Maroto to be the first Renaissance painter from the crown of Castile, Bermejo painted his image while in residence in Valéncia within the crown of Aragón. The topic of the *Virgen de la leche* was popular throughout the crown of Aragón in the fourteenth century as Valéncia was a leader in artistic and cultural traditions (Berg-Sobré 40).[37]

In studying these two images from Bermejo and Berruguete together, we have representations of the *Maria lactans* from both crowns on the cusp of unification, demonstrating the clear role that she had across the emerging Spanish nation. Alongside the increasingly prolific moralizing and medical treatises, contemporary Iberian artists created paintings and sculptures of the *virgo lactans* that were widely circulated and viewed by a large audience. At the same time, as Villaseñor Black states, these sacred images are influential due to their accessibility and power to communicate (179).[38] Many of these paintings were used in a religious context and displayed within churches. The images of the lactating Mary were public images throughout early modern Europe; people were not prudish about desexualized breasts. As Margaret Miles explains, in sixteenth-century Florence, pert, small breasts were the desired sexual breast; a swollen round breast used for nursing did not arouse desires.

Conclusion

In the texts written about breastfeeding and the visual works depicting a lactating Virgin, there are many contradictions. Alongside an idealized vision of a perfect mother and woman who is peaceful and loving, we also see a paranoia concerning the female body, female resistance, and the limits of masculine control. The female body is both controllable and troublesome. Whatever alternative models of belonging the milk sharing connote – where the Muslim other breastfeeds alongside the Christian deity – the discourse is simultaneously limited by accommodations to violence and masculinity. This is particularly highlighted in the cantigas that juxtapose a peaceful and loving scene of breastfeeding with a wartime crusading image. The narrative is of Muslim wartime spoils becoming a Christian Trojan horse and ultimately conquering a Muslim through righteous conversion. The Virgin Mary is the primary example of purity for Christendom; regular women could only aspire to be like her, and they relate to her through images that humanize her and add godly connotations to breastfeeding. However, simultaneously, this instructive model – as authored and annotated by men – also becomes an impossible ideal to achieve, existing in part outside their practical abilities and lifestyle, for both rich and poor.[39] The idea that the Virgin is a wet nurse to all of Christendom, combined with the power of milk to convert subjects, is a loose thread in a rigid paranoid Spanish state that looks to exclude all religious others. In a society that frequently used wet nurses, the streams of the Virgin's bountiful milk made sense, in that this divine milk allowed others to cross religious and ethnic lines.

As Alexandre-Bidon states, "la creencia en la virtud productora de la leche de María" ("the belief in the productive virtue of Mary's milk") was shared by those of both high and low birth (182). The popularity and the widespread nature of their audience reflect the importance of this figure and how people connected to her image. Although popularity faded as manuals were written directly opposing the creation of artistic interpretations of the *virgo lactans*, the question about how religious others responded to this figure has yet to be adequately considered. Jews and Muslims would not have seen these images within the space of a church, nor would they have their own religious iconography depicting religious subjects nursing. However, religious minorities were immersed in a context that both promoted this image and lived within a culture informed by contemporary behaviour guides. At the same time, their contact with the Christian majority became increasingly more restricted among lines of blood and breast milk.

It is clear that breastfeeding engages with early modern gender politics and presents tensions regarding social and racial purity. In focusing on the breastfeeding images and texts in the late medieval into the early modern period, we are emboldened to see the cracks that expose this counter-discourse. Breast milk becomes an important tool in the early modern period to create a homogeneous Catholic identity. Instead of focusing on traditional and patriarchal models of discourse where blood equates with lineage, this emphasis on maternal milk suggests a shift to everyday health practices and maternal care. Breast milk is simultaneously upheld as both life giving and miraculous and is proffered as an element of social control. This duality of celebration and regulation located in the female body is not an unfamiliar dynamic for women.

NOTES

1 According to Jutta Gisela Sperling, images are another form of speech that challenges normative discourse within the church and state (*Roman Charity* 348).

2 Carolyn Nadeau offers a comparative analysis of the advice literature in Fray Luis, Guevara, and Luján's texts in her article "Authorizing the Wife/

Mother in Sixteenth-Century Advice Manuals." She shows that these authors create a space for the mother as an authoritative figure in the early years of a child's life, especially seen through the lens of breast milk.

3 Magdalena Santo Tomás Pérez points out that it is not clear if the original was written in Castilian or Catalán given that the text was published in Palma de Mallorca and the original manuscript in Zaragoza (238). Many scholars consider it to be the first Castilian medical treatise as it was written in the vernacular to connect with female practitioners including midwives.

4 Various essays in this volume discuss the Galenic medical model and its impact on medical practice; see in particular the introduction and Mujica.

5 The image of the lactating Virgin first emerged in the thirteenth century (Villaseñor Black, "The Moralized Breast" 196).

6 We see the topics of conversion and religious identity of the *moriscos* found in Cantiga 48 having a continued relevance through the sixteenth century as shown in "Geneología y nacimiento de Mahoma" ("Geneology and Birth of Muhammad") in *Textos aljamiados sobre la vida de mahoma. El profeta de los moriscos* (ca.1500) (*Aljamiado Texts about the Life of Muhammad. The Prophet of the Moriscos*). In this text, the prophet Muhammad's wet nurse occupies a central role as does her breast milk. Consuelo López-Morillas shows that this text enjoyed great popularity and in reflecting the role of the Islamic prophet "nos ayuda a calibrar mejor la religiosidad de los moriscos ... la realidad vital del Siglo de oro español" ("helps us better understand the religiosity of the moriscos ... a vital reality of the Spanish Golden Age"; 15). Crucially for this study, we see the central role of milk sharing and the value that wet nursing had among Islamic populations. In fact, within Islam a series of legal prohibitions and rules according to marriage and milk sharing exist. Mohammed Hocine Benkheira shows that "milk kinship was rigourously modelled after the concept of blood kinship" (25). Since the nurse's husband transmits milk kinship, this patriarchal system is maintained and "connotes the passage of paternal blood" (56). This patriarchal system found in Islam is fundamental to this essay, in that male domination over the female body is heightened in the Counter-Reformation period.

7 Images celebrating the *virgo lactans* were created throughout Europe and over many centuries. In feeding her son, many scholars interpret that Mary is feeding the whole of Christendom.

8 Valerie Fildes in *Wet Nursing: A History from Antiquity to the Present* demonstrates that nursing was recommended for the first two years of the child's life within both Hebrew society as shown in the Talmud and for Muslims as recommended in the Koran.

9 Charlene Villaseñor Black in her article "Inquisitorial Practices Past and Present: Artistic Censorship, the Virgin Mary, and St. Anne" shows that

"babies were born unfinished" and in this way both mothers and wet nurses "influence [their] physical and emotional life" (179). Similarly, the Aristotelian tradition drew connections between psychological traits and body fluids (Martínez 48).

10 Carolyn Nadeau in "Blood Mother/Milk Mother: Breastfeeding, the Family and the State in Antonio de Guevara's *Relox de Príncipes*" demonstrates the central role that wet nurses had for principal figures in *Relox de Príncipes*, including the case of Philip II, who left his nurse a portion of his estate in his will. The wet nurse in this instance had a prominent place within the family structure.

11 I consider the figure of the wet nurse through the apt conceptualization proposed by Sperling that: "the lactating breast in all non-maternal milk relationships qualifies as a signifier of desire, power, and abundance" (*Roman Charity* 18). Complicating the role of wet nurses and the relationships of power and family, Rebecca Lynn Winer demonstrates that within a medieval context often slaves were used for wet nursing and slaves of childbearing age were the most expensive. The characteristics of the royal wet nurse were fundamental for Alfonso el Sabio (1252–84) in *Las siete partidas* (*The Seven Divisions*). The second *Partida* describes that a royal wet nurse should come from a good lineage, have good habits, be healthy, and have an abundance of milk. In this way the nurse would make healthy children and raise them well (Title 7, Law 3).

12 In the fourteenth century the female figure in religious art was humanized in order to connect with the population of practitioners, and the nursing virgin was made more real, more accessible. Villaseñor Black in "The Moralized Breast in Early Modern Spain" determines that these humanizing trends sought to highlight the Virgin as a credible mother (196).

13 Margaret Miles shows that the church controlled representations of the breast until the end of the fifteenth century; in the sixteenth century the medical profession and pornography industry would take over (*A Complex Delight: The Secularization of the Breast 1350–1750* 24).

14 As a substitution for human milk, *papilla* (pap), a mixture of water, bread, and animal milk fed through a cloth or a spoon, would sometimes be given to infants (Fildes, *Breasts, Bottles, and Babies* 224). Devices including shaped glasses filled with animal milk would be used as a replacement for human milk (142). Both of these substitutions yielded negative results for young babies. Miles comments that wet nurses who lacked milk would sometimes use the milk of a goat, a sheep, an ass, or another animal. As personality traits were transmitted through breast milk (through the mother or wet nurse), using animal milks would make the babies "vacant in the head" (*Complex Delight* 30).

15 Arabic medical treatises including the work of Avicenna had a huge impact on the late medieval world of the thirteenth century and would

continue to shape medical practice and the understanding of the body into the the early modern period.

16 Sperling shows that in early modern Italy, Italian humanists argued against the "contamination of elite offspring by vulgar habits of lower-class wet nurses" (*Medieval and Renaissance Lactations* 1). Olga Rivera aptly considers wet nurses "agentes de otredad social" (214) ("agents of social otherness"). Miles also discusses the role of famine in the breastfeeding practices in fourteenth-century Tuscany. Robert S. Gottfried shows that that Jews were often blamed for spreading the Black Death or plague in Iberia in the fourteenth century. The plague arrived in Iberia from a number of sources (North Africa, the Pyrenees, ships from Italy) between 1391 and 1457, and decimated between 20 and 40 per cent of the population depending on the region (51–3).

17 Gloria Gallego-Caminero et al. show that the Catholic king Fernando II de Aragón left an important sum of money to the family's midwife (603). Two extant midwifery books were written by women in England and Germany: Jane Sharp's A *Midwives Book* (1671) and Justine Siegemund in *The Court Midwife* (1737).

18 Other early modern humanists were advocates for maternal breastfeeding including Juan Vives, Fray Luis de León, Luther, Erasmus, More and Alberti (Villaseñor Black 176).

19 Guevara writes: "Deve assimismo la muger, en acabando de parir a la criatura, darle a mamar de su leche propria; porque parece cosa muy monstruosa aver parido ella el niño de sus entrañas y que le críen y den a mamar mugeres estrangeras. porque naturaleza no sólo hizo ábiles a las mugeres para parir, pero juntamente con esto las proveyó de leche para criar" ("In the same way, a woman having just given birth to a babe should nurse it with her own milk; because it is a monstruous act having given birth to a child from your own body and then giving it to unknown women to raise and nurse it, because the natural world not only made women able to give birth, but also provided them milk to nurse"; book 2, chapter 18).

20 Rivera points out that Vives in discussing contamination refers to it as "leche extraña" (foreign milk), which could result from adultery by the mother, or blood from a slave or crucially a barbarous (non-Christian) nation. She also shows that theologian Juan de Pineda asked Inquisitorial authorities to take action in condemning mercenary lactation as it could cause disasters "que medio cuarto que tenía de judío nunca dejaba de importer que se tornare judío" ("even a quarter Jewish blood matters because it could make someone become fully Jewish"; 209).

21 Mary Elizabeth Perry in *Gender and Disorder in Early Modern Seville* proposes that early modern Spain and particularly Seville represents a "patriarchy in crisis" and shifts a focus from official state accounts that mainly

focus on men and their role in the shaping of a new empire and instead looks at the fundamental role that women play in their society (13). She discusses how the purity of blood statutes affected female chastity and how "religious beliefs permeated gender ideology" and norms of enclosure and purity (6). Similarly, María Elena Martínez in *Genealogical Fictions* demonstrates how within the patriarchal system of Iberian rule "women are sources of contamination" (42). She proposes that the feminization of impurity shaped both purity of blood statutes in Spain and the caste system in the Americas. Peter Stallybrass in "Patriarchal Territories: The Body Enclosed" presents "the body as a site of conflict" in comparing the grotesque and unfinished body (feminine) with the classical body (read patriarchal power) (123). The female body in Renaissance discourse is associated with the grotesque/open body especially when seen through the lens of breastfeeding. The unfinished body "transgresses its own limits" and in this way interrogates hierarchies of gender and class (142). Breastfeeding women are seen as open because of the transfer of fluid. They transgress their own limits through milk production (that sprays out) as seen in the images of the lactating virgin. At the same time, Fray Luis in *La perfecta casada* theorizes that paternity is transmitted through the milk/blood connection and bypasses the role of the mother when a wet nurse is employed: "Pues el ama que cría pone lo mismo, porque la leche es sangre, y en aquella sangre la misma virtud del padre que vive en el hijo hace la misma obra" ("Well the wet nurse transmits the same, because milk is blood, and through that blood, the father's virtue lives in the child and has the same claim"; 137). In accord with Miles, "women, in this period we explore, did not own the breast" (3).

22 The *virgo lactans* had a prominent role in the conquest narratives, and there is a rich corpus of visual texts to study. Christa Irwin is currently investigating the numerous images of the lactating virgin in the colonial period in Peru.

23 María del Carmen García Herrero shows that a 1351 Ordinance from the archbishop of Toledo, the bishop of Cuenca, and the courts of Valladolid established this three-year period as optimal for receiving breast milk.

24 I worked with the excellent facsimile of this Códice Colección scriptorium (Madrid 2011) located at Tufts University Music Library. Quotations and images from this text come from this manuscript. I especially thank Michael Rogan for facilitating the manuscript and photographic access of this manuscript.

25 Heath Dillard through his work with *fueros* (codes of law) shows how these everyday practices are demonstrated throughout the *Cantigas*.

26 All the translations of this cantiga come from Kathleen Kulp-Hill's English-language edition of the *Cantigas de Santa María*.

27 Emilie L. Bergmann analyses Cantiga 122 wherein a wet nurse is distraught at the death of her charges and considers ending her own life before the virgin performs a miracle. In addition to the healing powers associated with breast milk that are referenced, another source of enquiry of the *Cantigas* includes other medical miracles that treat infertility and kidney stones, and restore amputated limbs among others.

28 See Miles's article "The Virgin's One Bare Breast" for a further discussion of the connection between the Virgin and the humanity of all mothers as an artistic trend in fourteenth-century Florence.

29 In the *Siete partidas* Alfonso the Wise places the central role of breastfeeding in the selection of the correct wet nurse and how she would raise the future king, "y los que primeramente deben hacer esta guarda han de ser el rey y la reina, y esto es en darles amas sanas y bien acostumbradas y de buen linaje, en manera que por su crianza de ellos no reciben muerte o enfermedad o malas costumbres" ("and it should be the king and the queen that do this first task, and that is to give them healthy and well-conditioned nurses from a good lineage, and in this way under their care they will receive neither death nor illness nor bad customs"; Título 7, Ley 3).

30 Miles demonstrates that before the fourteenth century, Italian images were created that featured an elite virgin, and in the fourteenth century a more humble image of the virgin began to be portrayed in order to connect with everyday people (*Complex Delight* 32). She was a model for all humanity and especially for women, she as the mother of Jesus had the power to nourish all of humanity (36).

31 Villaseñor Black points out that the earliest example of an illuminated miniature depicting a lactating virgin was created in 1269 in Aragón and was both abstract and hieratic ("Inquisitorial Practices" 180).

32 The row of pearls and the work with the transparent veil mark this painting within the Hispano-Flemish school according to Judith Berg Sobré and Eric Young.

33 There are at least three versions of the *María lactans* achieved by Berruguete, including *Virgen con el Niño* (Madrid Municipal), *Virgen Roda*, and *Virgen con el Niño* (Palencia, Museo Diocesano). The first is the most well-known and is the image that I focus on in this essay.

34 In the *Virgen Roda* the Christ child looks away and according to Mario Zucco rejects the breast. Instead of looking at his mother in this image, he gazes at two angels holding the cross and the crown of thorns.

35 Other scholars have analysed these paintings through important symbols; for example, Pilar Silva-Maroto shows that the glass vase filled with flowers (the version held by the Museo Diocesano in Palencia) represents the virginity of the virgin.

36 Fray Juan Interián de Ayala (*The Christian Painter* 1570) and Francisco Pacheco (*The Art of Painting* 1649) wrote treatises that forbid visual representations of nudity of the Christ Child and the Virgin Mother. Depictions of the lactating virgin were likewise condemned in the *Treatise on Sacred Images*: "Those breasts that nursed the creator of the world [should not be] exposed to everyone's view" (Villaseñor Black, "Inquisitorial Practices Past and Present" 181). Even prolific court painters including Murillo did not paint the *virgo lactans*.

37 In fact, within the tradition of *María lactans*, Bermejo was not alone in creating works within this topos. Another contemporary artist, Antoni Peris, created the *Retablo de la Virgen de la leche* (1415) upon its commission by the Capilla del Claustro del convento de Santo Domingo de Valéncia. By the sixteenth century, this topic would be much less common for artists (Berg Sobré 40).

38 García Herrero explains how early modern paintings capture their cultural reality and help teach us today about obstetrics (28).

39 There is a lack of texts authored by nursing women regarding their experiences and expectations for other women, but nuns in this period often discuss the miraculous effects of breastfeeding. Sarah E. Owens in *Navigating the Spanish Empire* shows how Sor Jerónima recalls visions in which she nursed from the Virgin's breast when she was ill. Owens shows that "religious women have manipulated images of milk and blood ... to invert traditional female roels and position themselves in a privileged position within the church's hierarchy" (110–11). Similarly, the nun Ana Bolea Francisca de Bolea Abarca describes breast milk as "lo esencial del ser humano" (32) in her *Catorze vidas de santas de la orden del Cister* (1655) when she eulogizes Ana Alyeda, a non-religious figure and mother of St. Bernard.

WORKS CITED

Alexandre-Bidon, Daniele. *La infancia a la sombra de las catedrales*. Translated by. Beatriz Pascual, Prensas universitarias de Zaragoza, 2008.

Berg-Sobré, Judith. *Bartolomé de Cárdenas "Bermejo": Pintor errante en la corona de Aragón*. International Scholars Publication, 1997.

Bergmann, Emilie L. "Language and Mother's Milk: Maternal Roles and the Nurturing Body in Early Modern Spanish Texts." *Maternal Measure: Figuring Caregiving in the Early Modern Period*, Aldershot, 2000, pp. 105–20.

– "Popular Balladry and the Terrible Wet Nurse: La Nodriza del Rey." *Medieval and Renaissance Lactations: Images, Rhetorics, Practices: Women and Gender in the Early Modern World*, Routledge, 2013, pp. 115–29.

Bolea Abarca, Ana Francisca de. *Catorze Vidas de Santas del Orden del Císter.* Biblioteca Universitaria, 1655.

Cantigas de Santa María. Edición facsímil del códice T-I-I de la Real Biblioteca de San Lorenzo de El Escorial Siglo XIII 2 Volumenes. Colección scriptorium, 2011.

Carbón, Damián. *Libro del arte de las comadres o madrinas y del regimiento de las preñadas y paridas y de los niños*, edited by Daniel García Guitiérrez, Anubar, 2000.

Dillard, Heath. *Daughters of the Reconquest: Women in Castilian Town Society 1100–1300."* Cambridge UP, 1984.

Fernández Fernández, Laura, and Elisa Ruiz García. "Quasi liber et picture: estudio codicológico del ms. T-I-I de la RBME." Edición facsímil del códice T-I-I de la Real Biblioteca de San Lorenzo de El Escorial Siglo XIII 2 Volumenes. Colección scriptorium, 2011, pp. 109–42.

Fildes, Valerie. *Breasts, Bottles and Babies: A History of Infant Feeding.* Edinburgh UP, 1986.

– *Wetnursing: A History from Antiquity to the Present.* Basil Blackwell, 1988.

Gallego-Caminero, Gloria, et al. "Las parteras y/o comadronas del siglo XVI: El manual de Diamiá Carbó." *Florianópolis*, vol. 14, no. 4, 2005, pp. 601–7.

García Herrero, María del Carmen. *Del nacer y el vivir.* Instituto Fernando el Católico, 2005.

Gottfried, Robert S. *The Black Death: Natural and Human Disaster in Medieval Europe.* The Free Press, 1983.

Guevara, Antonio de. *Obras Completas de Fray Antonio de Guevara*, tomo II. Ed. EmilioBlanco. *Biblioteca Castro* de la Fundación José Antonio de Castro, 1994. http://www.filosofia.org/cla/gue/guerp.htm.

Hocine Benkheira, Mohammed. "'The Milk of the Male'": Kinship, Maternity and Breastfeeding in Medieval Islam." *Medieval and Renaissance Lactations: Images, Rhetorics, Practices: Women and Gender in the Early Modern World*, edited by Jutta Gisela Sperling, Ashgate, 2013, pp. 21–36.

Klapisch-Zuber, Christiane. *Women, Family & Ristual in Renaissance Italy.* Translated by Lydia G. Cotrane, U of Chicago P, 1987.

León, Fray Luis de. *La perfecta casda.* Espasa Calpe, 1980.

López-Morillas, E. Consuelo, editor. *Textos aljamiados sobre la vida de mahoma. El profeta de los moriscos.* CSIC, 1994.

Luján, Pedro de. *Coloquios Matrimoniales.* Edited by Asunción Rallo Gruss, Biblioteca Virtual de Andalucía, Junta de Andalucía, 2010.

Martínez, María Elena. *Genealogical Fictions: Limpieza de Sangre, Religion and Gender in Colonial Mexico* Stanford UP, 2008.

Miles, Margaret R. *A Complex Delight: The Secularization of the Breast 1350–1750.* Berkeley UP, 2008.

– "The Virgin's One Bare Breast." *The Expanding Discourse: Feminism and Art History*, edited by Norma Broude and Mary D. Garroud, Westview Press, 1992, pp. 29–36.

– Miller, Naomi J. "Mothering Others: Caregiving as Spectrum and Spectacle in the Early Modern Period." *Maternal Measure: Figuring Caregiving in the Early Modern Period*, edited by Naomi J. Miller and Naomi Yavneh, Aldershot, 2000, pp. 1–5.

Nadeau, Carolyn. "Authorizing the Wife/Mother in Sixteenth-Century Advice Manuals." *Women in the Discourse in Early Modern Spain*, edited by Joan Cammarata, U of Florida P, 2003, pp. 19–34.

– "Blood Mother/Milk Mother: Breastfeeding, the Family, and the State in Antonio de Guevara's *Relox de Príncipes* (Dial of Princes)," *Hispanic Review*, no. 69, vol. 2, Spring 2001, pp. 153–74.

Owens, Sarah E. *Nuns Navigating the Spanish Empire*. U of New Mexico P, 2017.

Patton, Pamela A. *The Art of Estrangement: Redefining Jews in Reconquest Spain*. Penn State UP, 2013.

Pedro Berruguete: El primer pintor renacentista de la Corona de Castilla. Junta de Castilla y León: Consejería de Educación y Cultura, 2003.

Perry, Mary Elizabeth. *Gender and Disorder in Early Modern Seville*. Princeton UP, 1990.

Rivera, Olga. "La leche maternal y el sujeto de los descendientes en la *Perfecta casada*." *Hispanic Review*, no. 70, vol. 2, Spring 2002, pp. 207–17.

Siegemund, Justina. *The Court Midwife*. Edited and translated by Lynne Tatlock, U of Chicago P, 2005.

Simón Palmer, María del Carmen. *La cocina de palacio 1561–1931*. Editorial Castalia, 1997.

The Songs of Holy Mary by Alfonso X, the Wise: A Translation of the "Cantigas de Santa María." Translated by Kathleen Kulp-Hill, Arizona Center for Medieval and Renaissance Studies, 2000.

Sperling, Jutta Gisela. "Introduction." *Medieval and Renaissance Lactations: Images, Rhetorics, Practices: Women and Gender in the Early Modern World*, Routledge, 2013, pp. 1–20.

– *Roman Charity: Queer Lactations in Early Modern Visual Culture*. Transcript-Verlag, 2016.

Stallybrass, Peter. "Patriarchal Territories: The Body Enclosed." *Rewriting the Renaissance: The Discourses of Sexual Difference in Early Modern Europe*, edited by Margaret W. Ferguson, Maureen Quilligon, and Nancy J. Vickers, University of Chicago Press, 1986, pp. 123–42.

Tomás Pérez, Magdalena Santo. Reseña. Cárbon, Damián. "Libro del arte de las comadres o madrinas y del regimiento de las preñadas y paridas y de los niños." *Edad Media*, edited by Daniel García Gutierrez, 2001, pp. 236–8.

Villaseñor Black, Charlene. "Inquisitorial Practices Past and Present: Artistic Censorship, the Virgin Mary, and St. Anne." *Art, Piety and Destruction in the Christian West, 1500–1700*, edited by Virgina Chieffo Raguin, Ashgate, 2010, pp. 173–200.

– "The Moralized Breast in Early Modern Spain." *The Material Culture of Sex, Procreation and Marriage in Premodern Europe*, edited by Anne L. McLanan and Karen Rosoff Encarnación, Palgrave, 2002, pp. 191–219.

Vinyoles, Teresa, and Ximena Illanes Zubieta. "Treated as Sons and Daughters." *Adoption and Fosterage Practices in the Late Medieval and Modern Age*, edited by Maria Clara Rossi and Marina Garbellotti, Vielle Libreria Editrice, 2016.

Vives, Juan Luis. *Instrucción de la mujer Cristiana.* Espasa Calpe, 1944.

Winer, Rebecca Lynn. "The Enslaved Wetnurse as Nanny: The Transition from Free to Slave Labor in Childcare in Barcelona after the Black Death (1348)." *Slavery and Abolition*, vol. 38, no. 2, 2017, pp. 303–19.

Yaveneh, Naomi. "To Bare or Not Too Bare: Sofonisba Anguissola's Nursing Madonna and the Womanly Art of Breastfeeding." *Maternal Measure: Figuring Caregiving in the Early Modern Period*, Aldershot, 2000, pp. 65–78.

Young, Eric. *Bartolome Bermejo: The Great Hispano-Flemish Master.* Paul Elek, 1975.

Zubieta, Ximena Illanes. "Historias entrecurzadas: El período de la lactancia de niñas y niños abandonados en el mundo femenino de las nodrizas durante la primera mitad del siglo XV." *Anuario de estudios medievales*, vo. 43, no. 1, 2013, pp. 159–97.

Chapter Six

The Queer (Evil) Eye and Deviant Healing on the Early Modern Stage

SHERRY VELASCO

Throughout the early modern period Iberian physicians, theologians, writers, artists, and the general public were engaged in lively debates about "fascination" or what was commonly called the "evil eye" ("fascinación," "mal de ojo," and "aojamiento"). Dating back to classical antiquity, the evil eye was understood by many to be an infectious disease in which certain poisonous vapors issued from the eyes of one person, contaminated the air, and were absorbed into the body of another, thereby causing illness, disability, or death. The provocative discussion that emerged during the early modern period sought to determine whether the evil eye was merely a superstitious belief, the result of demonic intervention, or a life-threatening illness that required medical diagnosis, treatment, and prevention. Regardless of whether medical authorities believed in the existence of the evil eye, they found themselves obligated to address the topic seriously in light of its potential as a contagious disease and the general public's tendency to rely on unofficial health practitioners for solutions to what was often unexplained illness.[1] As people sought remedies and preventative measures deemed superstitious, religious authorities were likewise compelled to enter into the debate over the evil eye. The boom of anti-superstitious investigations and publications combined with the belief that demonic intervention might be at play in fascination created an ongoing discussion of the evil eye among theologians, frequently in dialogue with the medical community.

Given the pervasiveness of the belief in and debate surrounding the evil eye across all groups – not to mention the stories that people construct to make sense of misfortune in their lives – it would not be surprising that early modern audiences might relate to and find entertaining an *entremés* (dramatic interlude) focused exclusively on the topic. However, in light of how (non-procreative) women were the target of blame in most debates about the evil eye, it might seem unexpected that the anonymous one-act comedy *Entremés de los aojados* (*Victims of the Evil Eye*, published in 1680) is concerned primarily with male sufferers and their culpability in the vexing phenomenon.[2] As this essay aims to demonstrate, the interlude's provocative insight into the evil eye phenomenon is manifested through the ways in which it goes beyond the misogynist claims of most narratives on fascination to explore the role that men's deviant desires and behaviours played in the diagnosis, treatment, and prevention of visual contagion. In this way, *Los aojados* acts out some of the unspoken yet deeply unsettling anxieties and implications that fuelled the ubiquitous and steadfast belief in fascination. These fears, for the most part, signalled how men with "unnatural" desires and behaviours are the real cause (and not the victims) of the pervasive idea that women's toxicity is to blame for the evil eye.

The scientific explanation in the early modern period for why women, especially older women, were among those individuals considered most likely to infect others by means of the evil eye argued that their blood was toxic, even lethal. The belief in the venomous nature of women's bodies during menstruation and after menopause motivated theorists as well as poets, novelists, and playwrights to address the public's fear that women's physiology (toxic vapours from blood released through the eyes) could produce serious harm. The often repeated warnings regarding the health risk that menstruating and post-menopausal women posed to vulnerable recipients implied that older women were even more dangerous, primarily because, unlike younger women who only menstruate during limited days, post-menopausal women always carry the venomous toxins from the residue of menstrual blood in their veins. Physician Alonso López de Corella, in his 1547 encyclopedic collection of answers to a variety of scientific enquiries, *Secretos de philosophia y astrología y medicina* (*Secrets of Philosophy, Astrology, and Medicine*), poses the question in a chapter title, "How Can Old Women Give Children the Evil Eye?" The author first establishes that older women have an abundance of corrupt humours no longer purged through menstruation before he describes how their lack of intelligence leads to a more vivid imagination prone to evil, which makes the force of visual toxicity stronger (320). As Fernando Salmón and Montserrat Cabré explain, "in the cultural frame where the disease was located, fascination was thought to be produced by a harmful power that women naturally possessed" (61).

While Spanish physicians and theologians debated whether women could infect others inadvertently through a natural venom produced by menstrual blood, some early modern theorists also suspected women of voluntary harm due to their predisposition for demonic influence. In these cases, the Inquisition intervened in what was often personal rivalries, taking seriously the belief that women's propensity for negative emotions such as envy, hatred, and the desire for revenge could impact their physical bodies, and thereby provide the condition for the devil (working within the laws of nature) to utilize their ill-willed gaze to injure others.[3] Although men as well as women could experience the emotions associated with fascination (envy, desire, admiration, or ill will), after unexplained illnesses, deaths, or accidents, often the first to be suspected of visual toxicity was an old woman who may have been observed admiring the victim, as theologian Martín Del Río clarifies: "Every day plump, pretty little children attract such looks and praises, and since it is easy to find some wrinkled, misshapen old woman among their admirers, and since this kind of person is physically offensive, morose, and hateful, the harm is attributed to her rather than to anyone else" (125). As Del Río's commentary illustrates, the profile for individuals most at risk for visual infection are those with weak blood and fragile dispositions – mainly children and certain adults – as well as those who possess the attractive attributes of beauty and talent, thereby making them the target of desire and envy.

Early modern theatregoers might learn about the health risks of being beautiful, at times through lessons on humoral medicine as it relates to vulnerability to the evil eye. In Tirso de Molina's *El amor médico* (*Love the Doctor*), Doña Jerónima, disguised as a male physician, is not surprised that the beautiful Estefanía has fallen ill. The cross-dressed, fraudulent, yet learned "doctor" describes how the humoral physiology of beauty is composed of delicate blood, which justifies why women and children are susceptible to the evil eye: "cuando se proporcionan / de las cuatro humores, dan forma / a la belleza ... De aquí nace la belleza, / y esta tal consiste toda en la sangre delicada / ... Por esto niños y damas / tan fácilmente se aojan, / porque la fascinación / halla resistencia poca / en la sangre que penetra" ("when the four humours are balanced, they give shape to beauty ... From here beauty is born and consists of delicate blood ... That's why children and women are easily infected with the evil eye, because fascination finds little resistance from the blood it penetrates"; 61–2). The fear that beauty might attract the evil eye runs throughout Tirso's play. Indeed, numerous playwrights, including Lope de Vega, Luis Quiñones de Benavente, Antonio Mira de Amescua, and Lucas Fernández, among countless others, saw the dramatic potential of referencing the evil eye: the real or imagined positive qualities in an individual that attracted the admiration or envy of onlookers as well as the preventative or curative measures taken to avert harm.[4]

While aging women were most often blamed for illness or misfortune linked to the evil eye, their attempts to provide a cure for the condition were popular with many impacted yet met with suspicion by the medical and religious communities. At the start of the interlude we are introduced to the evileye-healing services of Manuela, whose business sign reads "Así dice: doña Fabia / santigua aquí, con licencia / a los que aojados vienen, / y cura con gran clemencia / a los ricos por dinero, / y a los pobres sobre prenda" ("It says: Doña Fabia blesses here, with licence, those inflicted with the evil eye; with great mercy she cures the rich for money and the poor on collateral"; Sanchez 372).[5] Manuela, as her sign indicates, works as a *santiguadora*: the faith healer who cures by making the sign of the cross over the patient while reciting certain prayers. Despite the general public's belief in their healing abilities, physicians and theologians warned against consulting the *santiguadoras*. Juan de la Torre y Valcárcel cautions in his 1668 medical treatise: "Otro remedio tiene comúnmente el vulgo por cosa muy santa (como ellos dicen) para curar este mal [*mal de ojo*], y es llamar a una vieja que santigüe a la criatura ... y si quien las llama, sólo pretende remedios espirituales para el mal, como son oraciones rogativas y signos, llame a sacerdotes, ministros inmediatos de Dios" ("Another remedy that the common person believes very holy (as they say) to cure this affliction is to call an old woman to say a blessing over the child ... and if one does contact one of them, only allow spiritual solutions for the ailment, such as supplicative prayers and gestures, call a priest, one of God's immediate ministers"; 369).

Scepticism about the efficacy of *santiguadoras* is dramatized by the two observers María Escamilla and Gálvez, who visit the shop to check out Doña Fabia and enjoy the entertaining stories told by customers recounting how they contracted the evil eye.[6] When Gálvez questions whether the evil eye infects more than just children, María Escamilla gives her friend (and the audience) a preview of the ailing customers who might consult the *santiguadora*: the afflicted include not only beautiful women but old and ugly ones as well. She goes on to exclaim that even men – especially those who pride themselves on being *lindos* – come to be cured.

As the audience was well aware, the term *lindo* meant more than just a handsome man; it held connotations of the effeminate man who may be inclined to fall into the sin of sodomy.[7] Early modern lexicographer Sebastián de Covarrubias exclaims in his definition of "lindo" that "decir el varón 'lindo' absolutamente es llamarle afeminado" ("to say that a man is 'lindo' is absolutely to call him effeminate"; 1201).[8] Male effeminacy, as physician Juan Huarte de San Juan posits, is recognizable through "ciertos movimientos que tiene, indecentes al sexo viril: mujeriles, mariosos, la voz blanda y melosa; son los tales inclinados a hacer obras de mujeres, y caen ordinariamente en el pecado nefando" ("certain movements that he has, which are indecent for men: they are feminine, unmanly, and have a soft and delicate voice. Such men are prone to do women's work and they usually fall into the sin of sodomy"; 609). The repetition of the term "lindo" throughout the brief interlude underscores the significance of male effeminacy (and the behaviours that accompany it) for understanding the complexities of visual toxicity. As the spectators will soon discover, what the parade of male sufferers who seek the services of the *santiguadora* have in common is their failure to conform to the social and sexual expectations for men, as dramatized through behaviours and vices such as an interest in fashion, excessive hygiene and tidiness, cowardice, unnatural sexual conduct including sodomy and bestiality, avoidance of or inability to perform procreative sex, attraction for repulsive women, and vain fantasies of their own attractiveness and sexual endowment.

The notion that men's failed masculinity and transgressive sexuality might be related to the evil eye is signalled through suggestive metaphors and wordplay throughout *Los aojados*. In particular, clock imagery or the eroticized image of the "hombre de reloj" (clock man), whose sexual body/mechanism might be faulty and in need of repair, was a topos that appeared in early modern literary works, especially on stage in the *entremeses*. As Rachel Schmidt observes, "satirical and humorous writers took full advantage of images of ill-adjusted, broken or even jerry-rigged clocks to poke fun at sexual relationships" (125).[9] Tellingly, Manuela's first lines foreshadow the theme of clocks and time: "¿Qué hora será ya? / ... Tarde me levanto, /¡cuánto los relojes vuelan!" ("What time is it? ... I got up so late, how time flies!"; 374). Those familiar with burlesque songs and poetry would have also recognized the erotic-phallic potential of clocks that either run on time or malfunction: "reloj con pesas sin mano, / vano; / y un impotente en el lecho, / sin provecho" ("a clock with weights but no hands is a waste. And an impotent man in bed, what's the use?"; Alzieu 197).

The image of time, whether measured in hours, days, seasons, or years, is what makes the first client Navarro both the object of interest and desperate for a cure. Navarro boasts of being ahead of the season in fashion: "soy un hombre que me precio / de traer las cosas nuevas, / tafetán me pongo un mes / antes de la primavera; / gasto en julio el terciopelo / y en agosto la bayeta, / en hacer fuera de tiempo / las cosas está mi tema" ("I am a man who prides himself on debuting new items; I put on taffeta a month before spring. I wear velvet in July and wool in August. I'm known for doing things in the off season"; 375). His admission that he attracted the toxic gaze of bystanders anxious to get an early peek at Easter when he appeared as a "disciplinante azotado de Valéncia" ("flogged penitent/criminal from Valencia") is satirically subversive.[10] A man with a penchant for debuting new outfits seen flogged in Valencia would surely conjure images of the sodomite punished with public lashings. Among the various sentences for "el delito nefando" ("the abominable crime") during the early modern period (such as execution, galley slavery, exile, confinement, whipping, fines, and absolution) the only two punishments that were public spectacles were death and lashing (Carrasco 70–3; Berco 76–7; Fernandez). Furthermore, as part of the Inquisition's elaborate punishment spectacles in the autos-da-fé, theologians delivered sermons that discouraged male effeminacy by linking it to sodomy. The priest Pedro de León, for example, endeavoured to instil fear among the male spectators by comparing the feminine costume required of sodomites forced to parade publicly with similar attire worn by the male aristocracy in attendance at the spectacle: "Some of you do not partake of the vice ... nonetheless some of you dress as if you do ... you too could be mistaken for one of them" (cited in Garza Carvajal 62). The need to reform men who seemed more interested in clothing and fabrics than in fulfilling the manly duties expected of noblemen persisted as an urgent social, moral, and political topic in a variety of venues throughout the seventeenth century. Fray Antonio de Ezcaray, for example, in his 1691 *Voces de dolor nacidas de la multitud de pecados ... trajes profanos* (*Voices of Pain Born from the Multitude of Sins ... Profane Clothing*) blames male effeminacy for Spain's decadence, even comparing it with the tragedy of being fascinated:

> Por nuestros pecados lo mas de esto se halla ya en los hombres, pues con tanta vileza ... O nacion española! *Quien te ha fascinado?* Quien ha hecho que degeneres de tu antiguo lustre, y valor? ... y ha llegado a tan exorbitante estremo la compostura en los hombres, que yo sé, que visitando un Medico a un enfermo, le halló con tantas Cintas, y compostura en la cama, que juzgó que era muger.

> Most of our sins are apparent in men nowadays with such evil ... Poor Spain, who has *fascinated* you? Who has made you degenerate from your past brilliance and courage? ... the affectation of men has come to such an extreme that when a doctor was visiting a patient, he found him with so many ribbons and daintiness in bed that he swore he was a woman. (22; emphasis mine)[11]

Navarro's perspective in *Los aojados*, however, counters the moralists' admonishing rhetoric by suggesting that the spectacles staged by the Inquisition to discourage sinful behaviour (such as *el pecado nefando* [the abominable sin]) may actually excite and create sadomasochistic voyeurs aroused by the lashings. When Manuela wonders why the sight of someone whipping himself would result in the evil eye ("¿Y aojan al que se pega?" [376]), Navarro responds that "el capricho, / aun martirizando, alegra" ("whims, even when martyred, bring pleasure"; 376), confirming the unorthodox enjoyment derived from painful practices.

Sexual vice that functions like clockwork continues with Doña Fabia's next client, Malaguilla, a man who claims he was stricken with the evil eye for "giving" to another. We soon learn that he prides himself on pampering his mules at all hours of the day: "antes de las siete y media / les sirven el chocolate, / y, en dando las nueve, almuerzan; / ... *lindos* platos de yerbas" ("before seven-thirty they are served chocolate; and when the clock strikes nine, they have lunch ... *dandy* plates of herbs"; 376, emphasis mine). Again, in the burlesque context of the *entremés* and erotic poetry, spectators would have recognized "dar" ("to give") (especially when referring to a clock that strikes on the hour) as a euphemism for the sex act: "ha dado más veces que un reloj" ("he has struck ["given it"] more times than a clock"; Alzieu 225).[12] When a confused Manuela asks for clarification – "¿Y os aojaron a vos, / por aojarlas a ellas?" ("So they gave you the evil eye because you had given it to your mules?"; 376) – the "lindo loco" believes that bystanders are envious of his relationship with his beasts. Like the client who preceded him, Malaguilla is indirectly accused of one of the "pecados nefandos" – in this case the sin/crime of bestiality – which was categorized and punished alongside sodomy (Carrasco 76).

After a fleeting appearance by a cowardly man (Pedro), who prides himself on his ability to run away (*huir*) from the manly activity of fighting, we meet the first female client to seek a remedy for her affliction.[13] Unlike the male clients, who are proud of the deviant attribute or talent that they believe attracted the evil eye, this woman is ashamed of being the unlikely contradiction of a "dueña aojada" ("fascinated matron"). While the stereotype of the *dueña* as an older, undesirable woman should protect her from any lustful or envious gaze, she explains her unbelievable predicament by calling out the perversion of those men who, like the client before her, "escape" from the norm: "en el mundo hallarás / hombre de tan buen humor, / que huya de las hermosuras, / y de las fierezas no" ("in the world you'll find men with such good humour(s) that they run from beautiful women but not from the ugly ones"; Sanz Hermida, *Cuatro tratados* 377).[14] Framed within humoral medicine, as

Huarte de San Juan confirms, this "good humor" might be diagnosed as an occasional deviation from the norm but one that could become more serious: "hay hombres que apetecen una mujer fea y aborrecen la hermosa ... si caen en la enfermedad del estómago que llamamos *malacia*, apetecen bestialidades nefandas" ("there are men who are attracted to ugly women and are repulsed by the beautiful woman ... if they become ill with the disease of the stomach that we call 'malacia,' they will crave perverse bestialities"; Huarte de San Juan 481).

Most cases of fascination typically seek to assign blame to a specific individual believed to have given the evil eye to the victim. This "history of blame," as Salmón and Cabré have described the epistemological framework of the evil eye and its implication of human agency in the production of sickness (53), is not a concern for most of the afflicted in *Los aojados*. This changes, however, when the blind man Escamilla assigns blame for his ailment to the blind woman whom he planned to marry, assuming perhaps that her desire for him triggered her toxic vapours. Echoing a recurrent question for specialists whether vision is necessary for giving the evil eye, Manuela wonders how his betrothed was able to fascinate him without the ability to see him.[15] Escamilla's response is comically suggestive: "me mató en un retrato / a tiento" ("she killed me when she felt my likeness"; 378). When Manuela again asks how, he quips with the familiar critique of inept physicians, but with an erotic undertone: "a tiento cura el dotor, / y mata con las recetas" ("Doctors heal with their hands but kill with medications"; 378). Surely Escamilla's earlier statement suggesting his sexual desirability and experience during his youth – "en mi edad tierna, / siendo yo como una rosa, / me desojaba por ciegas" ("in my youth, when I was as fresh as a rose, my petals were plucked with a blind eye"; Sanz Hermida, *Cuatro tratados* 378) – invited a more salacious interpretation of the blind person's malady. In this case, the audience might identify an impressive phallic endowment as the physical attribute that his partner discovered through her sense of touch. Consequently, his current health crisis would be understood as the result of the blind woman's treacherously voracious sexual appetite stimulated by his admirable physique.

The last male client, "Lazminito" (played by Villalba), also blames the evil eye for a recent onset of what seems to be a case of sexual dysfunction, since he has been unable to "atravesar una almendra" ("split an almond") for the past two days. Given that *aceite de almendras* (almond oil) was used in burlesque contexts as a metaphor for semen, Villalba's condition might have registered for some spectators as a temporary inability to achieve sexual satisfaction (Alzieu 84). Similarly, giving the evil eye was also one mechanism for "tying" someone and thereby preventing him from performing the sexual act. Theologian Pedro Sánchez Ciruelo, for example, begins his chapter "On the Evil Eye and Other Bewitchments" informing readers that the evil eye can be used to "ligar a los casados, que el marido y la mujer no se puedan conocer ni hacer generación" ("to tie or render a married couple impotent, so that the husband and wife can neither copulate nor conceive"; 315; 325). Villalba, however, attributes his sexualized woes to his unequalled fastidiousness and special talent for keeping tidy when "soiling" where he sits, especially the female space of the sitting area (*estrado*): "para ensuciar un estrado, / nadie ventaja le lleva. ... si viérais con la limpieza / y el aseo con que ensucia / cualquiera cosa en que se asienta" ("nobody is his equal in soiling a sitting room ... if you could see the cleanliness and hygiene with which he soils where his sits"; 379). Similar to the pattern established in the previous cases, Villalba's predicament hints at effeminacy and sexual transgression as the real poisons hidden beneath the evil eye superstition.

Undoubtedly familiar with both the risqué double entendres characteristic of the *entremés* genre and the gossip (and eventual public punishment) of women arrested by the Inquisition for heretical and superstitious practices, audience members would not have been surprised to see more than one male customer self-diagnose the evil eye as the cause of his sexual malfunctions. In effect, among the most common symptoms of *aojamiento* were differing forms of bodily paralysis or immobility, often described in terms of "drying up," including afflictions such as impotence and infertility, or the dried-up milk of a nursing mother (Tausiet, *Ponzoña en los ojos* 317–20). Referring to the apotropaic symbols (such as the fig-hand amulet) that protected against fascination and its manifestations of infertility, impotence, and drying up in general, cultural anthropologist Alan Dundes claims that "all these amulets or gestures signify the production of some form of liquid. Whether the liquid is semen or saliva" (276).

While this was often construed as a male problem, the individual most often suspected of colluding with the devil to prevent men (and some women) from participating in sexual relations was typically an envious or vengeful woman prone to evil (Tausiet, *Ponzoña en los ojos* 302–25). As Heinrich Kramer and James Sprenger reiterate throughout their highly influential witch-hunting manual *Malleus maleficarum* (*The Hammer of Witches*, 1486), far more witches are women than men, which explains why "men are more often fascinated than women ... and the venereal act can be more readily and easily fascinated in a man than in a woman" (167, translation modified). Villalba, for instance, identifies the *santiguadora* Manuela as the "mujer del demonio" ("demonic woman") who gave him the evil eye that resulted in his current limitations. Manuela defends herself from Villalba's accusation by crossing herself and pointing out his own vanity in believing himself to be "lindo" (379).

Although it may seem counter-intuitive, that Villalba consulted a *santiguadora* whom he also identifies as his perpetrator was not unheard of. Catalina Doyague, for example, was investigated by the Inquisition in Toledo (1557–8) for superstitious practices as a *curandera* (unlicensed medical practitioner) who claimed to diagnose and cure fascination. She was also known to give the evil eye. According to testimony against Catalina, she warned those who fell ill as a result of her malevolent gaze that they would not recover unless she provided the remedy (Sánchez Ortega 461–3). As María-Helena Sánchez Ortega notes, acting as both *curandera* and *aojadora* (giver of the evil eye) "was frequent among these women and consequently their personalities were ambiguous" (462). In a 1591 Inquisition case against Catalina García in Zaragoza, the defendant is accused of committing grave crimes and sins that injured many people – working as a "santiguadera, ensalmadora, hechicera y bruja" ("faith healer, charmer, sorceress, and witch"), making an explicit pact with the devil, and inflicting the evil eye, even causing death (cited in Tausiet, *Ponzoña en los ojos* 316; Tausiet, "*Un proceso de brujería*" 15).[16] Of course, religious treatises written in the vernacular, such as Martín de Castañega's 1529 *Tratado muy sotil y bien fundado de las supersticiones y hechizerías* and Sánchez Ciruelo's 1538 *Reprobación de las supersticiones y hechicerías*, discouraged the sick from going to *santiguadoras*: "No tengan recurso como suelen, a las viejas santiguaderas y hechizeras, salvo haganle sahumerios de yervas odoríeras y encienso y semejantes cosas aromaticas" ("Don't consult the old women faith healers or sorceresses. Instead the best remedy is to give aromatics with fragrant herbs and incense and other perfumed items"; Castañega, cited in Darst 310; translation modified). Not surprisingly, many physicians concurred with these theologians. Physician Tomás Ferrer de Esparça, for instance, informs his readers in 1634 that *hechiceros*, whom he claims are no different than the *saludadores* (charismatic healers), cannot cure the evil eye because they are the ones who cause it (96–7).

Inquisition records reveal that *santiguadoras* were, in fact, using many of the remedies recommended by both physicians and theologians (Cirac Estopañán 88–92). According to the Inquisition tribunals of Toledo and Cuenca, *santiguadoras* most often used prayers, aromatics, and powders to treat ailments caused by the evil eye (Sánchez Ortega 481). The ceremonies performed by *sanadoras* and *curanderas* in Galicia mostly involved short prayers and aromatics to heal cases of *mal de ojo*. Dominga Landeira, who was accused of being a sorceress who cast spells on those she would later cure, explained to inquisitors that she limited her healing practices to making the sign of the cross and using some herbs from the field (Sánchez Ortega 470, 474).

The *santiguadora* in *Los aojados*, on the other hand, does not perform any healing practices associated with her profession. She refrains from giving the sign of the cross over her clients (in fact, she crosses herself after being accused by Villalba) and at no point does she prescribe or administer aromatics, herbs, prayers, or any other remedy used by physicians, theologians, or non-traditional healers. Her clients in *Los aojados*, however, are well informed and willing to employ remedies commonly recommended by both official and unofficial healers. Villalba, for instance, enters with a pair of scissors to cut pieces of fabric from the clothing of the women who give him the evil eye "así para el sahumerio" ("to use in the aromatic"; 378). This action is a comical deviation from how female healers would take swatches from the clothing of the sick – not the guilty – to use for the aromatic, often mixing it with other substances such as the herb of Saint John (Sánchez Ortega 477). Manuela's female clients were also familiar with strategies employed to mitigate fascination – actions such as yawning or offering the blessing "¡Dios te bendiga!" ("may God bless you") when giving praise were believed to protect and ensure that there is no malice intended.

What Manuela does offer, however, is advice for how to change behaviours to avoid attracting potentially dangerous attention. For Navarro, whose talent for wearing the latest fabrics ahead of season (even when suffering lashes), Manuela recommends "si curarse desea, / procure mudar el tiempo, / tendrá salud muy entera" ("if you want to be cured, try changing time and you'll be completely healthy"; 376). In other words, to avoid unwanted attention he needs to change his timing or perhaps adjust the mechanism of his "timepiece." To Malaguilla, whose love for his mules is perversely excessive, she recommends that he treat himself as well as he does his mules to avoid such bestiality. Whether her advice implies that he should pleasure himself instead of his animals is left for the audience to consider. In the case of Villalba, who exhibits a disconcerting need for tidiness when committing a filthy or disgraceful act, Manuela characterizes his effeminate (unnatural) fastidiousness as bestial by recommending he take a lesson on hygiene from a dog (379).

Although Manuela offers personalized advice for her clients, she also understands that collective attitudes need to change before superstitious fears of the evil eye can be removed. The *santiguadora* indicates as much at the start of the *entremés* when she claims that her remedies won't take effect without a collective gathering: "Hasta haber aquí más gente, / no tiene el remedio fuerza" ("Until there are more people here, the cure will have no power"; 375). In light of the unexpected assembly of mostly male sufferers and their self-diagnoses, the collective healing seems destined for men who have deviated in some way from traditional notions of masculine actions and desires.

The effeminate vanity and sexual deviancy associated with *lindos* and *mariones* would not have been unexpected of the bawdy entertainment of the *entremés*. Yet there is an unsettling subtext rooted in the ancient origins of fascination that might provoke more nervous laughter. Curiously, what is absent from the anonymous comedy is the ubiquitous amulet deemed to be among the most effective in averting the evil eye: the *higa*, or fig-hand symbol. The *higa*, in fact, was an obscene phallic figure that dated back to antiquity and was believed to promote sexual potency and protect against impotence, infertility, or other carnal malfunctions. Covarrubias states as much in his definition of the *higa* gesture – a symbol of the ancient god Priapus, whose primary attribute was a hyperbolic erect phallus:

> Es disfrazada pulla. La higa antigua era tan solamente una semejanza del miembro viril, estendiendo el dedo medio y encogiendo el índice y el auricular ... [Y] también porque en quanto a la figura es supersticiosa, derivada de la gentilidad, que estava persuadida tener fuerça contra la fascinación la efigie priapeya, que como tenemos dicho era la higa.
>
> It is an obscene expression in disguise. The ancient fig gesture was an imitation of the male member by extending the middle finger while pulling back the index finger and third finger ... And with regard to the figure, it is superstitious, derived from the pagans, who were convinced that the effigy of Priapus (which, as we already mentioned, was the fig-hand) had power against the evil eye. (1053)

Not everybody was cognizant of the phallic origins of the amulet, and those who did know its history seemed keen to silence or prohibit its popular usage. Juan Eusebio Nieremberg, a natural scientist and theologian who took the evil eye seriously by devoting eighteen chapters to the topic in his work on the secrets of the natural world (*Curiosa y oculta filosofía*), was emphatic about his condemnation of the superstitious and idolatrous use of the *higa*: "La higa que traen los niños, es indigno que le usen los Christianos; y no dudo sino que si se supiese su principio, se dejara totalmente. Es su origen tan de supersticiosos, e idolatras y por otra parte tan sucio y abominable, que ni aun pensarla puede un pecho religioso" ("The fig-hand worn by children is improper for any Christian to use. No doubt that if they knew its origin, they would stop using it immediately. Its origin is not only superstitious and idolatrous but so lewd and abhorrent that a religious person can't even think about it"; 43v). What Nieremberg knew but silenced was the fact that Priapus was consistently associated with seed or semen and the male member as well as with aggressive sodomitical behaviours, which would become the basis for his controversial and contradictory icon. As the god who could assist anxious newlyweds to consummate the union, ensure descendants, and threaten enemies, Priapus had been worshipped and revered since antiquity.[17]

Given the history of angst over sexual functions that lurks beneath the controversial phenomenon, it is not by chance that the only dramatic work dedicated exclusively to the topic of fascination gestures towards some of the concerns regarding how to heal or correct men's social and sexual deviations. However, even as the *santiguadora* Manuela ignores medical and spiritual remedies (while her superstitious clients uncharacteristically forego the protection of the ever-present obscene *higa*), the interlude proposes instead behaviour modification to assuage widespread anxieties about fascination, sorcery, and the fear of sexual dysfunction – often construed as evidence of women's power to harm men. While Manuela might selfishly manipulate people's vanity and fears for her own economic gain, she refrains from actually performing what would have been deemed superstitious when practised by an unauthorized healer. Instead, she provides a service that directs her clients to change the behaviours that they proudly believe have attracted harm – namely, unmanly activities and "perverse" desires. In this way, the *santiguadora* in *Los aojados* is ironically both deviant healer and unofficial spokesperson for those who blame Spain's moral and political decline on a perceived deterioration of Spanish virility. Manuela claims to be an authorized *santiguadora*, yet her alternative healing methods give her clients the authority to heal themselves through behaviour (and belief) modification.

Of course, the anonymous playwright does not let Manuela have the last word. After she triumphantly boasts of her professional success ("Es mi oficio, señores, / muy *primoroso*, / pues en mí todos tienen / puestos sus ojos" ("In my profession, gentlemen, I am very skilled, so everyone has their eyes on me"), Gálvez re-establishes the guilt of old women who inflict visual harm: "De que aojen las viejas, / son muy *amigas*, / porque, al verse entre *ojos*, / parecen *niñas*" ("Old women are good 'friends' with the evil eye because when 'eyes' are on them, they turn into 'girls'"; emphasis mine; 380). The last joke, it seems, is on the *santiguadora*. Describing old women in terms of "amigas" (slang for lover or prostitute) and "niñas" (another euphemism for prostitute) who find themselves among "eyes" (a colloquial term for both the anus and female genitals) suggests that Manuela could also benefit from modifying her own sexual behaviour.[18] As "primoroso" indicates ("primor" refers to "skill" but is also slang for pretending to be one thing while being another), Manuela has presented herself as an expert healer but may be just as likely to infect those around her.[19] This is reinforced by the last word of the *entremés*: when the playwright leaves the spectators with the word "niñas" – it also refers to the pupils in her eyes – the audience is reminded that the infectious eyes of women have the power to harm, or as Kramer and Sprenger insist: "to fascinate them so that a man cannot perform the genital act with a woman" (115, translation modified).[20]

Perhaps the final and rapid shift from policing men's deficient virility to censuring the insatiable lust in women has more to do with the cultural nerve that the interlude strikes than it does with the exigencies of time and genre in the *entremés*. In the end what makes this *entremés* stand apart from other texts and performances focused on the phenomenon is how it reframes the evil eye debate by implicating the victim, specifically the risibly superstitious *lindo*. This temporary shift in blame away from aging women to deviant men surely sought to discourage spectators from identifying with the victim and instead consider the misguided nature of the popular beliefs and practices dramatized on stage.

NOTES

1 See Sanz Hermida (*Cuatro tratados médicos*) for a partial anthology of medical and theological texts addressing the evil eye. See also Elworthy.

2 Referring to women during menstruation and post-menopausal women, Maureen Flynn posits: "Ambos grupos de mujeres tienen un factor en común: éstas no están embarazadas" (Both groups of women have one factor in common: they are not pregnant) (30).

3 See Keitt; Campagne; and Henningsen.

4 See Caro Baroja 264–76.

5 All references to the *Entremés de los aojados* are cited from Sanz Hermida (*Cuatro tratados médicos*).

6 The list of characters to appear in the interlude likely refer to recognizable actors during the period of the 1680 publication: María de Escamilla, Antonio de Escamilla, Manuela de Escamilla, Isabel de Gálvez, Juan Navarro, Antonio de Villalba, Juan de Malaguilla, Alonso de Olmedo, to name a few. See Ferrer Valls; Shergold and Varey; and Oehrlein.

7 For early modern assumptions about "lindos" and sodomy, see Cartagena Calderón 254–324; Velasco 93–121; and Garza Carvajal.
8 *Diccionario de Autoridades*, vol. 4 (1734): "lindo": "el hombre afeminado, presumido de hermoso, y que cuida demasiado de su compostúra y aseo" ("the effeminate man who prides himself as handsome and who pays too much attention to his appearance and hygiene").
9 For medical satire in the *entremeses*, see Slater and López Terrada.
10 "Disciplinante" is a religious penitent while a "disciplinante de penca" is slang for a criminal flogged by the authorities (*Diccionario de Autoridades*, vol. 3 [1732]).
11 Like Ezcaray, Fray Tomás de Trujillo (in his 1563 *Libro llamado reprobación de trajes* [*Book on the Reform of Clothing*]) laments that men devote so much of their time, money, and interest in clothing and fashion.
12 See also Alzeiu 125, 128, and 263.
13 That "pendencias" and "peleas" ("fights") were also colloquial terms for sexual relations adds another layer of nuance to Pedro's unmanly behaviour (Chamorro 647; and Alzieu 191).
14 Covarrubias offers "la mujer fea" ("ugly woman") as one definition of "fiera" ("beast") (901).
15 According to Jacobo Sanz Hermida, the only two groups considered incapable of becoming "aojadores" or givers of the evil eye are children and the blind ("La literatura" 963). Some physicians and theologians, such as Juan Eusebio Nieremberg, opposed this common opinion, arguing that even without sight, one can expel infected vapours from the eyes (41–41v).
16 Slater and López Terrada define *ensalmadores* as charmers or "practitioners that cured using prayers or spells both written and worn as charms" (230).
17 Readers could learn about Priapus through the popular translations and commentaries of Ovid's *Metamorphoses* or the frequently reprinted and imitated *Priapea*, a series of eighty-some obscene poems dedicated to, spoken by, or about Priapus. See Parker; Hooper; and Richlin.
18 For "ojo," see Alzieu 74, 112, 167, 237, 250, 281, 290, 299; for "niña," see Chamorro 609; and Alonso Hernández 555; for "amigarse," see Chamorro 88.
19 For "primor," see Alonso Hernández 636.
20 For "niña de los ojos" as pupil, see Covarrubias 1313.

WORKS CITED

Alonso Hernández, José Luis. *Léxico del marginalismo del Siglo de Oro*. Universidad de Salamanca, 1977.

Alzieu, Pierre, Robert Jammes, and Yvan Lissorgues. *Poesía erótica del Siglo de Oro*. Biblioteca de Bolsillo, 2000.

Berco, Cristian. *Sexual Hierarchies, Public Status: Men, Sodomy, and Society in Spain's Golden Age*. U of Toronto P, 2007.

Campagne, Fabián Alejandro. "Witchcraft and the Sense-of-the-Impossible in Early Modern Spain: Some Reflections Based on the Literature of Superstition (ca. 1500–1800)." *The Harvard Theological Review*, vol. 96, no. 1, 2003, pp. 25–62.

Caro Baroja, Julio. *Algunos mitos españoles y otros ensayos*. Editora Nacional, 1944.

Carrasco, Rafael. *Inquisición y repression sexual en Valéncia. Historia de los sodomitas (1565–1785)*. Laertes, 1985.

Cartagena Calderón, José. *Masculinidades en obras: El drama de la hombría en la España imperial*. Juan de la Cuesta, 2008.

Castañega, Fray Martín de. *Tratado de las supersticiones y hechizerias y de la possibilidad y remedio dellas (1529)*, edited by Juan Robert Muro Abad, Instituto de Estudios Riojanos, 1994.

Chamorro, María Inés. *Tesoro de villanos. Diccionario de germanía*. Herder, 2002.

Cirac Estopañán, Sebastián. *Los procesos de hechicerías en la Inquisición de Castilla la Nueva: tribunales de Toledo y Cuenca*. Instituto Jerónimo Zurita, 1942.

Ciruelo, Pedro. *Pedro Ciruelo's "A Treatise Reproving all Superstitions and Forms of Witchcraft."* Translated by Eugene A. Maio and D'Orsay W. Pearson, Fairleigh Dickinson UP, 1977.

– *Reprobación de las supersticiones y hechicerías*. Pedro de Castro, 1538 [selection] in Sanz Hermida 2001, pp. 315–17.

Covarrubias, Sebastián de. *Tesoro de la lengua castellana o española*. 1611. Iberoamericana, 2006.

Darst, David. "Witchcraft in Spain: The Testimony of Martín de Castañega's Treatise on Superstition and Witchcraft (1529)." *Proceedings of the American Philosophical Society*, vol. 123, no. 5, 1979, pp. 298–322.

Del Río, Martín. *Investigations into Magic*. Edited and translated by P.G. Maxwell-Stuart, Manchester UP, 2000.

Diccionario de Autoridades. Real Academia Española (1726–1739). http://web.frl.es/DA.html.

Dundes, Alan. "Wet and Dry, the Evil Eye: An Essay in Indo-European and Semitic Worldview." *The Evil Eye: A Casebook*, edited by Alan Dundes, U of Wisconsin P, 1992, pp. 257–312.

Elworthy, F.T. *The Evil Eye. The Origin and Practices of Superstition*. Collier Books, 1970.

Entremés de los aojados in *Floresta de entremeses y rasgos de ocio a diferentes assumptos*. Viuda de Joseph Fernández, 1680 [selection] in Sanz Hermida 2001, pp. 372–80.

Ezcaray, Antonio de. *Vozes del dolor nacidas de la multitud de pecados que se cometen por los trages profanos, afeytes, escotados, y culpables ornatos*. Thomas López de Haro, 1691.

Fernandez, André. "The Repression of Sexual Behavior by the Aragonese Inquisition between 1560 and 1700." *Journal of the History of Sexuality*, vol. 7, no. 4, 1997, pp. 469–501.

Ferrer de Esparça, Tomás. *Tratado de la facultad medicamentosa*. Pedro Verges, 1634.

Ferrer Valls, Teresa. *Diccionario biográfico de actors del teatro clásico español*. Editional Reichenberger, 2008.

Flynn, Maureen. "La fascinación y la mirada femenina en la España del siglo XVI." *Historia silenciada de la mujer española desde la época medieval hasta la contemporánea*, edited by Alain Saint Saëns, Editorial Complutense, 1996, pp. 22–37.

Garza Carvajal, Federico. *Butterflies Will Burn: Prosecuting Sodomites in Early Modern Spain and Mexico*. Austin: U of Texas P, 2003.

Grajel, Luis. *Aspectos médicos de la literatura antisupersticiosa española de los siglos XVI y XVII*. Universidad de Salamanca, 1953.

Henningsen, Gustav. *The Witches' Advocate.: Basque Witchcraft and the Spanish Inquisition (1609–1614)*. U of Nevada P, 1980.

Hooper, Richard W. *The Priapus Poems: Erotic Epigrams from Ancient Rome*. U of Illinois P, 1999.

Huarte de San Juan, Juan. *Examen de ingenios*. Cátedra, 2007.

Keitt, Andrew. "The Miraculous Body of Evidence: Visionary Experience, Medical Discourse, and the Inquisition in Seventeenth-Century Spain." *Sixteenth Century Journal*, vol. 36, no. 1, 2005, pp. 77–96.

Kramer, Heinrich, and James Sprenger. *Malleus maleficarum*. Translated and Introduction by Montague Summers, Dover, 1974.

López de Corella Alonso. *Secretos de philosophia y astrología y medicina y de las cuatro matemáticas ciencias* [selection] in Sanz Hermida 2001, pp. 318–21.

Molina, Tirso de. *El amor médico*. Bibliobazaar, 2008.

Navarro, Gaspar. *Tribunal de superstición ladina*. Pedro Blusón, 1631 [selection] in Sanz Hermida 2001, pp. 348–9.

Nieremberg, Juan Eusebio. *Oculta filosofía de la sympatia y antipatia de las cosas...* Imprenta del Reyno, 1633.

Oehrlein, Josef. *El actor en el teatro español del Siglo de Oro*. Castalia, 1993.

Parker, W.H. *Priapea: Poems for a Phallic God*. Croom Helm, 1988.

Pérez Cascales, Francisco. *Liber de affectionibus puerorum ... Altera vero de Fascinatione*. Luis Sánchez, 1611.

Richlin, Amy. *The Garden of Priapus: Sexuality and Aggression in Roman Humor*. Oxford UP, 1992.

Salmón, Fernando, and Montserrat Cabré. "Fascinating Women: The Evil Eye in Medieval Scholasticism." *Medicine from the Black Death to the French Disease*, edited by R. French et al., Ashgate, 1998, pp. 53–84.

Sánchez Ortega, María-Helena. *Ese Viejo diablo llamado amor. La magia amorosa en la España moderna*. Universidad Nacional de Educación a Distancia, 2004.

Sanz Hermida, Jacobo. *Cuatro tratados médicos renacentistas sobre el mal de ojo.* Junta de Castilla y León, 2001.

– "La literatura de fascinación en la Península: una incursión por los tratados de mal de ojo de los siglos XV y XVI." *Anthropos*, vols. 154/155, 1994, pp. 106–11.

Schmidt, Rachel. "*Hecho reloj*: Human Clocks, Bodies and Sexuality in Early-Modern Spanish Humorous Literature." *Self, Other, and Context in Early Modern Spain*, edited by Isabel Jaén, Carolyn A Nadeau, and Julien Jacques Simon, Juan de la Cuesta, 2017, pp. 121–33.

Shergold, N.D., and J.E. Varey. *Genealogía, origen y noticias de los comediantes de España*. Tamesis, 1985.

Slater, John, and María Luz López Terrada. "Scenes of Mediation: Staging Medicine in the Spanish Interludes." *Social History of Medicine*, vol. 24, no. 2, 2011, pp. 226–43.

Tausiet, María. *Ponzoña en los ojos. Brujería y superstición en Aragón en el siglo XVI*. Turner, 2000.

– *Un proceso de brujería abierto en 1591 por el Arzobispo de Zaragoza (contra Catalina García, vecina de Peñarroya)*. Institución Fernando el Católico, 1988.

Torre y Valcárcel, Juan de la. *Espejo de la philosophia y comependio de toda la medicina theórica y práctica* [selection] in Sanz Hermida 2001, pp. 363–71.

Trujillo, Tomás de. *Libro llamado reprobación de trajes y de abuso de juramentos ...* Francisco Curteti, 1563.

Vallés, Francisco. *Libro singular de Francisco Vallés. Sobre cosas que fueron escritas físicamente en los libros sagrados o de la Sagrada filosofía*. Translated by Eustasio Sánchez F.-Villaran. Madrid: Cosano, 1971.

Velasco, Sherry. *Male Delivery: Reproduction, Effeminacy, and Pregnant Men in Early Modern Spain*. Vanderbilt UP, 2006.

Chapter Seven

Staging Women's Healing: Theory and Practice

MARGARET E. BOYLE

Representations of health practices in early modern Spanish literature are wide-ranging and pervasive, with the varied preoccupations and realities of health experiences tied intimately to the human condition, the daily grappling with bodies, ailing, healing, and mortality. While novels can provide a chance to escape these bodily preoccupations through fantasy and aspiration, they also frequently offer to readers the opportunity to wrestle with some of the central questions of their day-to-day lives. If we consider Miguel de Cervantes's seventeenth-century *Don Quixote* to be emblematic of the first modern novel and representative of the varied concerns and interests of its contemporary readers, we also acknowledge that part of its lasting appeal has to do with its ability to cut through to challenging and enduring questions relating to being and time and sense of self in relationship to these health experiences (see figure 10).

Wildly popular in Spain's sixteenth and seventeenth centuries, the three-act *comedia* appealed to a significantly more diverse audience than the *Quixote*, by virtue of its non-book form and propelled by playwright Lope de Vega's 1609 directive to make theatre that would both educate and entertain the masses.[1] Through frequently regulated by formulaic love triangles, scenes of confused identities, abrupt resolutions of multiple marriages, or sudden tragedy, these plays also provided a kind of escapism while engaging with the concerns most relevant and appealing to its audiences. The lucrative status of the comedia performances prompted moralists to regularly weigh in and attempt the regulation of form and content, while various taxation strategies on steady revenue streams from public theatres were also implemented. As Rachel Ball has argued, "The charitable function of playhouses" – meaning the taxation of theatre revenue as a way to fund a variety of social-charitable institutions, including hospitals – serves as a way to "legitimize and

Vol. I. p. 80.
W Hogarth Inv' et sculp
The Innkeeper's Wife & Daughter taking Care of ye Don after being beaten & bruised
Book 3rd Ch: 2nd

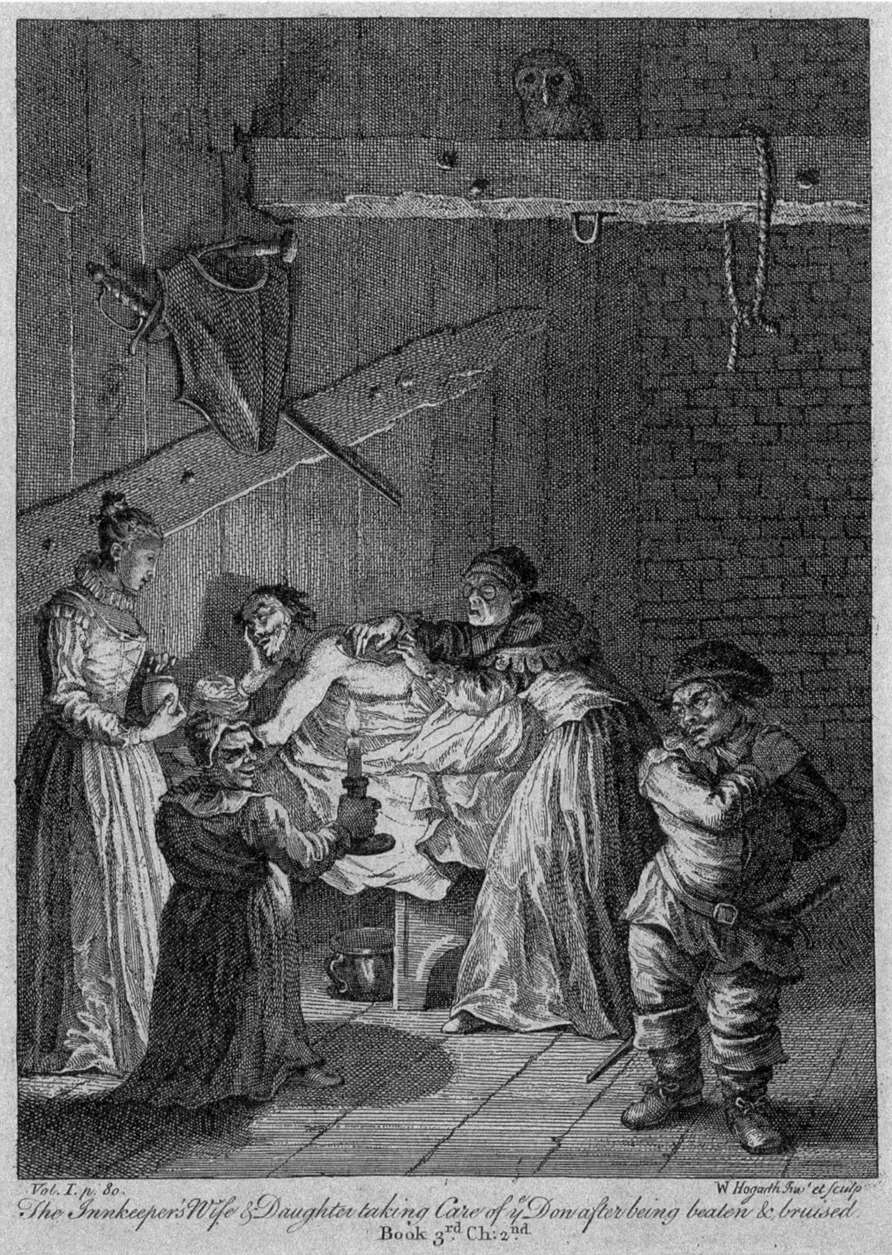

Figure 10. William Hogarth (1697–1764), *An old woman soothes a wound on Don Quixote's back,* engraving. Wellcome Collection.

popularize theater" (154).[2] In this way, both the spaces for and topics of health and healing were thus inextricably linked to public theatre, not only through this moral-financial tie but also by virtue of its ongoing dramatization of health practices as a trope or plot device.[3]

As one of the most well-known writers from his period, Spanish playwright Tirso de Molina (1579–1648) is recognized for his wide-ranging and provocative comedias, many celebrated for the variety of female characters depicted in his plays.[4] This essay explores a number of Tirso's plays as a way to explore the complex intersections between gender and health in the comedia. For example, consider a series of plays (here, chronologically): in *Marta la piadosa* (*Marta the Divine*, 1614?) the female protagonist feigns caretaking as an excuse to host her love interest in her home as she converts it into a pseudo-hospital; in *El amor médico* (*Love, the Doctor*, 1619–25) the female protagonist aspires to study medicine and disguises herself as a male doctor; in *La prudencia en la mujer* (*Prudence in a Woman*, 1621?) we encounter the stereotyped representation of the Jewish doctor as villain and coward; and finally, in *La venganza de Tamar* (*Tamar's Revenge*, 1624?), inspired by a well-known biblical story (from the Book of Samuel), Amnon feigns illness to lure Tamar to care for him, then rapes her. In all of these plays, Tirso openly negotiates the anxieties that surround the representation of marginalized identities (gendered, racial, religious) with concerns about the professionalization of medicine. The following kinds of questions emerge from this exploration: Who is allowed to practise medicine? What are the attributes of an effective physician or surgeon? What are the common stereotypes, anxieties, and desires held about the roles of physicians and surgeons? Where are the appropriate spaces for medical care? Is medicine effective? Who has access to treatment?

It should come as no surprise that comedias as text or performance do not provide standardized answers to these questions, but they do frequently make space for competing and contradictory answers.[5] It is also worth exploring how these kinds of questions are produced within the hybrid culture of the early modern period, which Pamela H. Smith describes with her term "techno-medico-science."[6] Or as John Slater et al. have argued persuasively for the case of the early modern Iberian Empire, "there were many medical cultures ... practices related to health and sickness were undertaken to a great extent by people without formal medical training who did not identify themselves as medical practitioners. This means that medical occupations and medical practices were not always related in discernible ways" (Slater et al. 13–14). Scholarship on gender in the early modern Hispanic world has also insisted on its dynamic and unstable nature. Allyson Poska, for example, has described the category of gender as subject to ongoing definition and redefinition, constant "adaptations, contestations, and negotiations" (211). With this framework of hybridity and plurality firmly established, it becomes possible to explore and contextualize the health questions raised by early modern Spanish comedia and the gendered dynamics posed by these relationships.

Sari Altschuler's *The Medical Imagination* creates a provocative axis between "both the various ways in which doctors and writers used their imaginations to craft, test, and implement their theories of health and the role literary forms played in developing that work" (Altschuler 8). Maríaluz López-Terrada has made an analogous argument particular to the function of comedias as a vehicle for understanding the social history of medicine, urging us to view both the production and the reception of a theatrical text. As she explains, "dramatists wrote on the basis of their own concept of illness and dramatized academic medicine, a point of contact with the public, since both sides shared concepts from the same Galenic humoral medicine" (López-Terrada 187). Thus, the comedia provides a more expansive and dynamic view of health practices from a variety of perspectives, demonstrating the reflexive relationships between fiction and readers, audiences and actors, health practices and practitioners.[7]

"Why should a woman study medicine?"

Early in the first act of Spanish playwright Tirso de Molina's three-act comedy *El amor médico* a provocative question is raised to the play's heroine: "Por qué ha de estudiar / medicina una mujer?" ("Why should a woman study medicine?"; 143–4). Here the protagonist's aspirations and practice of medicine within the world of the play provide insight into commonly held attitudes about women and medicine, both real and imagined. This essay will stress the importance of this question, the numerous and sometimes contradictory replies offered within this seventeenth-century play-text, the significance of the woman doctor – as both theatrical fiction and reality – as it relates to the professionalization of medicine across Spain from the late fifteenth century forward, and its impact on the topic of women's health management as well as women's work as healers, broadly defined, including educated physicians (*físicas*), doctors (*médicas*), midwives (*parteras*), and medicine women (*curanderas*). It also follows Monica H. Green's directive to conceptualize the study of women's health practices not in isolation but in ways that put "women *and men* in constant interplay over how knowledge of the female body was generated, disseminated and used" ("Gendering" 487).[8]

El amor médico was written somewhere between 1619 and 1625 and is set in the late fifteenth century. The plot of *El amor médico* is not without its complications. The first act takes place in Seville, and sets up the heroine Jerónima's romantic interest in Gaspar. In the second act, the play moves to Coimbra, Portugal.[9] There, Jerónima disguises herself as a male physician (Doctor Barbosa) and starts treating and courting Gaspar's current love interest, Estefanía (her father thinks she is ill with the plague).[10] Later in the act, when Gaspar is jealous that Estefanía has fallen in love with the doctor, he falls in love with a woman named Marta, who is, in fact, also Jerónima now dressed in woman's clothes. In act 3, Jerónima – through another series of tricks – eventually gets Estefanía to marry her brother Gonzalo, and Gaspar to marry herself. Her deceit is revealed, and she returns home to Spain and stops practising medicine. With this resolution, love is presented as the cure for its own disease (3626–8).[11] Although there is a certain conventionality in portraying the metaphor of love as a sickness that must be cured, the play sets the stage for important commentary about the practice of medicine, the gendering of illness, and the spaces and roles of women in relationship to healing.

Our heroine, Jerónima, stands out for her love of learning, an attitude the play attributes – somewhat conventionally – to her father's encouragement and praise: "Mi señor se recreaba / de oírme cuando estudiaba" ("My father enjoyed listening to me when I studied"; 971).[12] Here, the blame is placed on the father for the daughter's devious ways, emphasizing the importance of appropriate parental guidance. Jerónima also makes reference to an elite culture of women's learning, and specifically names Queen Isabel as well as her tutor Beatriz Galindo (1465–1534), or "La Latina," as examples of highly educated and powerful women: "Por esto quiero imitarla" ("For this reason, I wish to imitate her"; 117–25).[13] When her maid, Quiteria, suggests marriage as the next viable step in her imitation of Queen Isabel, Jerónima replies in the tradition of the *mujer varonil*: "El matrimonio es Argel, / la mujer cautiva en él. / Los artes son liberales / porque hacen que libre viva / a quien en ellas se emplea; / ¿cómo querrás tú que sea / a un tiempo libre y cautiva?" ("Marriage is an Algiers in which woman is held prisoner; the arts are called liberal, because they enable those who practise them to live in freedom. How do you expect me to be free and captive at the same time?"; 134–40). Her question puts her intellectual ambition at odds with marriage, pointing out the dilemma for women in her position.[14]

The particularities of the male dress and professional skills she assumes are what make this account of our *mujer varonil* compelling; Jerónima is not merely a nameless gentleman or wandering soldier as would be more conventional for the genre. Jerónima becomes Doctor Barbosa and applies her passionate study of science to medical practice. The play poses the question, "Why should a woman study medicine?" The play also offers several replies. First is the idea of imitation. In addition to her references to Queen Isabel and Beatriz Galindo, Jerónima alludes to a community of learned women. When, for example, she humorously asks the audience, "¿Siempre han de estar las mujeres / sin pasar la raya estrecha / de la aguja y la almohadilla? ¡Celebre alguna Sevilla / que en las ciencias aprovecha!" ("Must women always be tied to a needle and pincushion?"; 100–5), she subsequently cites women who pursue the challenges of scientific enquiry. In this way, the play insists on the establishment of women's participation in medical and scientific conversation.

Treatises on health and disease from this period frequently imparted medical advice through highly racialized and gendered moral norms. For a compelling example, consider the following entry on wet nurses from the anonymous fifteenth-century *Tratado de patología.*[15] In addition to offering extensive dietary advice (both foods to avoid and to consume) corresponding to humoral principles, the author provides a series of recommendations for selecting a wet nurse to best ensure the health of the infant:

> She should be young, not old, white, with a good body and form, nice arms and legs, a pretty face, polite, not easily angered, healthy, somewhat shapely; her breasts should be good, not big or small, soft not hard, with supple and widely shaped nipples, she should have a broad chest ... she should be from a good home, very sensible and in good health ... She should avoid eating salty, strong, constipating, or very spicy foods, such as leeks, onions, and garlic ... celery is especially bad as it can cause epilepsy in children; she should eat wheat, rice, well-marinated meat, good legumes, small fish, avoid indigestion, drunkenness, and be moderate in everything, even drinking water. (729–30)[16]

The dietary advice stands out in this passage for the specificity of the recommendations, not only with its interest in the properties or preparations of the various foods but also with its attention to physical descriptions. The passage also reveals an intersected construction of women's health as a product of class, race, age, beauty, education, and moral behaviour, which in this fascinating case of the wet nurse will be transmitted through her supply of milk to a dependent infant. This treatment of women by medical literature demonstrates the characteristic difficulties of both *being* and *treating* the female patient. It likewise points to an alternative reply to the question raised by Tirso's comedia of why women should study medicine, allowing audiences to contemplate the implications of women's participation in their own care and its impact on gendered advice and treatment models.

El amor médico also participates in current conversations about the professionalization of medicine, and the consequent restrictions placed on women's participation and ambition. Jerónima argues early in the play that women's contributions to medical conversation are essential for the protection of health. As she declares passionately in the first act: "Porque estimo la salud, / que anda en poder de ignorantes ... / ¿Piensas tú que seda y guantes / de curar tienen virtud? / Engañaste si lo piensas; / desvelos y naturales / son las partes principales / que con vigilias inmensas / hacen al médico sabio; / ... por ver si a mi patria puedo / aprovechar contra el miedo,/ que a la salud hace agravio" ("I value health, which is under the power of ignorant men. Do you think silk and gloves have healing powers? You are deceived if you think this"; 145–56). She points out the frivolity of women's proscribed material objects and preoccupations (that is, silk and gloves), and although she acknowledges that her commitment to study is perceived as "unnatural" for women, she emphasizes the urgency of her contributions.[17]

The tension surrounding the boundaries of women's medical expertise and practice even appears in Juan Luis Vives's widely circulated *Education of a Christian Woman* (1523). In the treatise, he anxiously delineates between women's roles as caretakers within the home and the practice of professional medicine. He emphasizes the limits of acceptable knowledge for women, as in the following recommendation concerning women's accumulation of medicinal knowledge:

> She will keep remedies on hand for common and almost daily maladies and will have them ready in a larder so that she may attend to her husband, small children, and the servants when required and will not have to send for the doctor often and buy everything from the apothecary. I should not wish that a woman dedicate herself to the art of medicine or have too much confidence in it ... She can learn this skill from the experience of other prudent matrons rather than from the advice of some nearby physician, or some simple handbook on the subject rather than from big, detailed medical tomes.[18]

On the one hand, Vives encourages women to have the knowledge necessary to nurse their families to good health; on the other hand, he advises against the accumulation of specialized medicinal knowledge outside of a woman's obligation to family. His gendered juxtaposition of the "simple handbook" against "big, detailed, medical tomes" and "prudent matron" over "nearby physician" is especially revealing for the way it pits the daily administration of the household against medical expertise, and the ways these ideas continue to shape both literary representations of health as well as the practice of medicine for centuries following the publication of the treatise.[19]

While there is ample time spent throughout the play discussing the place of women within medical theory, we also see Jerónima practising medicine in act 2 in her encounters with Estefanía, taking her pulse and offering potential diagnoses and treatments.[20] Jerónima, playing the part of Doctor Barbosa, moves quickly from a practised recitation of accepted medical knowledge, demonstrating education, authority, and expertise, to strategic and domineering moves of courtship, employing artful rhetoric designed to flatter and capture Estefanía. Even Gaspar remarks in an aside on the difficulty of distinguishing between medical practice and seduction: "Por Dios que soy, si se nombra/ medicina y no amor esto, / en uno y en otro idiota" ("By God, if this is medicine and not love, I'm an idiot in both"; 1878–80).[21] What is most important about the scene is the fact that we see Jerónima as a doctor not only in theory but also in practice.

In *La venganza de Tamar* (*Tamar's Revenge*]), a play written likely in the same years as *El amor médico*, Tirso also stages another scene that mixes seduction and a woman measuring a pulse. Instead of the devious courtship among two women, *La venganza* stages the incestuous desire of a brother towards his half-sister, anticipating the well-known end of act 2, in which Amnon rapes his sister Tamar (see Figure 11). Amnon pleads with his sister to remedy his illness as if she were a physician: "Advierte, que no siendo tú crüel, / sin piedras, montes o llanos, está mi vida en tus manos / y que en ellas la conservas. / Toma este pulso, en él pon (Tómale) / los dedos como instrumento, / a cuyo enciendo acento / conceptos del corazón / entiendas") ("No need for drugs or herbs or stones, / or minerals from hills or plains. / All I need's a little kindness. / Nonetheless, you do hold my life / in your hands. Take my pulse just there / [Tamar feels his pulse] / Decipher with your fingers / from this intense and fevered beat / the secret message of the heart"; 503–13). When Amnon asks Tamar if she understands his illness, she replies: "No sé yo que haya doctor / que tal gracia haya alcanzado. / Si hablando no me lo enseñas, / mal tu enfermedad sabré" ("No doctor that I know has that kind of skill. If I don't hear it from your lips, I'll never know what ails you"; 542–5). Finally, Amnon replies: "Pues yo del pulso bien sé, / que es lengua, que habla por señas. / Pero pues no conociste / por el tacto desvarío / en tu nombre y en el mío hermana,

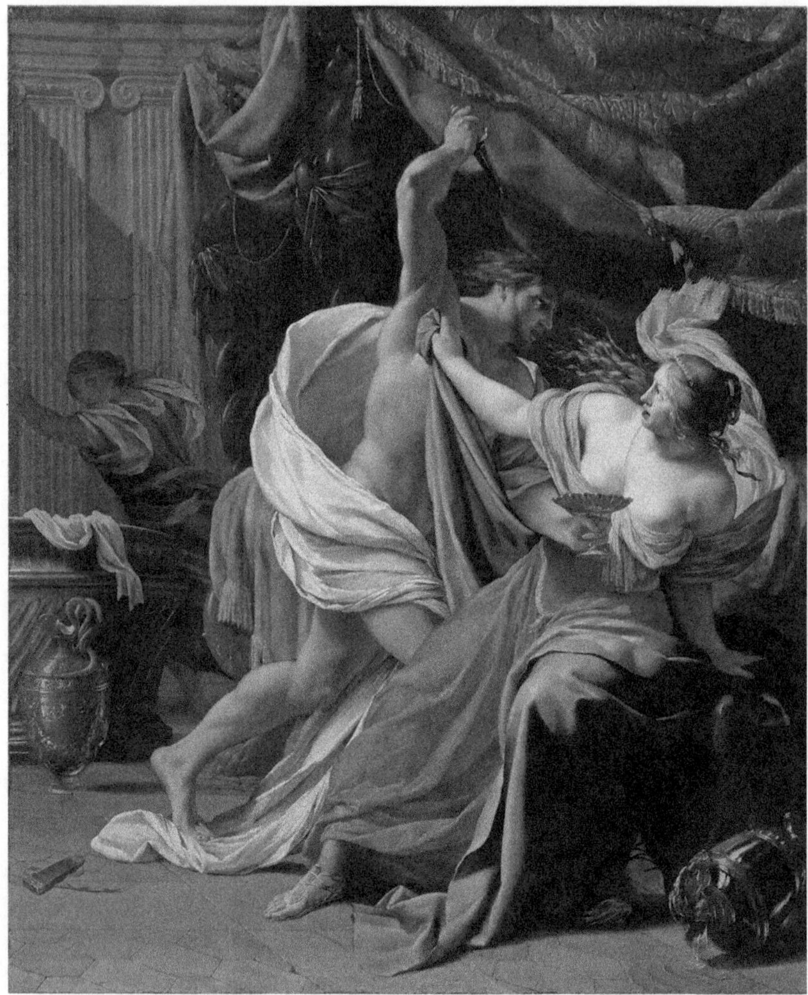

Figure 11. Eustache Le Seur, *Rape of Tamar,* circa 1640. Metropolitan Museum of Art, via Wikimedia Commons.

mi mal consiste" ("I know the pulse is a signal that speaks as loud as words. But since you could not diagnose by touch the fever that consumes the mind, I'll tell you"; 547–51). Once again, Tirso demonstrates his familiarity with a range of medical practices – drugs, herbs, stones, minerals, taking a pulse – while at the same time questioning their efficacy: the facility with which an untrained physician can step into the practices of the physician; the concept of love as illness; the association between medical practice, vulnerability, and manipulation (and subsequently violation), and of course the powered and gendered dynamics of practitioner and patient. This mixture of attributes presented in these scenes is likely reflective of personal or popular viewpoints in relation to the experience and stereotypes associated with medical practice.

As a distorted mirror of social reality, in *El amor médico* Jerónima is often a spokesperson for the greater regulation of medicine. For example, as she cites the unnecessary deaths caused by graduated but unlicensed physicians (calling out barber-surgeons in particular in one of many attacks against this profession), she speculates: "Quien no regula / estos peligros ¿no es necio?" ("Isn't it foolish not to regulate these dangers?"; 171–7).[22] With this question, might Tirso recognize the value of regulation for the increased efficacy of medical practice, but still argue for a place for women within this new configuration? Or perhaps the play's endorsement of regulation and standardization is merely a way to curry favour with legislators.

Jean Dangler has described the professionalization of medicine in Spain as a wave of four general developments, as a "concerted monarchical, municipal, ecclesiastical, and educational attempt to gain control of healing in the peninsular territory" (34). These four attributes include 1) the requirement of university study; 2) the enactment of laws regulating medical practice, which barred women, Jews, and Muslims from practice; 3) the establishment of licensing boards (including the Protomedicato); and finally, 4) the rise of hospitals and clinics (Dangler 35).[23] José M. López Piñero provides additional context for the ways in which the university education of physicians was "consolidated and developed" during the early modern period. Major changes included the way that anatomy was taught (the incorporation of the dissection of human corpses, usually one autopsy performed during winter months, designed to exemplify Galenist doctrines); the teaching of *materia medica*, the creation of chairs of botany, the teaching of "simples" (medicines derived from plants, animals, or mineral elements; López Piñero 66); and finally "clinical observation and environmentalist-oriented public health studies," resulting in what he describes as "'Hippocratic' Galenism developed from the mid-sixteenth century onward mainly in Italy, Spain, and France" (67).

It is widely argued that the professionalization and consolidation of medicine and medical practice did not completely obliterate the participation of women or the places for study and practice. As Meredith Ray argues, "early modern science was not studied and practised only in universities, laboratories, anatomy theatres, or other public spaces. Rather, natural enquiry unfolded in a variety of other contexts as well, many of which were more hospitable to the participation of women" (3). For example, women may have had access to some degree of formal education (often affiliated through associations with men: fathers, husbands, brothers, though sometimes also mothers). Many early modern women also had access to learning through experience in a range of locations, including leading or assisting home workshops, domestic or professional apothecary work, volunteer or paid caretaking responsibilities. The anonymous Spanish collection of culinary, cosmetic, and medical recipes *Manual de mujeres en el qual se contienen muchas y diversas recetas muy buenas* (*The Manual for Women in Which Is Contained Many, Very Good and Diverse Recipes*, 1475–1525) provides further evidence for women's interest and engagements in healing work.[24] The manuscript contains 145 recipes and is organized into medical remedies, fragrances, cosmetics, hair treatments, and recipes for food.

The actual layout of the book, however, frequently blends and confuses categories, placing, for example, a recipe for candying or preservation alongside medicinal ointments or tonics. Although the presumed audience of these early modern recipe collections were women – as managers of caregiving within their home – the explicit naming of both "women" and "manual" in the title is provocative for its segregation of knowledge and implications for the genre and form. The *Manual* operates as a comprehensive though somewhat unwieldy handbook with its divergent collection of recipes for the treatment of common physical ailments, the preparation of savoury and sweet foods, as well as a large number of cosmetic treatments. Similarly, the collection provides information about expectations placed on Spanish women concerning their own responsibilities to self and others, considering the circulation and use of recipe collections within households as models of practical and social education.

The long-term efforts to uncover and contextualize archival material testifying to women's ongoing experiences as both healers and patients continue to inform and challenge our understanding of health practices in early modern Spain. Anastasio Rojo Vega and Michele Clouse, for example, have unearthed the cases of seventeenth-century Spanish herbalists and bonesetters Elvira de Guevara, Catalina de Castresana, and María Hernández, including their new methods of treatment as well as their contributions to theories of medicine. Cristian Berco's *From Body to Community* tracks patient records from Toledo's Hospital de Santiago, including roughly eleven years and four thousand patients, more than half of whom were women. For a more comprehensive view of women's health within this period, it is critical to review and integrate these accounts from both the perspective of healer and patient. Through this kind of archival work, we can begin to construct a more nuanced and complete picture of early modern preventative and curative practices, recognizing the significant participation of Spanish women and the gendered dynamics that inform their treatment.

As a way to conclude, it is worthwhile to return to *Don Quixote*, not only for the ways that it emblematizes the health concerns from the period but also for the way it points to the enduring quality of these concerns, in conversation with theatre and through the manifestation of theatrical forms itself. Alonso Quijano is presented to us as a character made unwell by his unrestrained love of chivalric novels, but as readers we are put in a contradictory position; the reader is reminded of the plot's desire to cure the protagonist and at the same time begins to question the curative practices that would mean an end to the plot, or a closing of the book. In the second part of the novel, Don Quixote surprises readers with his straightforward description of a path towards health (chapter LX). He explains plainly to the bandit Roque Guinart:

> El principio de la salud está en conocer la enfermedad y en querer tomar el enfermo las medicinas que el médico le ordena: vuestra merced está enfermo, conoce su dolencia, y el cielo, o Dios, por mejor decir, que es nuestro médico, le aplicará medicinas que le sanen, las cuales suelen sanar poco a poco y no de repente y por milagro.
>
> The beginning of health lies in knowing the disease, and in the patient's willingness to take the medicines the doctor prescribes; your grace is ill, you know your ailment, and heaven, or should I say God, who is our physician, will treat you with the medicines that will cure you, and which tend to cure gradually, not suddenly and miraculously. (858)[25]

In a fusion of health practices both secular and divine, this description surprises readers, for it echoes the kinds of health advice routinely rejected by the protagonist throughout the novel. The episode reminds readers of the relevance of this kind of counsel, yet it is also likely that the reader has already developed enough affection for the protagonist to hold a reasonable amount of scepticism for these widely circulated claims.

Fast forward to the final scene of the novel, with Don Quixote on his deathbed (see figure 12). Sancho pleads, "No se muera vuestra merced, señor mío, sino tome mi consejo y viva muchos años, porque la mayor locura que puede hacer un hombre en esta vida es dejarse morir" ("Don't die, Señor; your grace should take my advice and live for many years, because the greatest madness a man can commit in this life is to let himself die"; 937). The aging Alonso Quijano reckons with mortality at the start of the novel and finds renewed purpose through

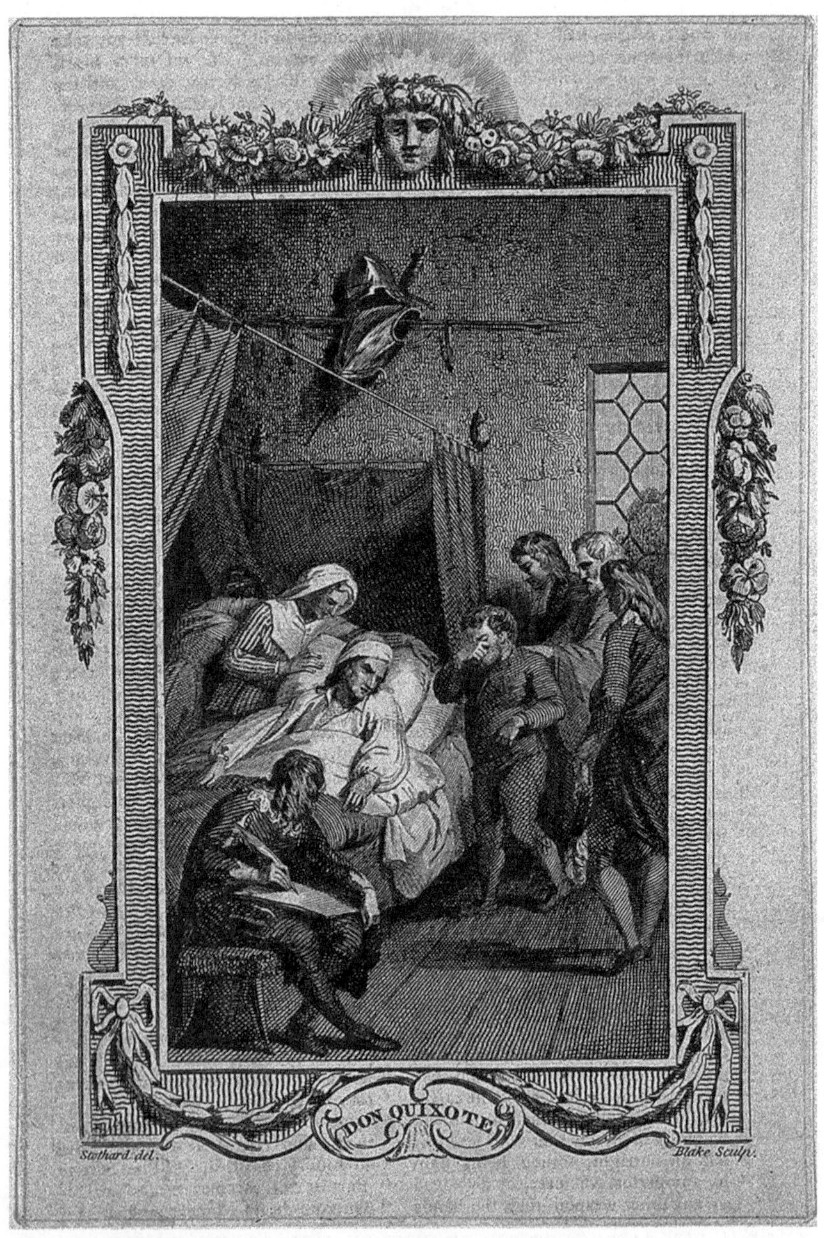

Figure 12. *The death bed of Don Quixote,* line engraving by Thomas Stothard, 1780–1789, after W. Hogarth. Wellcome Collection.

Don Quixote. Although the transformation is presented to us as a cautionary tale, the tragedy of this final scene also whispers furiously to readers about a vibrancy of living. It is the love for fiction and invention that permits Alonso Quijano and generations of readers to escape the limits of ailing bodies. In this way, the novel rejects conventional health advice and Don Quixote lives forever.

Putting *Quixote* into conversation with comedia, it is meaningful to consider to what extent women are permitted to stage role playing as a curative practice (invention as medicine, as healer, or as patient), and how these interventions are mediated by the limitations of the three-act play. Sustained focus on the gendered dimension of these staged relationships better allows for commentary on direct participation of patients in the construction of treatment plans as well as the impact of medical practices on health outcomes within these staged imaginations. Another question speaks more broadly to large-scale methodology: How might individual scholars or collaborative researchers best integrate text and motifs from comedia alongside contemporary performance, evidence of reception, and patient records? Certainly, this kind of expanded, ever more interconnected map can best provide insight into navigating the gendered dynamics of health care while highlighting the dynamism of theatre as text and practice and its ability to inform culturally relevant enquiry.

NOTES

1 To better understand this context it is worth consulting Lope's full treatise, "Arte nuevo de hacer comedias en este tiempo" ("The New Art of Writing Plays in This Age"), as an introduction to the ways that theatre was reimagined and energized during this time period. Cervantes's preoccupation with the *comedia* as genre is evident throughout both parts of the novel, both for the recurrent focus on theatricality and subterfuge and for the direct and sometimes envious commentary on the infamous and shape-shifting status of court-affiliated playwrights and actors. Chapter 11 of part two offers a particularly compelling example. For a rich exploration of the topic of "*Don Quixote* as theatre," see also Dale Wasserman.

2 I further explore this relationship in the introduction to my book *Unruly Women*, focusing on the ties between public theatre and Magdalen houses. J.E. Varey and Charles Davis's two-volume study is the first to catalogue the economic connections between Madrid's public theatres and hospitals. Emilio Cotarelo y Mori's *Bibliografía de las controversias sobre la licitud del teatro en España* is an excellent compendium for scholars seeking

information to contextualize these relationships. This volume considers not only the publication, presentation, and funding of various *comedias* but also the advice and protests of its contemporary moralists.

3 Medical treatment and practice frequently appeared as a plot or subplot of the period's literature. Playwrights sometimes wrote on the basis of their own concept of illness and often dramatized academic medicine as a way to display their own education. Nevertheless, the representation of health and healing on stage provides insight into the cultural and social image of medicine.

4 Fray Gabriel Telléz wrote under the pseudonym of Tirso de Molina, an extremely prolific writer engaged with a wide variety of themes. There are approximately eighty extant plays written by Tirso. The vast majority of criticism about the playwright focuses on the Don Juan character he popularized in *El burlador de Sevilla* (*The Trickster of Seville*).

5 There is a range of theatrical works we might also consider outside of the three-act genre in Spain. As an example, Elena N. Casey's presentation at the 2018 Modern Languages Association pointed to two short theatrical works by Pedro Calderón de la Barca: the interlude of *La melancólica* (*The Melancholic*, ca.1650) and the farce comedy *Segunda parte de la rabia* (*The Second Part of Rabies*, 1659), where lower-class women "serve as devious caregivers for the false melancholy afflictions of their female friends."

6 Luis S. Granjel's comprehensive introduction to medicine in early modern Spain locates a long tradition of hybrid approaches to medicine, linking pharmacological to manual practices, to miracles, religious beliefs, superstitions, and astrology frequently documented in popular literary texts, including *La Celestina* and *Retrato de Lozana andaluza* (Granjel 139–40).

7 Sujata Iyengar's working dictionary of medical language in William Shakespeare's plays is a comprehensive resource not only to scholars of early English theatre, but also a model text for building comparative work between other national theatres and language traditions.

8 Green clarifies the urgency of this point later in her argument, asking readers to continue "questioning our *assumption* that women, and only women, possess some 'natural' knowledge about the female body – we open up conceptual spaces for exploring how that knowledge might have been contested across gender boundaries" ("Gendering" 489). In this way, this essay aims to produce a "richer history of women's healthcare that shows medical epistemologies as various kinds of situated knowledge" (489). The study of women's health and healing in early modern Spain relies on the contextualization of these practices within existing power structures.

9 Anita K. Stoll has described the way that Portugal and Portuguese function as another layer of disguise throughout *El amor médico*. She writes: "Language itself is employed as one of the disguises. Since acts two and

three take place in Lisbon, Portuguese is a logical tool. Tello humorously misconstrues Portuguese words, confusing them with their Spanish meanings, such as the cognate *cagado*, which means something quite different in Portuguese. Appearing as the tapada with whom Gaspar will fall in love in Lisbon, Jerónima uses Portuguese to create this persona. She also uses it to pass herself off as Dr. Barbosa, as well as his sister, doña Marta, with whom Estafanía falls in love" (92).

10 The name "Barbosa" is likely referencing the profession of the *bárbaro*, the barber-surgeon.

11 In Tirso's *Marta la piadosa*, written just a few years prior to *El amor médico*, the topic of love as cure to illness is also a central focus of the play. The protagonist, Marta, convinces her lover, Don Felipe, to feign palsy in order to make the case that he requires individualized care within her family home. The play thus dramatizes the home transforming into hospital, with one amorous nurse tending to just one ailing patient. Marta persuasively begs her father to support her plan early in the play: "Padre y señor, ¿ve ese pobre? / Pues no sé qué compasión / las telas de corazón / no mueve para que cobre / remedio: si un hospital el cielo hacer me permite, / déjeme que me ejercite / en ése, y cure su mal" ("Father, do you see this poor soul? / I see him, and compassion parts / the very membranes of my heart, / and calls on me to help him. / Yes, if only heaven allowed / me to found a hospital, / I could nurse him back to health"; 1866–73).

12 English translations are from Sarah Brew's 2012 adaptation "Love, the Doctor." Note that translations provided throughout are not always literal translations but thematic ones.

13 Horst attributes linguistic success to two female instructors: Doña Lucia de Medrano, who is said to have publicly lectured on the Latin Classics at the University of Salamanca; and Francisca de Lebrija, daughter of famous historian Antonio de Nebjrija, who filled the chair of rhetoric at Alcalá (181).

14 Tello says such things as "el dotor desbarbado" ("the unbearded doctor") or "El Hipócrates capón" ("the [castrated] Hippocratic chicken").

15 The following passage is selected from the entry, "Cómo debe ser el ama que amamanta al niño." Teresa Herrera and Nieves Sánchez published a critical edition of the manuscript in 1997.

16 The translation into English is mine. The original reads as follows: "Debe ser joven y no vieja, blanca, de buen cuerpo, buenas carnes, buenos brazos, buenas piernas, de rostro agradables, educada, que no se enfade por cualquier cosa, sana y moderadamente gruesa; sus tetas deben ser buenas, ni grandes ni pequeñas, suaves pero no blandas, con pezones blandos y conductos anchos; debe ser ancha de pecho, que no haga ni mucho tiempo ni poco dese que haya parido y si ha tenido hija será mejor para el niño que va a amamantar que si ha sido hijo; si es posible que el ama sea familia

del niño, será mejor aún; escójase de buen lugar, de buen juicio y cordura y de buena salud. Evite comer el ama alimentos salados, fuertes, que constriñan o sean de cualidad muy caliente, como puerros, cebollas, ajos, oruga y menta; el apio es especialmente malo porque produce epilepsia en los niños; tome trigo, arroz, carne de animales jóvenes bien adobada, legumbres buenas, peces pequeños, extremidades de gallinas o de aves; no pase hambre ni se llene mucho, no tenga diarrea ni estreñimiento; trabaje con moderación; evite la indigestión, la borrachera, y sea moderada en todo; bebe agua también con moderación para que no se le cuaje la lecho, pues di esto sucede, el niño no podrá tomarla" (729–20).

17 "Pues por eso determino / irme tras el natural / que aprenden todos tan mal, / ya que en su estudio me inclino" (225–8).

18 It is worth consulting the latter half of chapter 9 of book 2 for fuller context and additional details regarding a married woman's responsibilities to maintaining her family's health.

19 While there is little evidence of female doctors working illegally, López-Terrada notes documentation of instances in which "extra-official healing practices were actively repressed" (8). In an exhaustive overview of women's ownership of medical texts, Green has also urged scholars to pay attention to women's interaction with "snippets of medical lore" found in personal correspondence or recipe books "as evidence for a much broader and wider medical discourse" ("Possibilities of Literacy" 48). Her table of individual female owners of medical books includes five fourteenth- and fifteenth-century Catalan women. She also lists the eight medical books collected by Margaret of Austria (1480–1530); the majority are French manuscripts or French translations of Latin texts. Upon Margaret's death, her medical books were inherited by her niece Marie of Hungary, regent of the Netherlands.

20 "También es enfermedad / el amor y, aunque es afecto / del alma cuyo sujeto / es, señor, la voluntad, / como obra por instrumentos / corporales y es pasión / que asiste en el corazón, / suelen los medicamentos / hallar cura en la experiencia, / que el alma espiritual / presa en el cuerpo mortal / obra siempre a su presencia. / *Tómale el pulso* / El pulso tenéis amante; / si Erasístrato viviera / fácilmente os conociera, / mas si el mal fuere adelante, / medios refrigerativos / habrá que ese daño aplaquen, / sangrías que el fuego saquen / y antídotos curativos" (2343–62).

21 Later Quiteria also equates love and science as kinds of madness: "Vamos, porque le asegures, y enferma para que cures / la ciencia que has estudiado, / que uno y otro es frenesí" ("Let's go, so that you find it out, and since you are ill, so that you can be cured, with the science that you have studied, for either is madness"; 318–20).

22 "Porque más hombres ha muerto, / prolijo de barba y capa, / en habiendo para mula / luego quede graduado, / antes de ser licenciado, / de doctor? Quien no regula / estos peligros ¿no es necio?" (171–7).

23 It would be incorrect to assume that women's medical activity was completely erased or absent during this period. For an introduction to medieval women's participation in medical conversation, see Green's edition of *The Trotula: A Medieval Compendium of Women's Medicine*.

24 See Alicia Martinez Crespo's 1995 edition of the manuscript.

25 English translation from Edith Grossman.

WORKS CITED

Altschuler, Sari. *The Medical Imagination: Literature and Health in the Early United States*. U of Pennsylvania P, 2018.

Ball, Rachel. *Treating the Public: Charitable Theater and Civic Health in the Early Modern Atlantic World*. Louisiana State UP, 2016.

Berco, Christian. *From Body to Community: Venereal Disease and Society in Baroque Spain*. U of Toronto P, 2016.

Boyle, Margaret. *Unruly Women: Performance, Penitence and Punishment in Early Modern Spain*. U of Toronto P, 2014.

Brew, Sarah A. "'Speak to Me in Vernacular, Doctor': Translating and Adapting Tirso de Molina's 'El Amor Médico' for the Stage." MFA thesis, University of Massachusetts (Amherst), 2012.

Clouse, Michelle. *Medicine, Government and Public Health in Philip II's Spain: Shared Interests, Competing Authorities*. Ashgate, 2011.

Cervantes, Miguel de. *Don Quixote*. Translated by Edith Grossman. Ecco, 2014.

– *Don Quijote*. Edited by Tom Lathrop. Cervantes, 2012.

Cotarelo y Mori, Emilio. *Bibliografía de las controversias sobre la licitud del teatro en España*. Est. de la "Rev. de archivos, bibliotecas y museos," 1904.

Dangler, Jean. *Mediating Fictions: Literature, Women Healers, and the Go-between in Medieval and Early Modern Iberia*. Bucknell UP, 2001.

Granjel, Luis S. *La medicina española renacentista*. Ediciones Universidad de Salamanca, 1980.

Green, Monica H. "Gendering the History of Women's Healthcare." *GEND Gender & History*, vol. 20, no. 3, 2008, pp. 487–518.

– "The Possibilities of Literacy and the Limits of Reading: Women and the Gendering of Medical Literacy." *Women's Healthcare in the Medieval West: Texts and Contexts*, Ashgate, 2000, pp. 1–76.

– editor and translator. *The Trotula: A Medieval Compendium of Women's Medicine*. U of Pennsylvania P, 2001.

Herrera, Teresa, and Nieves Sánchez, editors. *Tratado de patologia*. Editorial Arco/ Libros, 1997.

Horst, Robert Ter. "Aspects of Love and Learning in *El amor médico*." *Revista Canadiense de Estudios Hispánicos*, vol. 10, no. 2, 1986, pp. 279–98.

Iyengar, Sujata. *Shakespeare's Medical Language: A Dictionary*. Continuum, 2011.

López Piñero, José M. "The Faculty of Medicine of Valencia: Its Position in Renaissance Europe." *Universities and Science in the Early Modern Period*, Springer, 2006, pp. 65–82.

López-Terrada, Maríaluz. "'Sallow-Faced Girls, Either It's Love or You've Been Eating Clay': The Representation of Illness in Golden Age Theater." *Medical Cultures of the Early Modern Spanish Empire*, Ashgate, 2014, pp. 167–89.

Martinez Crespo, Alicia, editor. *Manual de mugeres en el qual se contienen muchas y diversas reçetas muy buenas*. Ediciones Universidad, 1995.

Molina, Tirso de. *El amor médico*. Edited by Blanca Oteiza, Revista Estudios, 1997.

– *La prudencia en la mujer*. Edited by Juana de Ontañon, Editorial Porrúa, 1975.

– *La venganza de Tamar*. Edited by John Lyon, Aris & Phillips, 1988.

– *Marta la piadosa/Marta the Divine*. Translated by Harley Erdman, Liverpool UP, 2012.

Poska, Allyson M. *Gendered Crossings: Women and Migration in the Spanish Empire*. U of New Mexico P, 2016.

Ray, Meredith K. *Daughters of Alchemy: Women and Scientific Culture in Early Modern Italy*. Harvard UP, 2015.

Rojo Vega, Anastasio. *Enfermos y sanadores en la Castilla del siglo XVI*. Universidad de Valladolid, 1993.

Slater, John, et al., editors. *Medical Cultures of the Early Modern Spanish Empire*. Ashgate, 2014.

Smith, Pamela H. "Science on the Move: Recent Trends in the History of Early Modern Science." *Renaissance Quarterly*, vol. 62, no. 2, Summer 2009, pp. 345–75.

Stoll, Anita K. "Cross-dressing in Tirso's *El amor médico* [*Love, the Doctor*] and *El Aquiles* [*Achilles*]." *Gender, Identity, and Representation in Spain's Golden Age*, edited by Anita K. Stoll and Dawn L Smith, Bucknell UP, 2000, pp. 86–95.

Varey, J.E., and Charles J. Davis. *Los corrales de comedias y los hospitales de Madrid: 1547–1615: Estudios y documentos. Fuentes para la historia del teatro en España*. Támesis, 1997.

– *Los corrales de comedias y los hospitales de Madrid: 1615–1849: Estudio y documentos. Fuentes para la historia del teatro en España*. Támesis, 1997.

Vega, Lope de. *Arte nuevo de hacer comedias*. Edited by Enrique Garcia Santo-Tomas, Catedra, 2006.

Vives, Juan Luis. *The Education of a Christian Woman: A Sixteenth-Century Manual*. Edited and translated by Charles Fantazzi, U of Chicago P, 2000.

Wasserman, Dale. "Don Quixote as Theater." *Cervantes: Bulletin of the Cervantes Society of America*, vol. 19, no. 1, 1999, pp. 125–30.

PART THREE

Faith and Illness

Chapter Eight

Work and Health in the Jesuit Province of Aragon (1617–1667)

PATRICIA W. MANNING

In considering early modern descriptions of mystics escaping their corporeal selves or the rigorous mortifications to which the devout subjected their bodies, it is possible to get the impression that the physical body could be a hindrance to the practice of Catholicism in this era. However, the Society of Jesus expected all of its members to take reasonable care of their physical selves. In order for Jesuits to be able to fulfil their "fourth vow," in which men promised to carry out mission work for the pope and therefore put themselves at his disposal for travel to distant locales (O'Malley 298), they would need robust health. This essay uses the order's foundational documents dating from the mid-1500s and correspondence between the Superior General and the Province of Aragon between 1617 and 1667 to study the manner in which the religious order attended to the health of Jesuits.[1] Like many early modern people, members of the Society of Jesus depended on the classical tradition and its subsequent reinterpretations for medical advice. In seeking to safeguard members' well-being, humoral medicine became such a fundamental practice in the Jesuit community that the order also employed it to analyse personalities for personnel decisions. As a corollary, Juan Huarte de San Juan's assertion that melancholy could be a sign of male intellectual gifts played a significant role in the order's treatment of melancholy men. Beyond temperaments, once very severe melancholy became pathologized, the order treated members accordingly. The community also sought to control external factors that could harm Jesuits and therefore followed medical theories regarding healthful locations, beneficial air, and avoidance of disease. In so doing, the order developed a definition of masculinity defined by work. Admittedly, the order's ultimate goal was gendered, namely, having physically and mentally healthy men available to carry out the duties of the all-male Catholic priesthood and healthy brothers (temporal coadjutors in the

Jesuits' system of grades) to support the work of the ordained. At the same time, the needs of aging and ill Jesuits were accommodated. Even though women were generally excluded from the order, its members nonetheless attended to women's religious needs.

Regulating Health in the Society of Jesus

Ignatius of Loyola's *Constitutions of the Society of Jesus* (1558–9) emphasize that Jesuits must "be ready at any hour to go to any part of the world" at the behest of their "superiors" or the pope (588).[2] In order to respond to such requests, particularly in the arduous travel conditions of the early modern world, Jesuits needed stamina. It therefore is not surprising that health is addressed explicitly in the Jesuits' governing documents. As A. Lynn Martin observes, a whole chapter of the *Constitutions* is dedicated to maintaining Jesuits' health (*Plague* 60; [lines 292–306]). Martin, echoing W.W. Meissner, posits that Ignatius of Loyola took such care with the well-being of his fellow Jesuits because he had damaged his own health through overly rigorous mortifications and did not wish others to do the same (Martin, *Plague* 59–60; Meissner 223). While Ignatius likely did want to protect others from his own errors, he also had the order's religious mission in mind. Explicit references to the need for "health" and "strength" to work in the order are reiterated at several points in the *Constitutions* (ll. 151 and 159) and applicants are questioned about their mental and physical health, in its initial section, the *General Examen* (l. 29). These documents also detail the circumstances in which a man could separate from the order for medical reasons (ll. 212–13, 216) and specify that the Society should construct its buildings in salubrious locales (l. 827) in keeping with Hippocratic ideas, which influenced thinking about the relationship between locations and infirmity. Besides these explicit references to well-being, as Cristiano Casalini suggests, Galenic theories underpin other facets of the community's policies, such as the *Formula of the Institute*'s interest in the physical appearance of potential members because of the belief that one's "appearance" also demonstrated one's "character" (195).

Gendering the Society of Jesus

Even within Roman Catholicism, which restricts the priesthood to men, the gender politics of the Society of Jesus are notable. In contrast to a number of other religious orders, including the Franciscans and Dominicans, the Jesuits do not have a sister community of nuns. As John W. O'Malley observes, at the behest of Pope Paul III, in 1545

Ignatius permitted a small number of women "to live in obedience to him," but this experiment ended after less than two years (75). Not only did Ignatius prevail in a legal dispute with Isabel Roser's family after she became affiliated with the community, but he also had Roser's and her companions' vows transferred to the local bishop and ensured that the Jesuits would not have to establish a female community (Simmonds 122; Soto Artuñedo 581–2).[3]

Beyond early negative experiences with female affiliates, there were more generalized tensions between the Jesuits' active ministry and potential women members. Due to the claustration of female religious in the Catholic Church, the peripatetic life of male Jesuits would not be possible for Catholic women of the cloth (Simmonds 121). Moreover, Ignatius feared that male Jesuits' ministerial obligations to the nuns in a potential female branch would take them away from missionary work (Simmonds 120; Soto Artuñedo 582). It is hardly incidental that paragraph 588 of the *Constitutions*, which prohibits Jesuits' supervision of nuns, begins with the phrase cited earlier concerning the need for Jesuits "to travel to any part of the world" on the church's behalf.

Medical Theory and the Society of Jesus

Even after the passing of its founder, the community continued to incorporate medical principles into its practices. Again according to Casalini, the Society implemented Juan Huarte de San Juan's theories on how humoral "temperaments" affected both "character" and abilities (190 and 197). Therefore, the triennial catalogues that were sent to Rome not only assess each member's "ingenium" ("talent") and "iudicium" ("judgment"), but also his "complexio" ("complexion"), or humoral characteristics.[4] Those of choleric disposition were considered most apt for pedagogical and leadership roles and melancholics excelled at scholarship (Casalini 203).

In this internal correspondence, Jesuits frequently emphasize the need for brothers and priests to be productive, as well as beneficial or useful to the community, avoiding the strident martial language often associated with the order.[5] Yet, language concerning productivity ties into other notions of masculinity, namely, the rhetoric concerning useful work that permeated seventeenth-century Spanish political and moral discourse about how to remedy the country's situation.[6] In Elizabeth A. Lehfeldt's analysis, a number of courtly writers proposed that the work of other men, such as that of farmers and artisans, would shore up the Spanish state (472–3). Meanwhile, as Lehfeldt and Shifra Armon note, men of noble birth generally were not industrious, but rather lack of productivity signalled their status (Armon 55; Lehfeldt 480).[7] However, Jesuits broke with this class-based expectation.

Melancholic Jesuits

For upper-class Spaniards of both genders, recourse to melancholy could justify their idleness; as Magdalena S. Sánchez observes, "melancholy was an acceptable explanation for inactivity, lethargy and boredom" (81). Yet, in the Society of Jesus, this temperament or diagnosis did not justify the neglect of one's obligations. In 1652, General Nickel lamented the state of "misery and poverty" into which the Jesuit *colegio* in Valencia had fallen. Nonetheless, the General maintained that "el ser melancolicos algunos sujetos" ("some subjects being melancholic") was no excuse for the "descuido" ("carelessness") that the Provincial noted during his visit (General Goswin Nickel to Vice Provincial Jacinto Piquer, 10 July 1652, Archivo Histórico Nacional (hereafter AHN), Jesuitas (hereafter J), legajo (hereafter leg.) 254 documento (hereafter doc.), 62).[8]

Rather than allow melancholy to fuel idleness, the high esteem in which the order held melancholics was intimately related to theories that associated this condition with male intellectual ability. According to Emilio García García and Aurora Miguel Alonso's research, each Jesuit house sought to have a few melancholics on hand to stimulate the "intellectual" atmosphere ("Conocimiento" 52).[9] Suggestions of a connection between melancholy and intellectual gifts in turn were linked inexorably to notions of male superiority.[10] According to Huarte de San Juan's 1575 *Examen de ingenios* (*Examination of Men's Wits*), it was "los melancólicos por adustión" ("the melancholics by adustion or adjustion"), whose combination of heat, coldness, and dryness fuelled both the intellect and the imagination, and therefore made them the most skilful at preaching (Huarte 458–60; trans. Carew 146). Moreover, Huarte opines that because of the preponderance of "phlegm" and "blood" in women, men had greater potential for intellect. The drier qualities, choleric and melancholic ones, which predominate in males, foment "la prudencia y sabiduría" ("prudence and sapience") of men (Huarte 365; trans. Carew 80).

In order to cultivate men who according to their humoral characteristics had the potential to be serious scholars, when Jesuits wrote to Rome alleging that their melancholy made them unsuitable for the order, they were encouraged in their vocations. Because a number of years elapsed between Jesuits' first and final vows, the order could dismiss men or Jesuits could petition to depart prior to making their final vows. Whereas the *Norms* to the *Constitutions* generally limited involuntary dismissal in this period to cases of "outstanding ineptitude," an exception was made for "poor health." If a man's medical issues made him "unsuited for leading his life in the Society" or if he hid his infirmities, he could be dismissed "against his will." However, if the individual's condition resulted from either "the Society's negligence" or from his service in the community, he could not be dismissed without his consent (*Norms*, in *Constitutions*, hereafter *CN*, 34).[11]

In 1632, General Vitelleschi informed Provincial Continente that Joseph Bonari's health was quite bad and that the order should consider what position would be best for him (General Muzio Vitelleschi to Provincial Pedro Continente, 12 July 1632, AHN J leg. 253 doc. 163).[12] Three years later, Vitelleschi informed Continente that Father Bonari "esta destemplado, y rendido a su melancolia" ("is unwell, and overcome by his melancholy") and asked to leave the order. Rather than accede to this request, Vitelleschi suggested that Continente "le aliente" ("is to encourage him") and to advise Rome of the Provincial's opinions on this individual (Vitelleschi to Continente, 16 April 1635, AHN J leg. 253 doc. 241). When Brother Francisco de Tapia asked to leave the community because of his poor health and "grandes melancolias" ("great melancholies"), Vitelleschi worried that "some temptation" motivated this request.[13] The nature of this temptation is not specified. Instead of agreeing to this departure, Vitelleschi asks that Provincial Ribas "le procure alentar" ("is to endeavor to encourage him") and if this does not improve Tapia's condition, to keep Rome apprised of the provincial officials' opinions on this individual (Vitelleschi to Provincial Luis de Ribas, 25 October 1636, AHN J leg. 253 doc. 281). Although Ribas writes to Rome that Tapia's condition has improved in a new position teaching grammar, Tapia himself informs the General that his state has worsened and "insta en que se le conceda dimissoria" ("[he] insists that he be given a dimissorial [a departure document from the order]"). Vitelleschi asks Ribas to meet with his consultants to decide on this petition (Vitelleschi to Ribas, 25 July 1637, AHN J leg. 253 doc. 305).

When Brother Cristóbal Bonaventura Exarnit requested to depart from the community, the order was "alentar, para que lleue con paciencia su falta de salud, y melancolias" ("to encourage [him], so that he may deal with his lack of health, and melancholies with patience"). Should attempts to "quietarle" ("calm him") prove unsuccessful, Fons could confer with his consultants and prepare dismissal paperwork if they believed this to be appropriate (Vitelleschi to Provincial Pedro Fons, 20 August 1639, AHN J leg. 253 doc. 360).

Encouragement was not the only treatment protocol for melancholic Jesuits. After unspecified "medios" ("means") to assist Father Marcos

Mirón, "para que se alegre, y diuierta de su melancolia" ("so that he may become happy, and turn away from his melancholy"), failed to alter his mood, Vitelleschi authorized Mirón's departure if the priest did not improve (Vitelleschi to Continente, 24 January 1635, AHN J leg. 253 doc. 232). Without referring to this specific case, Elena Carrera observes that the common prescription to urge melancholics to "experience joy" was based on the Hippocratic idea that this "sadness" could be "counteracted with its opposite" ("Introduction" 15). It seems that Mirón's melancholy was quite severe. The General's letter delicately alludes to the possibility that Mirón was close to desperation; it references the prospect of "algun desacierto" ("some bad choice") and Mirón's concern that he "se desespere" ("he may lose hope"). The gravity of Mirón's condition likely led to the General's willingness to allow for Mirón's departure if he showed no improvement. Despite these serious concerns, Vitelleschi stated that he would write to Mirón to encourage him to persevere (AHN J leg. 253 doc. 232).[14]

As the cases of Bonari and Tapia suggest, overwork or unsuitable work assignments could cause Jesuits' melancholy. The next case makes this suggestion more explicit. In 1638, Vitelleschi wrote to Ribas that Father Pedro Munt was profoundly unhappy in the position of procurator in the *colegio* in Barcelona: "representa tal desconsuelo, y melancholia, que confieso me a causado compassion" ("he depicts such despair, and melancholy, that I confess [that] it moved me to compassion" (Vitelleschi to Ribas, 30 June 1638, AHN J leg. 253 doc. 330). The procurator oversees the economic and legal affairs of the house (Olivares 2, 1757). Vitelleschi recalled that five or six years previously, Munt had experienced a similar condition under similar circumstances. The General requested that the Provincial "endeavour to console" Munt (AHN J leg. 253 doc. 330). As we will see in the case of Father Antioco Corta, this correspondence employs the verb "console" when Provincials are to remedy individuals' ills. But in contrast to other instances, here the General does not include a specific strategy. Given the importance of Munt's position, it seems unlikely that Munt could be relieved of it, at least not without a period of transition.

This is not to say that melancholic Jesuits never were dismissed. Subsequent references to Tapia and Mirón related their departures from the community (Vitelleschi to Ribas, 30 August 1637, AHN J leg. 253 doc. 307 and 16 October 1637, AHN J leg. 253 doc. 252). Rather, early career Jesuits with other health complaints were let go in shorter order without the same level of encouragement. (According to J.A. de Laburu, Pedro de Ribadeneira stated the Ignatius urged Jesuits to pay special attention to the health of those wanting to enter the community, particularly the young [79].) Brother Vicente Mut was to be dismissed "si VR no experimenta en el conocida mejoria de sus achaques espirituales" ("if Your Reverence does not experience a recognizable improvement in him of his spiritual aches and pains"; Vitelleschi to Continente, 25 March 1634, AHN J leg. 253 doc. 203). Mut's religious crisis was described in physical terms, and his dismissal for health reasons was not unique. When Brother Joseph Valls worried that his unspecified health condition would make him a burden to the community, he did not receive advice to persevere from Rome. Instead, Continente was told to speak with Valls and send Rome an assessment (Vitelleschi to Continente, 24 April 1633, AHN J leg. 253 doc. 177). A few months later, Vitelleschi wrote that "si el se rinde a sus achaques, y no a de ser de prouecho, instando en que le despidan" ("if he [Valls] gives in to his aches and pains, and he is not to be of use, insisting that he be dismissed"), this would be a good decision (Vitelleschi to Continente, 20 December 1633, AHN J leg. 253 doc 196).

Melancholics only were dismissed with similar swiftness when there were clear signs that melancholy was an initial symptom of a more serious illness. Drawing on classical sources, particularly Galen, early modern medicine began to classify melancholy so severe that it caused notable mental disturbances as a disease.[15] Andrés Velásquez and Tomás Murillo y Velarde prominently theorized about the disease they termed *melancholia morbus* (melancholy the illness or melancholia) in sixteenth- and seventeenth-century Spain; Velásquez 49v; Murillo y Velarde 83r and 88r–v). The two physicians concurred about the physiological origins of *melancholia morbus*.[16] Following Galen's thinking, both Velásquez and Murillo y Velarde posited similar possible origins for *atrabilis*, the "adjust melancholy, a pernicious form of putrefied blood or burnt bile" that caused the disease melancholia. The melancholic humours or the dregs of blood could putrefy and create "corrosive" *atrabilis* or, alternatively, retained bile could overheat and burn (Velásquez 48v–49v 52r; Murillo y Velarde 81r and 85v).[17]

In the Society, since the *Norms* to the *Constitutions* exempted those impacted by serious mental health crises from dismissal against their will (*CN* 34), in the seventeenth-century Province of Aragon, when individuals in the initial stages of their training showed signs of significant psychological issues combined with problematic behaviour, they were let go before their mental state made dismissal impossible. The melancholic Father Jerónimo Torres, who had behaved poorly enough that he was being punished, was dismissed promptly before his melancholy caused him to lose possession of his mental faculties (Vitelleschi to Continente, 16 April 1634, AHN J leg. 253 doc. 239). This approach was consistent with the order's attitude towards other misbehaving early career Jesuits; they were dismissed quickly to avoid providing others with negative role models.

As Laburu details, Ignatius required superiors to look after the health of their men and insisted that Jesuits assiduously follow their physicians' recommendations (76–7 and 117–18). And this advice is formalized in the *Constitutions*. Therefore, the Society's approach to treating melancholy reflected the medical assessment of this condition as a complex malady with several possible physiological causes, including *atrabilis* and excess bile.[18] Medical theory urged for early intervention for melancholy so that any built-up black bile would not "putrefy" and cause more serious mental problems (Carrera, "Understanding" 124). According to Elena del Río Parra, no overarching protocol existed for the treatment of melancholy; rather, practitioners tailored treatments to the specific delusions of each patient, thus continuing the treatment paradigm from the Middle Ages (113–14). Medical treatises suggested eliminating the built-up bile or melancholic humour through treatments, including purgation or bloodletting, and diet to balance the humours (Carrera, "Understanding" 133). In *Aprobación de ingenios* (1672), Murillo y Velarde prescribed bloodletting, purgatives, and dietary remedies (105r–108r and 136r–137r. As Carolyn Nadeau details, even popular dietary manuals assigned humoral qualities to food (143–6). Thus, the idea that particular foodstuffs could treat physical and mental illnesses brought about by humoral imbalances was commonplace.[19] Considering the repeated discussions about reimbursement rates for food costs for ill Jesuits residing away from their assigned residences (as in Vitelleschi to Ribas, 28 May 1638, AHN J leg. 253 doc. 327) and General Congregation 7's decree 18 (Padberg 254–5) to regulate this process, it seems logical to assume that most unwell Jesuits followed a special diet based on medical advice.

One prescription for melancholy would not have been officially available for celibates. According to classical medical authorities, including Galen and Hippocrates, regular – but not excessive – sexual intercourse was essential to good health and could prevent melancholy (Cadden 273–4). The retention of seed, produced by both males and females, unbalanced the humours and negatively impacted one's health (274). In Galen's assessment, men's humours were "hotter and drier" than their female counterparts (177). Therefore, the accumulated heat of retained male semen could pose greater risks to men's health (Cadden 274). Since the Jesuits' system for consulting physicians required that superiors, rather than patients, interact with physicians about treatments ([304]), it seems unlikely that Jesuits would receive prescriptions for masturbation. According to Joan Cadden's research, this cure for seminal retention appears in Galen, Avicenna, and others (275). But some evidence suggests that the chaste may have turned to herbal remedies to dry up excess semen and therefore maintain their humoral equilibrium. In Gregorio López's 1613 *Tesoro de medicina* in the entry titled "castidad" ("chastity"), following a list of plant products that stop blood flow, López suggests: "La raiz del lirio cardeno, bebida con vinagre, consume el semen" ("The root of the iris, drunk with vinegar, consumes semen"; Losa 353).[20]

Admittedly, the earliest Jesuits did not appear to be highly receptive to using herbal remedies to help them resist sexual temptation. As historian of the Society of Jesus Antonio Astrain relates, an often-repeated tale concerning Jesuits Peter Favre and Antonio de Araoz recounts that courtiers in Valladolid, impressed with the Jesuits' virtue, clamoured to learn what "yerba" ("medicinal plant") they took to curb their sexual impulses. Araoz replied that only "the fear of God" fortified his continence (vol. 1, 250–1). As Astrain admits, this anecdote may be apocryphal (1, 251n1), but its retelling nonetheless speaks to the level of belief in such products. By the seventeenth-century, the Society may have felt differently about the use of such plants as medicinal remedies to balance the humours.

Beyond a humoral trait or a disease, melancholy also was a fashionable affliction and a cultivated affectation. Following in the footsteps of Raymond Klibansky, Erwin Panofsky, and Fritz Saxl, Teresa Scott Soufas asserts that many distinguished men either fancied themselves melancholics or were perceived as such (3). Such feigned or exaggerated symptoms were not met with sympathy in the Jesuit community. When Brother Juan Geriz sought to leave the order due to the poverty of his family and because his assigned work aggravated his "melancholies," General Oliva judged Geriz's reasons to be insufficient and asked for the Provincial's assessment (General Giovanni Paolo Oliva to Provincial Domingo Langa, 30 July 1665, AHN J leg. 255 doc. 125).

Place, Disease, and Productivity

Sometimes, in order for Jesuits to be productive, changes of venue and other accommodations were required. According to Hippocrates's treatise "Airs, Waters, Places," the climate of a particular locale, like its prevailing winds and water sources, could negatively affect health in a myriad of ways (for example, 149–52). Therefore, if a particular climate caused health problems, changing locales could bring about improvements.

At the individual level, Jesuits frequently allowed unwell men to move, motivated in part by compassion and in greater part to maximize their performance. In 1633, Brother Casanova "tiene necessidad de que le muden a puesto mas seco donde puede repararse, y cobrar salud" ("is in need of being moved to a drier place where he can restore himself, and recover health"). In asking Continente to do what he can for this man, the General emphasizes the contributions Casanova could make if he were healthy: "porque es Hermano que puede acudir con satisfaccion a los officios de su vocacion si la tiene" ("because he is a Brother who can attend with satisfaction to the tasks of his vocation if he has it [his health]"; Vitelleschi to Continente, 24 April 1633, AHN J leg. 253 doc. 178). In a similar fashion, Father Miguel Palacios informed the General that "dessea tener empleo conforme sus fuerças y le parece que haria mas en Çaragoça donde estaria mejor con los ayres naturales" ("he desires to have a job in accordance with his strength and it seems to him that he would do more in Zaragoza where he would be better with his natural airs"). Agreeing with Father Palacios' self-assessment, Vitelleschi left the matter to his Provincial's "great charity" (Vitelleschi to Provincial Juan Sanz, 8 December 1617, AHN J leg. 253 doc. 44). Like Palacios, many Jesuits hoped that they would recover by returning to their home regions. As Martin observes in studying Jesuits in France, "native air was practically the panacea for every ailment" (*Jesuit* 163).

When dealing with epidemic disease, namely, the pest, now commonly known as the plague, the order employed a similar strategy. Since air could be a vector for the spread of this malady in the medical thinking of the era, medical authorities like Girolamo Fracastoro advised departure from stricken areas (Martin, *Plague* 125).[21] According to Martin's research, in the early years of the community, many Jesuits ministered to those sickened by the plague, but by the mid-1550s, the order's policy shifted to leave only a small number in affected zones (*Plague* 119–21). For example, when pest threatened Barcelona and Zaragoza respectively in 1651 and 1652, Nickel requested that only those needed to tend to the spiritual needs of the ill should stay (Nickel to Fons, 27 July 1651, AHN J leg. 254 doc. 27 and to Provincial Francisco Franco, 26 September 1652, AHN J leg. 254 doc. 67).[22] Not only did Jesuits evacuate those in their care, like students and novices, during outbreaks, but also Juan Alfonso de Polanco suggested that those deemed "more important for the common good" should depart (Martin, *Plague* 122–3). As a result, the rector frequently left with the novices (123).

The discussion surrounding the Jesuits' evacuation of their *colegio* in Perpignan (then Perpinyà and still part of Catalonia) in 1632 offers insight into how evacuating those with leadership roles along with students and novices helped carry out the order's mission. During their time away from the school, Vitelleschi requested that Continente not allow the group to be divided up among the second homes of nobles, but instead that the men reside "en algun puesto apropiado a donde viuan con el orden, y obseruancia que se pudiere" ("in some appropriate place where they may live with the order and observance that they can"; Vitelleschi to Continente, 27 February 1632, AHN J leg. 253 doc. 159). The presence of at least some of the superiors in the community would be necessary to maintain standards and practices.

This is not to say that Jesuits abandoned the infected. General Gottifredi expressed his gratitude for the "charity" with which Jesuit priests administered the sacraments to the infected in Huesca (General Alesandro Gottifredi to Piquer, 24 February 1652, AHN J leg. 254 doc. 43). In the same year, Gottifredi was impressed by the "edification and good zeal" with which Father Pedro Lassus, the rector of the *colegio* at Vic, "consoled" plague victims in that locale. At the same time, Gottifredi was pleased that the rector had departed from Vic "in time," presumably before the town was quarantined. Due to his timely departure, Lassus was able to continue his ministry by preaching Lenten sermons in Perpignan (Gottifredi to Fons, 19 February 1652, AHN J leg. 254 doc. 42). Even as the pest quarantined certain communities, the order wanted to have personnel available to minister in other areas, especially during the penitential season of Lent.

Criteria for determining who should stay in place during outbreaks varied among Jesuit communities. Martin's research found reference to the use of individuals' humoral temperaments, "complexio" ("complexion") in the triennial catalogues, to determine which Jesuits would be more "vulnerable" during epidemics, but the documents did not detail how this information was used to assess susceptibility (*Plague* 121, 123–4). In the Province of Aragon, Jesuits apparently could volunteer. During the outbreak of pest in Vic, Father Carlos Estales, who had evacuated because of the epidemic, offered to return to minister to the ill (AHN J leg. 254 doc. 42).

Accommodations, Luxuries, and Jesuit Masculinity

Despite the close connection between health and work in the Jesuit community, those whose infirmities hindered their ability to keep up with their obligations were treated with empathy. When his fellow Jesuits were facing illness, Ignatius urged them to treat infirmity as a divine "gift," to use their malady as an opportunity for growth and to model "edifying" behaviours for others (ll. 89 and 272). In the post-Ignatian community, the funerary sermon that Father Manuel de Nájera gave for fellow Jesuit Father Juan Eusebio Nieremberg recounted the manner in which Nieremberg used his final illness to share Christ's suffering (16r).

The treatment of the elderly and ill people also followed Ignatius's approach. The sick were encouraged to follow medical advice for their conditions, regardless of whether doing so would take them away from their assigned tasks. When Father Juan de San Juan's doctors prescribed yearly trips to mineral baths to relieve his aches and pains, Vitelleschi asked Provincial Pedro Gil to allow San Juan to do so (Vitelleschi to Provincial Pedro Gil, 23 March 1620, AHN J leg. 253 doc. 96). In 1658, when Nickel learned that physicians warned Provincial Piquer that travel to Aragon in wintertime could endanger Piquer's life, Nickel readily conceded that Piquer should follow this medical advice and postpone his trip (Nickel to Piquer, 16 July 1658, AHN J leg. 254 doc. 202).

Such concessions were available only to those with genuine health concerns.

Throughout this correspondence, Jesuit authorities deemed fashionable protective commodities, like gloves and eyewear to shield travellers' skin and eyes, unseemly for members. Other domestic luxuries, like the two mattresses used by Jesuits in Valencia without medical need to do so, were not permissible (Vitelleschi to Ribas, 31 January 1636, AHN J leg. 253 doc. 258). However, Jesuits' objections to these superfluous possessions went beyond concerns about decorum and into gendered expectations. In advising future rulers and ministers in his 1657 emblem book, Spanish Jesuit Andrés Mendo maintained that "too many" "delicias" ("delicacies"), including food, expensive clothing, and "los adornos domesticos superfluos" ("superfluous domestic adornments"), "afeminan los animos, enflaquecen los brios, y abaten los pensamientos" ("feminize the spirits, weaken the energies, and dishearten the thoughts"; 138 and 37). In this spirit, Roman Jesuit authorities attempted to curtail members' indulgence in several alimentary crazes, including drinking beverages cooled with snow, and chocolate.

Within the order, the medicinal use of chocolate was supposed to be tightly controlled; correspondence from Rome emphasized that chocolate could only be consumed by Jesuits with a special licence from the General (Oliva to Langa, 30 January 1660, AHN J leg. 255 doc. 135). Licensed Jesuits were to take cacao products secretly (AHN J leg. 255 doc. 135), presumably to avoid tempting others to ask for permission. Yet, by 1663, Oliva observed that chocolate drinking was motivating Jesuits' desire to say Mass early. Oliva demanded that Langa remedy this "disorder;" Oliva only had issued a few licences for chocolate consumption in the province (Oliva to Langa, 18 November 1663, AHN J leg. 255 doc. 76).

If Oliva found Jesuits' requests to use chocolate to treat a variety of medical conditions worthy of consideration, the General then requested that Piquer, who knew the men's "edad, trabajos y meritos" ("age, works, and merits"), examine their cases with his consultants and advise the General (Oliva to Piquer, 22 August 1666, AHN J leg 255 doc.148). When young Father Mathias Ortiz requested permission to drink chocolate because he found it "effective" in easing "his aches and pains," the General decided that Ortiz should find another remedy and offer up the lack of chocolate as a sacrifice. Oliva explained that he wished to limit the use of chocolate among the young so that the practice did not become an "abuse" (Oliva to Piquer, 26 August 1667, AHN J leg. 255 doc. 184). While Oliva also wished to curb the use of tobacco among Jesuits, he was far more vehement about restricting the consumption of chocolate (see AHN J leg. 255 doc. 135). This firm desire to restrict cacao consumption likely related to the long-standing belief that this product incited sexual desire.[23] Since the ensuing build-up of semen could damage men's health, chocolate was not merely a "feminizing" luxury, but also a potential threat to wellness.

In contrast, when an older Jesuit, like former Provincial Ginés Vidal, asks to take chocolate, the General decides without the need to consult the Province that Vidal "merece" ("deserves") a licence for it. But even in this situation, Oliva warned about medicinal chocolate's pernicious side effects. The General noted that a Cardinal and deceased General Piccolomini both stopped taking chocolate on the advice of their physicians because it caused urinary difficulties (AHN J leg 255 doc. 148).

Permission to consume chocolate was not the only privilege earned with age. Although Martin notes that the *Constitutions* do not regulate the treatment of elderly members (*Jesuit* 177), Jesuits nonetheless made allowances for health challenges due to advancing age by reallocating positions or changing established procedures. In 1635, Vitelleschi suggested that Continente allow older men who grew uncomfortable when seated during recreation to walk around in order to warm themselves or to take their recreation in a different location (AHN J leg. 253 doc. 232). If elderly Jesuits found that the harsh winters in the Pyrenees aggravated their infirmities, they were permitted to move to houses in more temperate climes, as were Brother Juan Samarán and Father Valentín Matheo (Vitelleschi to Fons, 22 January 1639, AHN J leg. 253 doc. 338 and AHN J leg. 253 doc. 307).

Moreover, duties were modified due to the elderly's health concerns, as in the case of infirmarian Brother Domingo Matheo (Vitelleschi to Ribas, 21 January 1636, AHN J leg. 253 doc. 259). When Father Antioco Corta, afflicted by "his age and aches and pains," needed assistance to make his bed and clean his room, the General asked the Provincial to "console" Corta, perhaps by allowing him to live in the *colegio*, where presumably some household assistance already was available to boarding students. Vitelleschi recognized the difficulty of this request, but asked that Ribas arrange whatever seemed reasonable (Vitelleschi to Ribas, 12 March 1638, AHN J leg. 253 doc. 322).

Jesuits and Women

Although another admission criterion of the early Society, namely, the acceptance of *conversos* (those with Jewish or Islamic lineages) was later reversed, this was not the case with the exclusion of women. But one subsequent exception was made, the largely secret admission of Juana de Austria, Philip II's sister, in 1554.[24] Whereas the princess became a full-fledged Jesuit, a number of *beatas* attached themselves to the community, with what Carlos A. Page describes not as "vows to the Society of Jesus, but rather [...] simple and private vows," which the women professed to themselves (8). However, in at least one instance, the relationship between the Jesuit order and María Antonia de San José, a Jesuit "beata profesa" ("professed *beata*") in what today is Argentina, appears more ambiguous. As Alicia Fraschina observes, no records survive regarding to whom San José professed (260). Part of the ambiguity regarding this particular *beata*'s status stems from the timing of her relationship with the order. Following the expulsion of the Society from Spain's territories beginning in 1767 and the order's subsequent papal suppression in 1773, no one was available to clarify San José's status. But in the order's absence, San José continued some Jesuit practices. According to Fraschina's research, San José received permission to "organize" the *Spiritual Exercises* (215).

Despite the significant role that theories based on male superiority played in the Society of Jesus, the order did not isolate itself from women's religious needs. Elizabeth Rhodes posits that Teresa de Ávila's writings about her positive experience with Jesuits encouraged other women to turn to Jesuit priests for spiritual guidance (Rhodes 41). Unfortunately, the subsequent need to preserve the Society's standing circumscribed the relationships between Jesuits and women seeking direction from them (42–3). Nonetheless, after limiting young priests' contact with female confessants, Jesuits continued to look after the souls of women, both lay and of the cloth, in the seventeenth-century Province of Aragon and beyond it. At least in part, they were able to carry out this and other work because they cared for their own health.

To this end, the order's foundational documents not only enquired about the health of potential applicants but also mandated that the Society actively protect the wellness of members, including by constructing buildings in salubrious locations. In addition to the classical medical authorities whose work underpins the *Constitutions'* approach to protecting Jesuits' wellness, the Society's thinking about health evolved along with medical thought. After physicians such as Girolamo Fracastoro advised the healthy to evacuate areas impacted by epidemics, Jesuit policy evolved and thereafter most of the order's personnel left zones affected by outbreaks of disease. Moreover, the Society's approach to melancholics was influenced by Juan Huarte de San Juan's theories linking melancholy to superior intelligence in men. At the same time, as medical theory pathologized serious melancholy, treatment was sought for gravely melancholic Jesuits. Admittedly, some potential treatments for melancholy would have been unavailable to celibates. Beyond melancholy, the order limited treatments that did not infringe on members' vows when remedies were perceived as luxuries or fads. A number of these, including the use of multiple mattresses, chocolate, and tobacco, were not only deemed inappropriate, but also considered potentially emasculating. Ultimately, this zealous interest in safeguarding the health of members was motivated by the desire to have personnel available to carry out the order's mission.[25]

NOTES

1 The three *legajos* in the Archivo Histórico Nacional cited here contain 1,299 letters, written between 1616 and 1681. Since this correspondence briefly mentions large numbers of individuals, this essay necessarily duplicates its source texts and therefore references a number of Jesuits.The Province of Aragon encompasses the peninsular territories of the formerly independent crowns of Aragon, Catalonia, and Valencia, including the Balearic Islands.

2 Citations from the *Constitutions* reference bracketed paragraph numbers.

3 See Simmonds 122 for an overview of this episode and Ignatius, *Fontes* 696–713 for documents concerning Roser's relationship with the Jesuits.

4 All unattributed translations are mine. See Batllori 174–5 for transcriptions of these assessments for the writer Baltasar Gracián.

5 See Rhodes 35 for an analysis of this martial imagery in terms of "traditional masculinity."

6 I deliberately avoid the label "decline" in acknowledgment of Kamen's critique of "the myth of [Spain's] perpetual decline" (172–205).

7 Armon questions whether Spanish masculinity underwent a "crisis" during the early modern period, as scholars such as Donnell have argued (Armon 10–14). Regardless of how one characterizes this cultural moment, it cannot be denied that Spanish society reflected deeply on masculinity.

8 Citations from documents and rare books maintain their original orthography.
9 Those of other temperaments generally were relegated to less distinguished tasks (Casalini 203).
10 Although a number of Neo-Aristotelian theorists developed this point, I focus on Huarte because of his influence on the Society of Jesus. See García García et al. "El *Examen*" for an analysis of Huarte's impact on Antonio Possevino's work and Casalini (190–1) for Jesuits who dialogued with Huarte's work.
11 The *Norms* are referenced by paragraph number.
12 While I standardize the spelling of names of individuals and places in my text, I do not alter first names when I have no evidence about whether a particular individual would have used a Spanish or Catalan form.
13 The final digit of the date is difficult to read; it may be an 8.
14 Correspondents' names and dates are included in the first reference.
15 See Gowland 86–93 for an overview of this process in Europe.
16 Other terms also were used for this infirmity. Another physician, Alonso de Freylas, termed it "melancholia negra" ("black melancholy"; Bartra, *Cultura* 60).
17 My text and the list of works cited modernize the spelling of authors' names, but orthographical variants beyond accent marks are noted in brackets in the works cited. Otherwise, I leave all other elements of rare imprints in their original forms to facilitate electronic searches.
18 As a number of scholars, including Orobitg (25–7), Soufas (46–7), and Bartra (*Cultura*, 49–63) indicate, medieval and early modern sources considered possible demonic origins for melancholy. Both Velásquez and Murillo y Velarde's treatises examine this question in detail. While this Jesuit correspondence references the melancholy of a number of Jesuits as well as a very small number of cases of possible demonic influence on members, I have not found any that connect melancholy with demonic sources. As Bartra explains, Catholic exorcists developed protocols to differentiate melancholy from diabolical possession ("Arabs," 65), which Jesuits might well have incorporated into their thinking.
19 See Carrera, "Understanding" 113–21 for an overview of the role of diet in treating mental illness.
20 I thank Elizabeth Rhodes for this reference. At least one member of the clergy was interested in López's advice: the handwritten inscription in the Biblioteca Nacional de España's Raro U 1339 indicates that it belonged to a man of the cloth.

In 1613, Francisco Losa published a biography of López accompanied by López's writings. Losa's work was republished in Spain on several occasions; and López came to be so respected that several Spanish monarchs supported his case for sainthood (Rodríguez-Sala et al. 404 and 406).

21 See Tuchman 101–2 for the medical theory as to how the air spread this malady.

22 The precise date in July is difficult to read. This approach was not without controversy. During a 1576–7 outbreak in Italy, the archbishop of Milan Carlo Borromeo took issue with this Jesuit practice (Martin, *Plague?* 175).

23 As Norton notes, in addition to Bernal Díaz del Castillo's reference to Moctezuma's use of chocolate to enhance his sexual performance, this cacao product also "was used in ritual contexts associated with sexuality and domestic unions" in Mesoamerica (15 and 30). Norton also demonstrates that both European medical authorities, like Francisco Hernández, and popular culture as evidenced by tile paintings, believed that the consumption of chocolate increased sexual desire (126 and 179).

24 See Soto Artuñedo for other women who wanted to affiliate themselves with the Society of Jesus and the vows Juana de Austria took and O'Malley for the problems that ensued following Juana's admission (Soto Artuñedo 581–6; O'Malley 75–6 and 318).

25 This research was supported by the University of Kansas General Research Fund allocations 2166082 and 2301038. I thank the editors and readers for their comments in refining this essay.

WORKS CITED

Archivo Histórico Nacional. Madrid. Jesuitas. Legajos 253, 254 (positive microfilm 1359) and 255 (positive microfilm 1360).

Armon, Shifra. *Masculine Virtue in Early Modern Spain*. Ashgate, 2015.

Astrain, Antonio. *Historia de la Compañía de Jesús en la asistencia de España*, vol. 1, Administración de Razón y Fe, 1912.

Bartra, Roger. "Arabs, Jews, and the Enigma of Spanish Imperial Melancholy." Translated by Amanda Harris Fonseca, *Discourse*, vol. 22, no. 3, Fall 2000, pp. 64–72.

– *Cultura y melancolía. Las enfermedades del alma en la España del Siglo de Oro*. Anagrama, 2001.

Batllori, Miguel. *Gracián y el barroco*. Edizioni di Storia e Letteratura, 1958.

Cadden, Joan. *Meanings of Sex Difference in the Middle Ages: Medicine, Science and Culture*. Cambridge UP, 1993.

Carrera, Elena. "Introduction. Madness and Melancholy in Sixteenth- and Seventeenth-Century Spain: New Evidence, New Approaches." *Bulletin of Spanish Studies*, vol. 87, no. 8, December 2010, pp. 1–15.

– "Understanding Mental Disturbance in Sixteenth- and Seventeenth-Century Spain: Medical Approaches." *Bulletin of Spanish Studies*, vol. 87, no. 8, December 2010, pp. 105–36.

Casalini, Cristiano. "Discerning Skills: Psychological Insight at the Core of Jesuit Identity." *Exploring Jesuit Distinctiveness: Interdisciplinary Perspectives on Ways of Proceeding within the Society of Jesus*. Edited by Robert Aleksander Maryks, Brill, 2016, pp. 189–211.

Donnell, Sidney. *Feminizing the Enemy: Imperial Spain, Transvestite Drama, and the Crisis of Masculinity*. Bucknell UP, 2003.

Fraschina, Alicia. *Mujeres consagradas en el Buenos Aires colonial*. Eudeba, 2010.

Galen. *De semine. On Semen*. Edited and translated by Phillip de Lacy, Akademie Verlag, 1992.

García García, Emilio, and Aurora Miguel Alonso. "El conocimiento psicológico de la Compañía de Jesús y el *Examen de ingenios* de Huarte de San Juan." *Revista de Historia de la Psicología*, vol. 26, nos. 2–3, 2005, pp. 45–53.

– "El *Examen de ingenios* de Huarte de San Juan en la Bibliotheca Selecta de Antonio Possevino." *Revista de Historia de la Psicología*, vol. 25, nos. 3–4, 2003, pp. 387–96.

Gowland, Angus. "The Problem of Early Modern Melancholy." *Past and Present* 191, May 2006, pp. 77–120.

Hippocrates. "Airs, Waters, Places." *Hippocratic Writings*, edited by G.E.R. Lloyd and translated by J. Chadwick et al., Penguin Classics, 1983, pp. 148–69.

Huarte de San Juan, Juan. *Examen de ingenios para las ciencias*. Edited by Guillermo Serés, Cátedra, 1989.

– *The Examination of Men's Wits*. Translated by Richard Carew, Scholars' Facsimiles and Reprints, 1959.

Ignatius of Loyola. *The Constitutions of the Society of Jesus and their Complementary Norms: A Complete English Translation of the Official Latin Texts*. The Institute of Jesuit Sources, 1996.

– *Fontes documentales de S. Ignatio de Loyola*. Edited by Candidus de Dalmases, Institutum Historicum Societatis Iesu, 1977. Monumenta Historica Societatis Iesu vol. 115.

Kamen, Henry. *Imagining Spain: Historical Myth and National Identity*. Yale UP, 2008.

Laburu, J.A. de. *La salud corporal y san Ignacio de Loyola*. Editorial Mosca Hermanos, 1938.

Lehfeldt, Elizabeth A. "Ideal Men: Masculinity and Decline in Seventeenth-Century Spain." *Renaissance Quarterly*, vol. 61, no. 2, Summer 2008, pp. 463–94.

Losa, Francisco. *Vida del siervo de Dios Gregorio Lopez, escrita por el Padre Francisco Losa, cura de almas, que fue de la Iglesia Mayor de Mexico, y su compañero en la soledad. A que se añaden los escritos de Apocalypsi, y Tesoro de Medicina, del mismo siervo de Dios Gregorio Lopez*. Madrid, Imprenta de Juan de Ariztia, 1727.

Martin, A. Lynn. *The Jesuit Mind: The Mentality of an Elite in Early Modern France*. Cornell UP, 1988.

– *Plague? Jesuit Accounts of Epidemic Disease in the Sixteenth Century*. Sixteenth Century Journal Publishers, 1996.
Meissner, W.W. *Ignatius of Loyola: The Psychology of a Saint*. Yale UP, 1992.
Mendo, Andrés. *Principe perfecto y ministros aivstados, docvmentos politicos, y morales*. Leon de Francia, A costa de Horacio Boissat y George Remevs, 1662.
Murillo y Velarde, Tomás [Thomas] de. *Aprobacion de ingenios, y cvracion de hipochondricos, con observaciones, y remedios mvy particvlares*. Zaragoça, Diego de Ormer, 1672.
Nadeau, Carolyn A. *Food Matters: Alonso Quijano's Diet and the Discourse of Food in Early Modern Spain*. U of Toronto P, 2016.
Nájera, Manuel de [Manvel de Naxera]. *Sermon qve predico el padre Manvel de Naxera predicador de sv Magestad en las piadosas exeqvias, qve consagrò a la memoria del P. Ivan Evsebio Nieremberg*. Madrid, Andres Garcia de la Iglesia, 1658.
Norton, Marcy. *Sacred Gifts, Profane Pleasures: A History of Tobacco and Chocolate in the Atlantic World*. Cornell UP, 2008.
Olivares, E. "Gobierno local." "Procurador o ecónomo." *Diccionario histórico de la Compañía de Jesús*. Edited by Charles E. O'Neill and Joaquín María Domínguez, Institutum Historicum, S.I., Universidad Pontificia Comillas, 2001, vol. 2, p. 1757.
O'Malley, John W. *The First Jesuits*. Harvard UP, 1993.
Orobitg, Christine. "Melancolía e inspiración en la España del Siglo de Oro." *Bulletin of Spanish Studies*, vol. 87, no. 8, December 2010, pp. 17–31.
Padberg, John W., et al. *For Matters of Greater Moment: The First Thirty Jesuit General Congregations*. The Institute of Jesuit Sources, 1994.
Page, Carlos A. "De beatas y beaterios jesuitas de la provincia del Paraguay, siglos XVII–XVIII." *Región y sociedad* vol. 30, no. 73, 2018, pp. 1–22.
Rhodes, Elizabeth. "Join the Jesuits, See the World: Early Modern Women in Spain and the Society of Jesus." *The Jesuits II: Cultures, Sciences and the Arts 1540–1773*, edited by John W. O'Malley et al., U of Toronto P, 2006, pp. 33–49.
Río Parra, Elena del. *Materia médica. Rareza, singularidad y accidente en la España temprano-moderna*. North Carolina Studies in the Romance Languages and Literatures, UNC at Chapel Hill Department of Romance Studies, 2016.
Rodríguez-Sala, María Luisa, and Rosalba Tena-Villeda. "El venerable varón Gregorio López, repercusiones de su vida y obra a lo largo de cuatrocientos años, 1562–2000." *Gaceta médica de México*, vol. 139, no. 4, 2003, pp. 401–8.
Sánchez, Magdalena S. "Melancholy and Female Illness: Habsburg Women and Politics at the Court of Philip III." *Journal of Women's History*, vol. 8, no. 2, Summer 1996, pp. 81–102.
Simmonds, Gemma. "Women Jesuits?" *The Cambridge Companion to the Jesuits*, edited by Thomas Worcester, Cambridge UP, 2008, pp. 120–35.
Soto Artuñedo, Wenceslao. "Juana de Austria, ¿de la compañía de Jesús?" *V Reunión científica Asociación española de historia moderna*. Tomo I, *Felipe II y*

su tiempo, edited by José Luis Pereira Iglesias, Servicio de Publicaciones de la Universidad de Cádiz, Asociación Española de Historia Moderna, 1999, vol. I, pp. 579–88.

Soufas, Teresa Scott. *Melancholy and the Secular Mind in Spanish Golden Age Literature*. U of Missouri P, 1990.

Tuchman, Barbara W. *A Distant Mirror: The Calamitous Fourteenth Century*. Alfred A. Knopf, 1978.

Velásquez, Andrés. *Libro de la melancholia, en el qval se trata dela natvraleza desta enfermedad; assi llamada melancholia, y de sus causas y simptomas*. Sevilla, Hernando Diaz, 1585.

Chapter Nine

Chronicles of Pain: Carmelite Women and Galenism

BÁRBARA MUJICA

Illness was feared in early modern convents because contagious diseases could spread throughout the community, putting the entire house in danger. Although nearly all early modern medical writing was produced by men, including that dealing with women's health, women religious also wrote about disease and healing, sometimes offering detailed accounts of their own illnesses and those of their sisters. Teresa de Ávila, founder of the Discalced Carmelite order, and her disciples María de San José and Ana de Jesús all described their own suffering and that of others, either in *Vidas* [spiritual memoirs] or in letters or both. Often nuns who wrote about health provided advice about cures for ailments as diverse as melancholia and rheumatism.

Although Andreas Vesalius challenged Galen's anatomical theories in the 1530s, Galenic medicine remained the basis of diagnosis and treatment throughout the sixteenth and early seventeenth centuries.[1] Nuns shared a belief in Galenic principles with male medics, but their commentaries differ radically in focus from those of university-trained physicians and offer valuable insight into how these women experienced pain and disease. While traditional medical men tended to focus primarily on the body, especially the uterus, as the primary source of women's physical and psychological discomfort, these women demonstrate how faith enabled them to sublimate pain into spiritual experience. Rather than conventional medical treatises, they looked to the writings of "mystical medics," notably Bernardino de Laredo (1482–1540), who saw the body as a vehicle for spiritual enlightenment.

Conventional Galenism

In order to grasp how radically different the Carmelite approach to illness was from that of conventional medicine, it will be valuable to review some basic tenets of Galenism and their impact on women's health care. As the introduction to this book has already demonstrated, Galenic theory viewed physical and mental disease as the result of fluctuations in humours and their impact on overall constitutional make-up, including assessment of individual temperaments.

Melancholia, a common diagnosis in early modern Europe, was considered a serious ailment caused by a humoral imbalance and was associated with many physical conditions, including malfunctions of the organs. Physicians thought that the melancholia humour, or black bile, could be brought into balance through diet modification, medication, or phlebotomy. Teresa Soufas notes that for some doctors, melancholia was simply a natural phenomenon, a consequence of bile produced in the liver to facilitate digestion. When it occurred in excess, a person began to experience inexplicable sadness, negative thoughts, and fear (6). For others, melancholia was an abnormal state caused by a strong emotional or physical reaction.[2] Thus, physical health and spiritual occurrences often merge into the experiential in the writings of the devout.

While melancholia could affect either men or women, in men it was usually associated with creativity and genius, while in women it was associated with fragility, disequilibrium, loss of control, nervousness, and excessive emotionalism. Melancholic women were routinely diagnosed with hysteria, also known as "woman's disease" (*hysterika* means "uterus" in Greek), a manifestation of which was inarticulateness – the kind of hesitance we see in some female mystic writers. While melancholy in men was viewed as a sign of divine inspiration that generated great works of art or philosophy, the "babbling" of melancholic women was either ignored or else attributed to demonic intervention (Schiesari 15).

For conventional Galenist medics, the seat of nearly all female disorders was the uterus, and menstruation was key to women's physiology (Green 25).[3] The 1569 treatise *Dignotio et Cvra Affectvvm Melancholicorvm* (*Sobre la melancolía*), by the physician/philosopher/cartographer Alonso de Santa Cruz, exemplifies this approach to medicine. Santa Cruz offers seventeen case studies, including several of women.[4] One involves a young woman suffering from *furor uterino* – normally translated "nymphomania," but here more like manic depression – who was not menstruating regularly. Graceful and charming although a bit hirsute, she was old enough to *recibir varón* (receive a man). Her symptoms included bouts of sadness, exhaustion, irrational fear, and violent behaviour. The best remedy, explains Santa Cruz, is cohabitation with a man, but in the meantime, cures such as bleeding, a diet of light, moist foods, and cold-water sprays can help. The Galenic tradition taught that women generated female semen (unused or putrefying menses) that blended with male semen during intercourse. Santa Cruz describes how many women, young and old, virgins and widows, suffer from retention of semen, causing them terrible hallucinations or bouts of sadness. In one example, a nun in her sixties suffered from pain in her eyes. Eventually, her brain dried up, leading to insomnia, unhealthy thoughts, fear, and sadness. Santa Cruz cured her with warm baths and donkey's milk, along with a weekly dose of an an Arabic compound known as hamech.[5]

Santa Cruz believed that the lack of menstrual flow drove women mad, and without medical care, many of his female patients would have committed suicide (109). When women remain virgins past their sexual prime, they may suffer from irregular menstrual flow, believed Santa Cruz. For nubile women, the most effective means of avoiding physical and psychological health problems was marriage. Since, according to Santa Cruz, sexual activity was essential to cleanse the uterus, widows and nuns were particularly vulnerable to illness – a notion shared by most physicians. Sharon Strocchia points out that medical experts thought that the celibate life of nuns exacerbated melancholia by obviating the "health-giving purgative effects of sexual intercourse" ("Melancholic Nun" 92). The mental health of women, particularly nuns, became a vital subject in the sixteenth century because of the growing fear of demonic possession. Priests called on doctors to diagnose physical symptoms such as pain, sweating, quaking, and seizures to determine whether these were caused by diabolical or natural causes. If medical treatments proved ineffective, clerics assumed that the ailment was probably due to possession or witchcraft (Sluhovsky 194–6).

Oliva Sabuco de Nantes Barrera (1562–1629?), author of the *New Philosophy of Human Nature*, offers an alternative to the prevailing male perspective. Sabuco is credited with being the first to posit that the brain controls the body. She elucidated the material relationship between mental and physical health and the effects of absorption of nutrients through digestion on both the body and the mind.[6] Sabuco does not automatically classify women as hysterical. Although she concedes that women are sensitive and therefore suffer from "angry grief" (depression) more than men, she believes that this is because they are overwhelmed by the demands of motherhood (*New Philosophy* 51). She prescribes the same treatment for melancholic men and women: avoidance of solitude and of certain "melancholic foods" such as shad, horse mackerel, codfish, animal brains, and milk products (*New Philosophy* 80).

Aside from Sabuco's, female voices are mostly absent from early modern medical literature, although some Spanish women did work as physicians, usually without official authorization (Clouse 24).[7] Women played an important role in the fields of gynaecology and obstetrics, although by the mid-sixteenth century, even these areas became increasingly dominated by men. As training became more professionalized, male midwives gradually replaced women, particularly in urban areas. In 1566 Hans Kaspar Wolf and Conrad Gesner published in Basel the *Gynaeciorum libri*, a Pan-European compendium of texts on women's medical issues. It went through several editions and played an important role in the eventual triumph of the male midwife and the masculinization of gynaecology and obstetrics,[8] although, as Lianne McTavish notes, women continued to dominate these fields in rural areas of France and elsewhere.

One vehicle for proliferating Galenism was the medical manual in the vernacular. From the fourteenth through the sixteenth centuries, basic medical information became increasingly available in Spain to laypeople, including women, as respected physicians produced treatises in Castilian as a means of enhancing their reputations among the populace. They actively publicized these writings, emphasizing how useful, accessible, and effective they were (Solomon 13). Works such as the *Sevilla medicina*, by the Spanish-Jewish physician Juan de Avignon (1381–1418), stressed the importance of diet and provided recipes for cures using household ingredients.

Bernardino de Laredo's Mystical Medicine

While conventional medieval and early modern Galenic medicine focused on symptoms and therefore on the body as the source of pain, "mystical medics" (often reformed Franciscans) took a broader view of human physiology. The best known of these is the *converso* physician Bernardino de Laredo, whose *Subida del Monte Sión* (*Ascent of Mount Sion*) Teresa de Ávila not only read but also underlined (Kavanaugh 35). Laredo began practising medicine around 1507 and was so skilful that he was called upon to treat King John III of Portugal. He became a reformed Franciscan lay friar and apothecary at a small convent near Seville.

For Laredo, the spiritual could be reached only through the corporeal, thus physical pain served to help the individual identify with the Passion.[9] Through sophisticated medical reasoning, he shows that the human body stems from earth and water moulded by God, which makes it the starting point for self-knowledge and spiritual meditation. Jessica Boon contends that "medieval theories of cognition made the divorce of the body from the soul impossible for a Galenic doctor" (7). For Laredo, the *entrañas* (entrails) are the "seat of God in the soul" (Boon 6). Laredo built on optical epistemologies to show that a physical devotional object seen with the external senses and a vision seen with the mind's eye both affect the body with equal force. Thus, argues Boon, "physicality, spirituality, and optically based cognition cannot be fully separated in any discussion of Franciscan mysticism" (143). Rather than endeavouring simply to cure pain, as conventional Galenists did, Laredo focused on the cognitive process that linked vision, memory, and pain, thereby transforming pain into spiritual experience.

Laredo constructs his system on the "optics of intromission," which posits a physical relationship between the seer and the thing seen. According to this theory, vision results from something representative of the object physically entering the eye, allowing the viewed object to transform the eye of the beholder into the viewed object (148). "In intromission, a viewed object is momentarily imprinted on the devotee's optic nerve" (Boon 156). By contemplating physical or mental images of Christ's pain, the devotee actually *melds into* or *becomes* the suffering Christ. Laypeople and nuns were particularly receptive to this means of achieving intimate knowledge of Christ, as their spirituality tended to be affective rather than intellectual.

In *Ascenso*, Laredo describes how reflecting on Christ's scourging will cause the devotee to feel blows, while reflecting on the crowning will cause the thorns to pierce the devotee's skin and draw blood (Laredo 222). Thus, Christ's physical suffering becomes one with the devotee's and vice versa. Instead of rejecting the physical body in traditional *contemptus mundi*, Laredo's method relies on the body to intensify the visual impact of Passion events (Boon 156). Although Laredo shared with conventional Galenists the notion of the mind-body-spirit connection, he differed from them in that he stressed physiology as a foundation for meditation.[10] Boon notes that Laredo "provides a list of patients he cured with prayer rather than pharmaceuticals" and reputedly cured an epileptic nun with a special cross that worked against the devil (61).

Teresa de Ávila surely did not read Laredo's *Metaphora medicinae* (Seville 1522 and 1536) or *Modus faciendi cum ordine medicandi* (Seville 1527, 1534, 1542, 1627), two of the first pharmacopeia written in Spanish, although we do know that *Subida del Monte Sión* (*Ascent of Mount Sion*), Seville 1535, 1538) was one of her favourite readings. She writes in *El libro de su vida* (*The Book of Her Life*), "Mirando libros para ver si sabría decir la oración que tenía, hallé en uno que llaman *Subida al monte*, en lo que toca a unión del alma con Dios, todas las señales que yo tenía en aquel no pensar nada, que esto era lo que yo más decía: que no podía pensar nada cuando tenía aquella oración" ("Looking through books in order to see if I could learn how to explain the prayer I was experiencing, I found in one they call *Ascent of the Mount*, where it touches on the union of the soul with God, all the signs I experienced in not thinking of anything. This was what I was most often saying: that when I experienced that prayer I wasn't able to think of anything"; *Vida* 300; *Life* 23:12, *CWST 1*, 205).[11] This "not thinking of anything" is the key to Teresa's recollective meditation, which requires the numbing of the senses and faculties. In *Life*, she describes her efforts to practise a purely apophatic spiritual path, one that dispensed with all images, only to realize the centrality of the humanity of Christ, the Word made visible and therefore representable, to her own spiritual journey.[12]

Chronicles of Pain and Paralysis

Belief in the inseparability of the body and spirit coincided with Teresa's propensity to view illness through the lens of spiritual experience. Although, like conventional Galenists, Teresa often treated physical ills through dietary modifications and herbs, for her and for many other devout men and women, both lay and religious, who were influenced by spiritual reform movements, ailments were spiritual trials that enabled the individual to identify more closely with Christ. However, the early Discalced Carmelite nuns are of particular interest because they chronicled their illnesses in their letters and memoirs. The Discalced expansion compelled these women to travel, and they maintained contact with friends and family through missives in which they detailed fluctuations in their health, enquired about the well-being of their correspondents, offered remedies for diverse maladies, and counselled on ways of dealing with pain. The Discalced Carmelites also fostered life writing, and some, such as Teresa and her nurse Ana de San Bartolomé, left *Vidas* (spiritual memoirs) in which they discuss health.

Sickly most of her life, in her writing Teresa mentions diverse ailments such as digestive and heart problems; headaches; toothaches; jaw pain; paralysis of the limbs and tongue; and vomiting. Although she provides myriad homeopathic remedies for diverse illnesses,[13] because of her theistic ethos, she often turned to prayer, *lectio divina*, and Holy Communion. In her rare mention of doctors, she notes that they were sometimes flummoxed by her situation or that their treatments (bleeding, purging, or diet changes) aggravated matters. Significantly, she always describes her ailments as spiritual trials.

As a *doncella de piso* (boarder) at an Augustinian convent during her adolescence, Teresa became so ill that she had to be sent home. The event is significant not because of the symptoms, which she does not enumerate, but because of its transcendental implications. Teresa saw her ordeal as part of God's plan: because God was preparing her to become a nun, she says, He sent her a serious illness to test her endurance (*Vida* 3:3, 130). The following year, she underwent terrible inner struggles accompanied by high fever and fainting spells while discerning her vocation: "Poníame el demonio que no podría sufrir los trabajo de la religión" ("The devil was suggesting that I would not be able to suffer the trials of religious life," she explains, and she was afraid that he might be right"; *Vida* 3:6, 132; *Life* 3:6, *CWST 1*, 63). She explains that her fondness for good books was her salvation: "leía en las Epístolas de San Jerónimo, que animaban de suerte que me animé a decirlo a mi padre, que casi era como para tomar el hábito" ("reading the *Letters of St. Jerome* so encouraged me that I decided to tell my father about my decision to take the habit"; *Vida* 3:7, 132; *Life* 3:7, *CWST 1*, 63). She entered the convent on 2 November 1536.

Two years later, she was so ill with heart and digestive problems that her father sent her to Becedas to see a famous healer: "Comenzáronme a crecer los desmayos y dióme un mal de corazón tan grandísimo, que ponía espanto a quien lo vía ... pasé el primer año con harto mala salud . casi me privaba el sentido siempre, y algunas veces del todo quedaba sin él" ("My fainting spells began to increase, and I experienced such heart pains that this frightened any who witnessed them ... I passed the first year with very poor health ... [often she] nearly lost consciousness, and sometimes lost it completely"; *Vida* 4:5, 136; *Life* 4:5, *CWST 1*, 66). Teresa's primary concern during this time was having the patience to endure her trials without offending God. She writes about another nun who was "enferma de grandísima enfermedad y muy penosa, porque era una boca en el vientre, que le habían hecho de opilaciones, por donde echaba lo que comía; murió presto de ello ... a mí hacíame gran envidia su paciencia. Pedía a Dios que, dándomela ansí a mí, me diese las enfermedades que fuese servido" ("afflicted with the most serious and painful illness, because there were some holes in her abdomen which caused obstructions in such a way that she had to eject through them what she ate. She soon died from this ... I envied her patience. I asked God that, dealing with me in like manner, He would give me the illnesses by which He would be served"; *Vida* 5:2, 141; *Life* 5:2, *CWST 1*, 70). For Teresa, pain was a gift that enabled her to share Christ's suffering; enduring pain gracefully was a form of service to God.

According to Teresa, God acquiesced: "antes de dos años estaba tal que, aunque no el mal de aquella suerte, creo que no menos penoso y trabajoso" ("within two years I was so sick that, although this sickness was not the same as the nun's, I don't think it was any less painful or laborious"; *Vida* 5:2, 142; *Life* 5:2, *CWST 1*, 71). After being bled excessively in Becedas, Teresa returned home in July 1539. In August, she fell into a coma that lasted four days, after which began years of a paralysis.

> Quedé de estos cuatro días de parajismo de manera que sólo el Señor puede saber los incomportables tormentos que sentía en mí. La lengua hecha pedazos de mordida; la garganta de no haber pasado nada y de la gran flaqueza, que me ahogaba, que aun el agua no podía pasar; todo me parecía que estaba desconyuntada, con grandíamo desatino en la cabeza; todo encogida, hecha un ovillo ... sin poder menearme ni brazo, ni pie, ni mano, ni cabeza ... todo estaba tan lastimado, que no lo podía sufrir. En una sábana, una de un lado y otra de otro, me meneaban. (*Vida* 6:1, 149)

> Such were these four days I spent in this paroxysm that only the Lord can know the unbearable torments I suffered within myself: my tongue, bitten to pieces, my throat unable to let even water pass down – from not having swallowed anything and from the great weakness that oppressed me; everything seemed to be disjointed; the greatest confusion in my head; all shriveled up and drawn together into a ball ... I was unable to stir, not an arm or a foot, neither hand nor head ... I was so bruised that I couldn't endure it; they moved me about in a sheet, one of the nuns at one end and another at the other. (*Life* 6:1, *CWST 1*, 76)

She also experienced severe chills and loss of appetite. According to Diego de Rivera, Teresa's first biographer, when she finally came out of the coma, she asked why they had awakened her, as she had greatly profited from that experience. She described visions of heaven and hell, as well as of her future foundations and of death (*Vida* 111). The paralysis required her to "andar a gatas" ("go about on hands and knees"; *Vida* 6:2, 150; *Life* 6:2, *CWST 1*, 77). Yet she saw the episode as a blessing: "estaba muy conforme con la voluntad de Dios") ("I was very conformed to the will of God"; *Vida* 6:2, 150; *Life* 6:2, *CWST 1*, 77). She sought consolation in solitude, prayer, and confession. By 1562, when she began her *Life*, Teresa had clearly absorbed the main tenets of Laredo's *Subida*, of which she owned the 1538 edition.

Today, many scholars have seen Teresa's raptures as manifestations of mental or physical illness,[14] while others challenge this notion.[15] Efrén de la Madre de Dios and Otger Steggink mention some modern diagnoses, such as tuberculosis (124, 131), malnutrition (127), psychosis (129), neurosis (130), malaria (131), trigeminal neuralgia (131), dysmenorrhea (menstrual cramps) (131), and angina (132). Marcelle Biro Barton suggests that Teresa could have had epilepsy, possibly temporal lobe seizures, which caused her mystical raptures. Encarnación

Juárez-Almendros agrees that Teresa suffered from epilepsy resulting from a lesion in the temporal lobes and argues that Teresa's paroxysm was clearly an epileptic seizure. Francisco Alonso-Fernández concludes that Teresa suffered from a serious depressive disorder associated with hysterical comorbidity of the psychomotor type. A sixteenth-century medical examiner who assessed her condition when she was sixty-seven years old remarked that it was impossible to pinpoint the source of her maladies, as her whole body was "un arsenal de enfermedades" ("an arsenal of illness"; Efrén and Steggink 125). Teresa never attempted to analyse her illnesses in physio-medical terms. Yet even in her own time, some authorities questioned the notion that physical suffering was essential to bring one closer to Christ. Fray Gaspar Dávila thought that illness had to be treated by doctors, while spiritual purity required obedience and prayer, not bodily pain.[16]

Because clerics often attributed ecstatic experience to hysteria, Teresa was reluctant to assert the authenticity of her own mystical experiences. She constantly urged her confessors to evaluate them and used expressions of uncertainty such as *puede ser, paréceme* (it may be, it seems to me) when describing them.[17] Similarly, she assessed her nuns' claims to supernatural experience with prudence. Although we do not know exactly how medical contemporaries of Teresa diagnosed her, she did display symptoms then associated with hysteria – seizures accompanied by intense pain, convulsions, powerful, unsettling emotions – and in the nineteenth century was actually diagnosed as hysteric (Bache "Reappraisal"). Hysteria has fallen from use as a diagnosis, yet even in the twentieth century, some medical authorities were still debating whether mystical raptures were, in fact, manifestations of this disease.

Teresa herself hardly mentions hysteria at all except to say that sarsaparilla water helps alleviate the effects of *mal de madre* (menstrual problems), one of which was believed to be hysteria (*Epistolario* 276; *Letters I*, 317).[18] However, she did write at length about the broader medical classification, melancholia. Most medics considered melancholia a mental illness, and mental illness was associated with sin. A letter about a melancholic nun that Teresa wrote to her friend María de San José, prioress of the Seville Carmel, illustrates what a touchy subject this was. Teresa says that the priest told her "loca me dijo claramente" ("clearly she is insane, so I said no more"; *Epistolario* 275; *Letters I*, 316).[19] Apparently, María was reluctant to share information about this woman, who was "melancholic in the extreme, for she lost her mind," so Teresa had to urge her to "speak of this matter plainly" (*Letters I*, 322).[20] Yet Teresa recognized symptoms of melancholia in herself, and in a letter to her friend María Bautista she mentions a syrup that helped relieved the symptoms (*Epistolario* 158; *Letters I*, 159).

Teresa's writings on melancholy reflect much of the prevalent thought on the subject. Her comments on women, whom she describes throughout her works as fragile, weak-minded, and excessively emotional, suggest she shared society's views on female volatility.[21] Like the physicians of her time, she considered melancholy a psychosomatic medical condition resulting from humoral imbalances that could be treated with diet and changes in routine. Aggravating factors could be excessive prayer, unmitigated solitude, extreme fasting, or sleep deprivation (Soufas 41). Like many of her contemporaries, Teresa believed that such activities could weaken a woman's spirit and leave her vulnerable to the machinations of the devil. In one case, she refused to take an aspirant whom her collaborator Jerónimo Gracián described as a "melancholic *beata*" ("holy woman"), even though the archbishop was promoting her admission (*Epistolario* 452; *Letters I*, 552). Jennifer Radden notes that Teresa's understanding of the seriousness of the disease and the threat it posed to a closed community, such as a convent, was unusual for her time (31). Teresa grasped that melancholy could be contagious, spreading from nun to nun and putting an entire convent at risk for investigation by the Inquisition, always wary of spurious claims of mystical rapture. Once Teresa wrote to Gracián about a woman of ill repute he was trying to help: "mucho se me ha asentado que no es tanto melancolía como demonio" ("I am convinced that it is due not so much to melancholy as to the devil"; *Epistolario* 321–2; *Letters I*, 400). She cautions Gracián that the devil may try to entrap him as well, "así es menester andar con gran recato en este negocio y no ir vuestra paternidad a su casa en ninguna manera" ("so you must proceed with great discretion in this matter and by no means go to her house"; *Epistolario* 321–2; *Letters I*, 400). Teresa believed that this woman was not a true melancholic, but a seductress.

Many young nuns suffered from melancholia, perhaps because they suddenly found themselves in an unfamiliar environment, far from family and friends. In her discussion of melancholic nuns in *Foundations*, Teresa shows compassion. She does not automatically assume these nuns are possessed or hysterical. Rather than ostracize them, she regulated their diet, typically recommending meat to fortify their bodies. She assigned them domestic tasks to distract them and limited the time they spent in prayer, confession, and mortification. Like Sabuco, she recognized that men were as susceptible to melancholia as women and displayed the same symptoms. She also suggests the same mind/body, holistic treatment for men and women as Sabuco. She wrote to Bishop Teutonio de Berganza, who was experiencing bouts of the disease: "La melancolía congójase de parecer se le ha de hacer premio, procure vuestra señoría algunas veces, cuando se ve apretado, irse adonde vea cielo, y andarse paseando" ("Melancholy dislikes being treated with severity. It is best to use less severe means and at times relax outdoors where you can walk and see the sky"; *Epistolario* 169; *Letters I*, 172).

Teresa did not automatically attribute nuns' melancholia to uterine or menstrual disorders, and, in fact, rarely mentions such matters. This does not appear to be due to reticence about the subject, however. Ana de San Bartolomé, Teresa's nurse, dealt with menstruation in a very straightforward way. She wrote to a friend who was suffering from cramps: "Esto hago para enviarla unos parchecillos, que creo que es stodo lo más que tiene mal de madre; de ahí veine la desgana de comer. Si la hubieran puesto una ventosa al vientre cuando la sangraron, estudiar mejor. Y si tienen una pequeña escudilla que sea redonda y que no esté el borde roto, caliente y úntela con una gota de aceite y un ajo, y verá cómo le hace provecho; y si esta escudilla fuese de madera, sería mejor. Hágala hacer ... que ha de ser de roble; mas en tanto que la hacen, traiga este parchecillo, y no coma cosa de vin[agre ni de queso] cuando está así" ("Here I'm sending you some little poultices, as I think all that's wrong is menstrual cramps. That's why you don't feel like eating. If they had put a suction cup on your belly when they bled you, you would have felt better. If they have a small beaker, one that's round and deep and doesn't have broken edges, heat it up and rub it with a little oil and some garlic, and you'll see what great good it will do you. If the beaker is wooden, all the better. Have one made ... and make sure it's oak. In the meantime, wear this poultice and don't eat anything with vinegar or cheese while you're in this state"; 1290–1; trans. mine). Ana makes no mention of the possible psychological consequences of her friend's malady. Although their awareness of the mind-body connection is evident in their use of diet modification to treat illness, including melancholia, Ana and Teresa, unlike male physicians like Santa Cruz, did not automatically link the uterus to the emotions.

Following her example, Teresa's disciples often provided detailed accounts of their health in their writing. María de San José and Ana de Jesús, both prioresses, were two of Teresa's closest friends. After Teresa died in 1582, they became embroiled in a controversy to preserve the 1581 Constitutions of the Order, which the Provincial Nicolás Doria was manoeuvring to change. The matter came to a head in 1590, when the nuns petitioned Pope Sixtus V to maintain the 1581 Constitutions. Although Sixtus acquiesced, he soon died, and in the end, Doria got what he wanted. Both women were deprived of voice and vote, and María was imprisoned incommunicado in the convent of São Alberto, in Lisbon, which she had founded in 1584.[22]

As a result of her quarrel with the Discalced authorities, nearly all of María's letters were burned. However, a missive María wrote in January 1597 to an unidentified Carmelite nun survives. In it, she describes the tribulations of the past ten years, including the physical and emotional effects of her incarceration.[23] By the time she wrote this letter, María was in failing health. The ordeal that Doria and his men put her through left her depressed and physically weakened.[24] Unlike physicians' case studies, María's report contains no analyses of causes or descriptions of cures. It is a candid testimony regarding her physical decline, which she sees as God's will. Here, as in her treatise *Ramillete de mirra* (*Bouquet of Myrrh*), she describes her suffering as a bond with the Saviour that enabled her actually to feel His pain in the way Laredo describes.

In prison, María developed stomach problems and vertigo:

> Como avía estado aquellos tantos meses sentada en un cabo sin menearme de un lugar, criáronme piedras en el stómago ... Y fue que me dio una tan rezia enfermedad de un vaguido, que estuve muchos meses y aun cerca de un año padeciendo los maiores tomentos que en mi vida he padecido, porque me dio un fluxo de piedras y en vómitos. Estuve aquí affligidísima, porque me quitó Dios el gusto que toda me vida he tenido en todas las cosas con sólo pensar que era la voluntad de Dios.

> Because I sat in one place for so long without moving, stones grew in my stomach. ... And I [also] became afflicted with terrible fits of dizziness. For many months, in fact, nearly a year, I suffered the most horrible torments of my life, because I threw up a stream of stones and vomit. I was extremely afflicted, because God took away all the pleasure I have had during my whole life in all things just by thinking they were God's will. (*MHCT* 21, Doc. 122, p. 653; trans. mine)

María says that she had never feared death before, but now that the doctors appeared convinced that she would not recover, she was overcome with terror. Yet, she explains, she is grateful for the experience, which has brought her to a new understanding of Christ's agony.

In addition to these infirmities, María was suffering from eye problems: "comencé con tan poca vista que quasi no veÿa, porque como V.R. sabrá, por remate de mis enfermedades estuve un mes ciega sin poder rezar el officio divino ni ver letra ni casi por dónde andava; sin tener mal ni dolor en los ojos, vine a cegar" ("I started off with so little sight that I almost couldn't see anything, for, as Your Reverence probably knows, on top of all my other illnesses, I was blind for a month. I couldn't even pray the Divine Office or see the letters. In fact, I couldn't even see where I was going. I didn't feel pain or discomfort in my eyes, but I went blind"; *MHCT* 21, Doc. 122, p. 656; trans. mine). However, María finds consolation in visions of Jesus and Teresa, who assure her that the blindness will not be permanent, and gradually her sight does return to her. Although temporary blindness was considered a symptom of melancholy or even hysteria, María attributes her eye problems to the pressure that the archbishop of Evora is bringing on her to reform the convent of Saint Monica. Although she is clearly exhausted and frail, she is determined to soldier on and obey his command: "Aquí estoy; haga el Señor en mí su eterna voluntad" ("Here I am. May the Lord use me according to His eternal will"; *MHCT* 21, Doc. 122, p. 657; trans. mine). For both men and women religious, obeying superiors was not only an obligation but a service to God.

In contrast with María, Ana de Jesús went on to have a long career after her confrontation with Doria. In 1594, she left Madrid and became prioress in Salamanca. In 1604, at age fifty-nine, she went to Paris to found the first Discalced Carmelite convent in France. Three years later, she founded convents in Brussels and Louvain. She did not write an autobiography, but nearly a hundred of her letters survive.

Ana's early missives exude enthusiasm for the Carmelite expansion, although clashes with clerics in France and the Low Countries later caused her to temper her zeal. Much of her late epistolary writing is concerned with her health. Towards 1608, her tone becomes increasingly sombre as mention of her declining strength becomes more frequent. Her last letters constitute a veritable chronicle of her physical deterioration. During this period, her motor skills degenerated rapidly, depriving her of control of her bodily functions. For this once-active prioress, accustomed to micromanaging every detail of convent life from finding appropriate housing to procuring firewood, this must have been devastating. Ana's epistolary corpus and an account of her last days by her close friend Beatriz de la Concepción, which covers the period from 1590 until her death in 1621, afford us a glimpse into the means by which this early modern nun dealt psychologically with her physical decline and imminent death.

During her last years, Ana experienced throat infections, gout, pleurisy, sciatica, paralysis, dropsy, tumours (especially a particularly painful one in her left cheek), and diverse body aches.[25] Although her physicians surely sought humoral causes for these illnesses, Ana saw her material and social surroundings as at least partially responsible. From her perspective, conditions in Belgium were not conducive to good health. The intense cold aggravated her joints. She wrote to a friend that it was so cold that the wells and irrigation ditches froze, making it impossible to bathe. The bitter temperatures contributed to frequent colds, lung congestion, and sore throats. A second factor was the predominance of Protestants in parts of the country, which depressed Ana, for she was terrified that she would die alone among heretics. Although contemporary scholars might scoff at this fear, Ana's feelings of isolation clearly affected her mental health and her ability to cope with her ailments.

Her declining physical condition and the omnipresence of Protestants go hand in hand as dominant themes in her late correspondence. The burden of coping with Protestants exhausts her. She complains to her friend Fray Diego de Guevara in a letter dated 4 July 1609:

> If you could see how they mistreat our good God in these lands ... I would like for them to take out on me all the disdain they heap on Him, and for them to esteem the One who watches over us. We should not pay attention to anything that happens to us, only to His Majesty, who was held to be worse than Barabas ... Today I don't have the energy to be in a place where they make such a show of behaving this way. I can't wait to return [to Spain]. (*Cartas* 77)[26]

On 28 December 1609, she writes again to Guevara: "Although I have few friends left in Spain, I want to be with them again ... my soul is tired of being surrounded by people who don't know my good Jesus" (*Cartas* 83).[27]

In her letters of this period, Ana complains constantly of weariness and pain. On 24 January1608, she tells Beatriz that she is "tired because of her aches and pains and countless other things" (*Cartas* 68).[28] On 10 June 1610, she explains a lapse in her letter writing to Fray Diego: "Because I was very ill, I haven't attended to this until now" (*Cartas* 90).[29] She repeats the point on 29 July 1611, attributing her silence to "my lack of health" (*Cartas* 93).[30] On 21 January 1612, she writes: "my lack of health doesn't allow me to write as often as I would like" (*Cartas* 95).[31]

During the months that follow, descriptions of her ailments become increasingly graphic: "I speak with so much difficulty,"[32] she writes to Juana del Espíritu Santo, Beatriz's sister (22 September 1612, *Cartas* 97). According to Beatriz, Ana's mouth was so swollen that she couldn't articulate clearly and drooled incessantly (*Écrits* 550). A letter from the Infanta Isabel Clara Eugenia confirms that Ana had completely lost the faculty of speech: "It seems Our Lord wants to mortify us with this, that you can't speak" (*Écrits* 536).[33] We have no medical diagnosis from the period, but today these symptoms are associated with stroke and lung or nerve disorders.[34]

According to Beatriz, Ana was gradually losing control of her limbs. She was unable even to "wipe a tear with her hands or lift a bit of food to her mouth" (*Écrits* 550).[35] In a letter to an unknown recipient Ana complains: "Look what a state your poor mother is in. I can't give the blessing because I can't move my hand. I am giving it in my heart, for I haven't been able to make the sign of the cross in three years" (*Cartas* 101).[36] However, instead of feeling sorry for herself, she is mortified that she is inconveniencing others. On 8 September 1617, she explains to an unidentified priest: "I can do nothing but make work for these sisters, with the grave illness and impediments that I have" (*Cartas* 105).[37] A letter of 22 March 1617 to Juana del Espíritu Santo reveals her appalling physical state and growing sense of isolation: "These are the most awful pains a human being has ever suffered. From head to toe I'm a prisoner, so that I can't help myself using any of my limbs, and I'm so exhausted that sometimes I can't even speak" (*Cartas* 104).[38] Incredibly, she manages to make a joke about her condition: "I can't lie in bed naked even for a minute. They throw me on the floor and pick me up like a rag doll. These people who help me have it hard, because I weigh more than a dead body" (*Cartas* 104).[39] Beatriz explains that Ana's skin was so sensitive that even wearing a habit caused her pain, so at night the nuns dressed her in a light cloth. In order to lay her down or sit her up, they had to pull her by the arms, which, because of her weight, was agonizing (*Écrits* 551). Ana complied with her duties as prioress as long as she could, and even when she had lost complete control of her limbs, she asked to be carried to wherever the nuns were enjoying their hour of recreation so she could be near them.

Ana apparently had no hope that doctors could help her, and indeed, when Duke Albert and Duchess Isabel Clara Eugenia sent her the royal physician, he admitted that because of her age and number of infirmities, there was nothing he could do (*Écrits* 551). She was given an ounce of expectorant to clear up the phlegm, but the relief was fleeting. Ana, however, was not expecting relief from the doctor. She wanted to see him only to ask whether it was time for her to receive extreme unction. She was terrified of dying without the last rites.

Ana had dreamt for years of returning to Spain, but during her last years it became clear that she would die in what she continued to see as a hostile, pagan land. Death now began to occupy her thoughts. She writes to Juana del Espíritu Santo on 13 December 1616: "Look, daughter, heaven is where we'll be happy, and not here, where if you turn your head, what you love the most disappears" (*Cartas* 102).[40] She repeats the same thought in a letter written around 1619: "May we be together again in heaven. That is what I most desire and to see myself free of this body. My suffering is unbelievable" (*Cartas* 107).[41] In her last letter, dated 15 February 1621, seven days before her death, she tells her brother, Cristóbal de Lobera: "I'm suffocating with pain. I've never in my life had such agonizing pain as today. I beg your Lordship to have some masses said for me, whether I'm dead or alive" (*Cartas* 110).[42]

Ana's letters chronicle how paralysis slowly overtook her body and plunged her into dejection, affecting her ability to think clearly and perform basic human functions without help. Yet, like her sisters in religion, Ana believed in the salutary spiritual effects of physical suffering.[43] Although she clearly resented her growing dependence on others, she saw physical torment as a grace that enabled her to identify with Jesus. In her letter to Fray Diego of 1 November 1607, she complains of pain that is torturous but welcome, for it purifies the soul. She writes that her suffering is the punishment she deserves for her sins, and indeed, she craves punishment for them: "May God grant me peace in all this suffering I endure; the pain is so terrible that I feel like a heap of bones, and although I crave it and see my sins clearly, it is [actually] very little for the punishment I deserve for the very least of my sins" (*Cartas* 56).[44] Suffering likens us to Christ, she explains, and so when God sends pain, we should rejoice. One senses that Ana, dying and increasingly disillusioned with Flanders, is coming to terms with her own end – finding meaning in her misery and taking stock of her life.

Beatriz describes the patience with which Ana bore her suffering as "supernatural," and the royal physician concurred (*Écrits* 550, 551). Given her age and condition, he thought it was a "miracle" that she still lived (*Écrits* 551). For Ana, death was a spiritual experience for which she prepared. She took communion daily and sometimes heard mass even more often. Although her facial muscles were paralyzed, at the moment of receiving the host, "she avidly opened her mouth, writes Beatriz" (*Écrits* 552).[45] Right before her death, she blessed her spiritual daughters and then, looking them each in the eye, left her imprint on their souls.

Beatriz imbues her description of Ana's death with a sense of the mystical: her face regained the smoothness of alabaster and her feet, their original whiteness; her hands became lovely and supple (*Écrits* 553). Afterward, her funeral was celebrated with great pomp and veneration. During the ceremony, a woman who had been paralyzed for over fourteen years miraculously stood and walked, an occurrence the provincial decided to keep secret until it could be revealed for maximum dramatic effect (*Écrits* 553–4).

Human Pain, Christ's Pain

In the sixteenth century, as today, physicians often analysed the causes and consequences of illness without considering how their patients actually experienced it. When the patient was a woman, conventional Galenic principles traced myriad physical and emotional ailments to the uterus. However, "mystical medics" such as Laredo saw the body as inseparable from the spirit. For Laredo, the suffering body was a conduit to Christ that actually enabled us to feel Christ's pain. What unites the writings of the three nuns discussed here is the sense that illness and pain are gifts that make spiritual union possible. The individual becomes one with God by experiencing pain. While these women understood and modified their behaviors in response to relationships between food, environment, and health, they nevertheless experienced pain not just in the context of the physical body, but as part of the body-spirit continuum. While they sometimes called on doctors, in their writings about pain, they mention them only passingly, if at all. For them, more desirable than simply alleviating pain was to experience it to the fullest in order to live Christ's Passion.

NOTES

1 After the publication of *De humani corporis fabrica libri septem,* Vesalius entered the Spanish court and became a court physician to Charles V, Holy Roman Emperor, starting in 1543; he later moved to Spain to attend to King Philip II in 1559.

2 Some did make a distinction between the physical and the spiritual, for example, Gaspar Dávila. See Laningham. Elena Carrera points out that "melancholia" was associated with "excess, scorching or putrefaction of bodily fluids, darkness, corruption of mental faculties and helplessness ("Madness and Melancholy"). Jennifer Radden explains that in the sixteenth century, it embraced a much broader register of symptoms than what we now call depression or bipolar disorder (30). The notion of the disordered imagination characteristic of the melancholic "cannot easily be understood in terms of any faculty-psychology division between feeling and thinking," as these distinctions were clarified only in the eighteenth and nineteenth centuries, writes Radden (30). Thus, physical health and spiritual occurrences often merge into the experiential in the writings of the devout.

3 Women were thought to be of cold temperament, a consequence of which was that they could not process their nutrients adequately. Because, it was assumed, they did not engage in physical labour, they could not expel

their nutrimental waste through sweat and other means, as men did. Thus, they had to purge it through menstruation. Otherwise, waste material would accumulate in their bodies and lead to a humoral imbalance resulting in disease (Green 21).

4 Curiously, in some case studies, he refers to women as *el enfermo*, the generic word for patient, while in others, he uses *la enferma* (female patient).

5 A compound of different fruits and flowers given to patients with ulcers.

6 Until recently, the author of the *New Philosophy* was thought to be Sabuco's father, who claimed to have penned it. Furthermore, early modern medical authorities argued that the work was beyond the aptitude of a woman. However, Sabuco's modern editors assert that the book represents not only a feminine but even a feminist voice (Waithe et al. 13). The evenhandedness of Sabuco's treatment of female issues such as menstruation and pregnancy, her use of female exemplars, and her focus on human health rather than on gendered symptoms distinguish her writing from that of her male colleagues, they argue.

7 Women also worked as healers, convent infirmarians, midwives, and barber-surgeons. Sometimes healers did serious damage to their patients – for example, the medicine woman who treated Teresa de Ávila in Becedas as discussed later in this essay. However, because of the high fees of university-trained doctors and the fear many people had of them, medical help was sought elsewhere. Many nuns served their convents and the greater community by proffering medical advice. See Whaley; Mujica ("Healing on the Margins"); and also Strocchia ("The Nun Apothecaries of Renaissance Florence")."

8 See Helen King, *Midwifery, Obstetrics and the Rise of Gynaecology*.

9 For a full explanation of Laredo's notions of the embodied soul and the Passion, see Jessica Boon.

10 See Boon 85–107.

11 All English translations of Teresa's *Book of Her Life* are from Kavanaugh and Rodríguez and are found in *The Collected Works of Saint Teresa of Ávila*, which is cited parenthetically in the text with the abbreviation *CWST*.

12 See my article "Beyond Image: The Apophatic-Kataphatic Dialectic in Teresa de Ávila."

13 See Mujica, *Religious Women* 150–6.

14 See Efrén de la Madre de Dios and Steggink 133–4.

15 See Newberg et al., *Why God Won't Go Away*.

16 See Laningham.

17 See Weber, *Teresa of Avila*.

18 Curiously, Kavanaugh translates *mal de madre* as "hysteria," although the term could refer to several symptoms, for example, menstrual cramps.

19 All translations of Teresa's letters are from *The Collected Letters of St. Teresa of Avila*, trans. Kieran Kavanaugh, O.C.D.

20 "Había estado tan en extremo melancólica, que había perdido el juicio ... Trátalo con llaneza" (*Epistolario* 278).

21 See Weber, *Teresa of Avila*; and Mujica, "Was Teresa of Ávila a Feminist?"

22 See Moriones, *El P. Doria y El Carisma Teresiano*. Also, Mujica, *Religious Women and Epistolary Culture in the Carmelite Reform: The Disciples of Teresa de Ávila*, which contains a detailed account of the controversy along with María letters on the subject.

23 In María de San José, "María de San José (Salazar)."

24 In 1585, Doria was elected the second provincial of the order, replacing Gracián, who had been the first. Teresa had given prioresses considerable power in her original Constitutions, and Doria thought they were too independent. When Doria moved to modify the Constitutions to bring the prioresses under the control of clerics, María and Ana de Jesús appealed to the pope, in what came to be known as "the nuns' revolt." Doria and his allies not only imprisoned María in the dungeon of her convent, they accused her and Gracián of immoral behaviour and of stirring up unrest in the order. Doria commanded María to refrain from all from further contact with Gracián and harassed her incessantly, circulating letters to turns other nuns against her. She wrote to Carmelite authorities trying to clear both their names, but the pressure and her imprisonment took their toll on her health. For an in-depth study of María de San José and her conflict with Doria, see my forthcoming book, *Religious Women and Epistolary Culture in the Carmelite Reform: The Disciples of Teresa de Ávila*.

25 Beatrix de la Conception, in Anne de Jésus, *Écrits et documents* 549.

26 "Si viese quan maltratan en estas tierras a n(uestr)o buen Dios ... Quería que içiesen en mí todo el despreçio y estimasen al que nos vió y no hay q(ue) açer caso sino de lo q(ue) nos llegare más a su Mag(estad) que fue tenido por peor q(ue) Barabás ... Oy día ya me falta el ánimo pa(ra) estar donde con tanta publicidad se açe esto, y no veo l ora de volverme allá" (trans. mine).

27 "aun(que) me an q(ue)dado pocos (amigos) en España, deseo verme con ellos ... mi alma, q(ue) la tengo fatigada de verme donde ay tantos q(ue) no conocen ami buen Jesús" (trans. mine).

28 "estava fatigada de mis dolores y otras mil cosas q(ue) son sin quento (cuenta)" (trans. mine).

29 "Por aver estado muy mala no echo ésto asta aora" (trans. mine).

30 "La culpa de tanto silençio es la falta de mi salud" (trans. mine).

31 "mi falta de salud no me da lugar açer esto (escribir) las veçes q(ue) lo deseo" (trans. mine).

32 "Ablo con tanta dificultad" (trans. mine).

33 "Il me semble que Notre Seigneur veut nous mortifier tous en cela que vous ne pouvez parler" (trans. mine).

34 See Mayo Clinic website: www.mayoclinic.org/diseases-conditions/dysarthria/symptoms-causes/syc-20371994.

35 "elle ne pouvait même pas s'essuyer une larme avec ses mains, ni approcher une bouchée de sa bouche" (trans. mine).

36 "¡Miren qué estado está su pobre m(adr)e, que para echar la bendizión no puedo menear la mano. Echosela con el corazón, que a más de tres años que no me persino" (trans. mine).

37 "ya no puedo, sino dar trabajo a estas ermanas con la grabe enfermedad inpedimento que tengo" (trans. mine).

38 "Los [trabajos] más rrigurosos que emos bisto en persona umana. Desde la cabeza asta los pies estoy aprisionada, de manera que no me puedo ayudar de ninguno de mis mienbros, y tan fatigada que muchas bezes me quita el abla" (trans. mine).

39 "No es possible estar en un punto desnuda en la cama, por estos suelos me echan y me lebantan como desconyuntada. Arto padezen los que me me ayudan y peso más que un cuerpo muerto" (trans. mine).

40 "Mire, yja mía, que en el zielo es donde emos de gozar y no donde a buelta de cabeza se desapareze lo que queremos" (trans. mine).

41 "En el zielo lo [juntas] estemos; muchísimo lo deseo y berme fuera de este cuerpo. Es increíble lo que padezco" (trans. mine).

42 "Estoy apretadísima con mis dolores; en mi bida los e tenido tan grandes como oy. Suplico a V(uestra) S(eñorí)a me diga unas misas por muerta o por biba" (trans. mine).

43 References to the spiritual benefits of physical and emotional suffering are widespread not only in Spain, but throughout Europe. It is the crux of María de San José's *Ramillete de mirra* (1595). (See my *Religious Women* for an in-depth discussion of this issue.) Teresa tells her friend Jerónimo Gracián, that God orders physical ailments as an expression of His love (*Letters 2*, 131ff; 15 October 1578). Both in and out of convents, the devout practised mortifications as a means of inducing physical suffering that would help them identify with Christ. In *Fragmentation and Redemption,* Caroline Walker Bynum explores female somatic asceticism and the role of the body in late medieval female piety. She notes that "torture of the flesh ... was a horrible yet delicious elevation" that gave the individual "access to the divine" (182). Both men and women engaged in self-torture, including whipping, in order to experience the Crucifixion psychosomatically. Heinrich Seuse, the fourteenth-century German Dominican, wrote that "If suffering brought with it no other gain than that by our griefs and pains we grow in likeness to Christ, our prototype, it would still be a priceless benefit" (qtd. Bynum 184). David Fletcher

Tinsley provides examples of extreme asceticism in fourteenth-century Germany, where Dominican nuns practised mortification of the flesh. In *Holy Anorexia,* Rudolph M. Bell cites the example of Catherine Benincasa, the fourteenth-century Florentine Dominican tertiary, who starved and flagellated herself with iron chains until her back was bloody (43). Bell also studies the cases of other Italian female votaries, among them Catherine of Siena, who practised extreme fasting and self-flagellation in order to share Christ's pain. He notes that the woman who engaged in such self-imposed affliction "rebels against passive, vicarious, dependent Christianity; her piety centres intensely and personally upon Jesus and his crucifixion, and she actively seeks an intimate, physical union with God" (116). Such mortifications continued well into the seventeenth century. Writing about Parisian convents, Barbara B. Diefendorf notes that "Les Filles de Sainte-Elisabeth, for example, scourged themselves three times a week during Advent and Lent and twice a week at other times of the year" (146). Ulrike Strasser notes the example of Clara Hortulana, a Poor Clare in Munich, who carried the imitation of Christ to an extreme: on 14 October 1689, Hortulana committed suicide by plunging from the choir in order to die "like a true martyr, shedding her blood for Christ" (39). This intimate, physical union with God was the objective of the re-enactments of martyrdom in the Discalced Carmelite convents of the sixteenth and early seventeenth centuries. See Mujica, *Religious Women.*

44 "Con paz ... ruegue que se la tenga yo en las fatigas tan grandes que padezco con estos dolores tan terribles que me tienen descoyuntada, y aunque los apetezco y beo claros, es muy poco para el castigo que merezía el menor de mis pecados" (trans. mine).

45 "elle ouvrit la bouche avec une grande avidité" (trans. mine).

WORKS CITED

Alonso-Fernández, Francisco. *Historia personal de la monja Teresa de Jesús.* Hoja del Monte, 2013.

Ana de Jesús (Lobera). *Cartas (1590–1621).* Edited by Concepción Torres, Ediciones Universidad de Salamanca, 1996.

– *Écrits et documents.* Edited by Antonio Fortes and Restituto Palmero, Édition du Carmel, 2001.

Ana de San Bartolomé. *Obras completas.* Edited by Julián Urkiza, Brugos, 1988.

Bache, Chistopher. "A Reappraisal of Teresa of Avila's Supposed Hysteria." *Journal of Religion and Health,* vol. 24 no. 4, Winter 1985, pp. 300–15.

Barton, Marcella Biro. "Saint Teresa de Ávila: Did She Have Epilepsy." *Catholic Historical Review,* vol. 68, no. 4, October 1982, p. 581.

Béatrix de la Conception. "Béatrix de la Conception sur Anne de Jésus, récit de la maladie et de la mort." In *Ana de Jésus, Écrits et documents* 549–55.

Bell, Rudolph M. *Holy Anorexia.* U of Chicago P, 1985.

Boon, Jessica A. *The Mystical Science of the Soul: Medieval Cognition in Bernardino de Laredo's Recollection Method.* U of Toronto P, 2012.

Bynum, Caroline Walker. *Fragmentation and Redemption.* Zone, 1992.

Carrera, Elena. "Madness and Melancholy in Sixteenth- and Seventeenth-Century Spain: New Evidence, New Approaches." *Bulletin of Spanish Studies*, vol. 87, no. 8, 2010, pp. 1–5. DOI: 10.1080/14753820.2010.530832.

Clouse, Michele L. *Medicine, Government and Public Health in Philip II's Spain: Shared Interests, Competing Authorities.* Ashgate, 2011.

Diefendorf, Barbara B. *From Penitence to Charity: Pious Women and the Catholic Reformation in Paris.* Oxford UP, 2004.

Efrén de la Madre de Dios and Otger Steggink. *Tiempo y vida de Santa Teresa.* Biblioteca de Autores Cristianos, 1996.

Green, Monica H. *The Trotula: A Medieval Compendium of Women's Medicine.* U of Pennsylvania P, 2013.

Juárez-Almendros, Encarnación. "Hallucinations, Persecutions and Self-Defense: The Autobiography of Teresa of Ávila." *Arizona Journal of Hispanic Cultural Studies*, vol. 17, 2013, pp. 177–92. *JSTOR*, www.jstor.org/stable/24582275.

Kavanaugh, Kieran. "Introduction." *The Collected Works of Saint Teresa of Ávila*, Translated by Kieran Kavanaugh, O.C.D., and Otilio Rodríguez, O.C.D, vol. 1, Institute of Carmelite Studies, 1980–7, pp. 15–51.

King, Helen. *Midwifery, Obstetrics and the Rise of Gynaecology: The Uses of a Sixteenth-Century Compendium.* Ashgate, 2007.

Laningham, Susan. "Maladies up Her Sleeve? Clerical Interpretation of a Suffering Female Body in Counter-Reformation Spain." *Early Modern Women*, vol. 1, 2006, pp. 69–97.

Laredo, Bernardino de. *Subida del Monte Sión.* Edited by Alegría Alonso González, Mercedes García Trascasas, and Bertha Gutiérrez, Fundación Universitaria Española, 2000.

López-Terrada, Marialuz. "'Sallow-faced Girl, Either It's Love of You've Been Eating Clay'": The Representation of Illness in Golden Age Theater." *Medical Cultures of the Early Modern Spanish Empire*, edited by John Slater, et al., Ashgate, 2014, pp. 167–87.

María de San José. "María de San José (Salazar) a una Camelita Descalza." *Monumenta Hieronymi Gracián: Expulsión del Padre Gracián*, vol. 3, edited by Juan Luis Astigarraga, *Monumenta Historica Carmeli Teresiani*, 21, 2004, pp. 649–57.

– *Ramillete de mirra.* In *Escritos Espirituales*. Edited by Simeón de la Sagrada Familia, Postulación General O.C.D., 1979, pp. 281–340.

Mayo Clinic. "Dysarthria." www.mayoclinic.org/diseases-conditions/dysarthria/symptoms-causes/syc-20371994.

McTavish, Lianne. *Childbirth and the Display of Authority in Early Modern France.* Ashgate, 2005.

Moriones, Ildefonso. *El P. Doria y el charisma teresiano.* Orden de los Padres Carmelitas Descalzos, 1994.

Mujica, Bárbara. "Beyond Image: The Apophatic-Kataphatic Dialectic in Teresa de Avila." *Hispania,* Dec. 2001, pp. 741–8.

– "Healing on the Margins: Ana de San Bartolomé: Convent Nurse." *Early Modern Studies Journal,* vol. 6, 2014. https://www.earlymodernstudiesjournal.org/wp-content/uploads/2014/10/5.-Mujica.pdf.

– *Women Religious and Epistolary Exchange in the Carmelite Reform: The Disciples of Teresa of Ávila.* Amsterdam UP, 2020.

– *Teresa de Ávila, Lettered Woman.* Vanderbilt UP, 2009.

– "Was Teresa of Ávila a Feminist?" *Approaches to Teaching Teresa of Ávila and the Spanish Mystics,* edited by Alison Weber. The Modern Language Association, 2009, pp. 74–82.

Newberg, Andrew B., Eugene G. D'Aquili, and Vince Rause. *Why God Won't Go Away: Brain Science and the Biology of Belief.* Ballantine Books, 2008.

Radden, Jennifer. *Moody Minds Distempered: Essays on Melancholy and Depression.* Oxford UP, 2009.

Ribera, Francisco de. *Vida de Santa Teresa de Jesús.* Gustavo Gili, 1908.

Sabuco de Nantes Barrera, Oliva. *New Philosophy of Human Nature: Neither Known to nor Attained by the Great Ancient Philosophers, Which Will Improve Human Life and Health.* Edited and translated by Mary E. Waithe, María C. Vintró, and C. Ángel Zorita, U of Illinois P, 2007.

Santa Cruz, Alonso de. *Sobre la melancolía: Diagnóstico y curación de los afectos melancólicos (1569).* Translated by Raúl Lavalle, edited by Juan Antonio Paniagua, EUNSA, 2005.

Schiesari, Juliana. *The Gendering of Melancholia.* Cornell UP, 1992.

Sluhovsky, Moshe. *Believe Not Every Spirit: Possession, Mysticism, & Discernment in Early Modern Catholicism.* U of Chicago P, 2007.

Solomon, Michael. *Fictions of Well-Being.* U of Pennsylvania P, 2010.

Soufas, Teresa. *Melancholy and the Secular Mind in Spanish Golden Age Literature.* U of Missouri P, 1990.

Strasser, Ulrike. "Clara Hortulana of Embach or How to Suffer Martyrdom in the Cloister." *Female Monasticism in Early Modern Europe: An Interdisciplinary View,* edited by Cordula van Wyhe, Ashgate, 2008, pp. 39–57.

Strocchia, Sharon T. "The Melancholic Nun in Late Renaissance Italy." *Diseases of the Imagination and Imaginary Disease in the Early Modern Period,* edited by Yasmin Haskell Tournhout, Brepols, 2011, pp. 139–58.

– "The Nun Apothecaries of Renaissance Florence: Marketing Medicines in the Convent." *Renaissance Studies*, vol. 25, no. 5, 2011, pp. 627–47.

Teresa of Ávila (Teresa de Jesús). *The Collected Letters of St. Teresa of Ávila*. Translated by Kiernan Kavanaugh, O.C.D., Institute of Carmelite Studies, vol. 1 2001, vol. 2 2007.

– *The Collected Works of Saint Teresa of Ávila*. Translated by Kieran Kavanaugh, O.C.D., and Otilio Rodríguez, O.C.D., Institute of Carmelite Studies, 1980–7. 3 vols.

– *Epistolario*. Edited by Luis Rodríguez Martínez and Teófanes Egido. Espiritualidad, 1984.

– *Libro de su vida*. Edited by Dámaso Chicarro. Cátedra, 1993.

Tinsley, David F. *The Scourge and the Cross: Ascetic Mentalities of the Later Middle Ages*. Peeters, 2010.

Waithe, Mary E., and María C. Vintró. "Posthumously Plagiarizing Oliva Sabuco: An Appeal to Cataloguing Librarians." *Cataloging & Classification Quarterly*, vol. 35, nos. 3–4, 2003, pp. 525–40. https://www.tandfonline.com/doi/abs/10.1300/J104v35n03_11.

Weber, Alison. *Teresa of Avila and the Rhetoric of Femininity*. Princeton UP, 1990.

Whaley, Leigh. *Women and the Practice of Medical Care in Early Modern Europe, 1400–1800*. Palgrave/MacMillan, 2011.

Waithe, Mary E., et al. Introduction. Sabuco de Nantes y Barrera. *New Philosophy of Human Nature: Neither Known to nor Attained by the Great Ancient Philosophers, Which Will Improve Human Life and Health*. U of Illinois P, 2007.

Chapter Ten

Sacred Embryology: Intrauterine Baptisms and the Negotiation of Theology and Health Sciences across the Eighteenth-Century Spanish Empire

GEORGE A. KLAEREN

Almost every Thursday in eighteenth-century Seville, physicians, natural philosophers, and theologians could be found meeting at the Royal Society of Medicine and Other Sciences to hear papers presented and to discuss topics of interest (Valera Candel and López Fernández).[1] On 20 February 1772, an address was given by Father Vicente de la Asumpción, a member of the society, a Mercedarian priest, and a theological evaluator for the Inquisition. His topic, "A Theological Dissertation on the Baptism of the Fetus within the Uterus," might seem to modern readers to be unrelated to medicine, or indeed to any scientific discipline (de la Asumpción 66).[2] Yet in Enlightenment Spain, this dissertation touched directly upon a sensitive nexus of scientific, medical, theological, and moral concerns. In the eighteenth-century Hispanic world, new advancements in anatomical knowledge and instruction prompted unprecedented progress in embryology and obstetrics. In surgical colleges, in hospitals, and in academic societies across the Spanish Empire, these developments forced theologians and philosophers to re-examine important moral and spiritual questions, especially those regarding generation and conception, ensoulment, and baptism.

These topics represented an epistemic joint venture between natural philosophy and theology. The two disciplines worked both independently and in dialogue to create knowledge and craft public policies regarding embryology and obstetrics throughout the Hispanic world. Emblematic of the overlapping nature of the field of enquiry is the title of one of the leading embryological publications from the period, which labelled the topic "sacred embryology" (Cangiamila).[3] More broadly considered, "sacred embryology" represented part of a larger concern in the eighteenth century about medico-moralism, or what might be called today bioethics or medical ethics – a field which was beginning to develop as a genre and which was still in the process of self-definition.[4] The medical-moral realm included questions of importance to both science and theology and was discussed by physicians and theologians alike. Within this field, sacred embryology serves as a particularly rich case study.

This chapter briefly explores the debates over intrauterine baptisms generated by the field of sacred embryology as an example of the dialogical relationship between science and theology in the eighteenth-century Hispanic world. After introducing the historiography of early modern Spanish obstetrics, it is possible to summarize the role that the natural sciences had in informing and reassessing theological opinions and doctrinal discussions in Spain by demonstrating that advances in embryology and the health sciences prompted theological reconsiderations of ensoulment and animation.[5] Reciprocally, theological decisions provided the context, initiative, and demand for new scientific research in obstetrical surgery, anatomical study, and embryology, particularly in the development of techniques for intrauterine baptisms. The field of "sacred embryology" in eighteenth-century Spain thus helps in understanding the deeper, fundamental dialogue between science and theology during the early modern period. Finally, the case study of intrauterine baptisms may aid in understanding notions of gender and identity, particularly for pregnant women, in the early modern Hispanic world.

A Historiography of Spanish Embryology and Obstetrics

To date, historical surveys of Spanish medicine in the eighteenth century focus more on the development of obstetrics than on embryology. Previous studies have connected the development of embryology and obstetrics in the eighteenth-century Spanish Empire with the professionalization of the medical field and the reform of surgical colleges, hospitals, and universities, and the evolution of the role of the midwife. They have likewise assessed the development of obstetrics in relation to the state regulation of medical practices by the office of the Protomedicato.[6] These studies have especially examined obstetrics in eighteenth-century colonial Latin America (M.E. Rodríguez; Reid; Cook; Warren, *Piety and Danger*; Warren, "Foreign and Local"; Rigau-Pérez; Valle).

Teresa Ortiz, for example, has demonstrated how scientific advancements accompanied with "a complex process of reorganization of the medical professions" sublimated midwifery in early modern Spain, gradually replacing midwives with male surgeons and obstetricians (Ortiz 95). Martha Few, writing about the Kingdom of Guatemala, describes the maturation of obstetrics as a project of state expansion that "construct[ed] colonial fetuses," encouraged medical surveillance of a once-private pregnancy and birth process, and medicalized and claimed the womb – particularly of colonial subjects – as the lawful jurisdiction of the Spanish government (Few 96). In a similar study, Nora Jaffary has described the dramatic professionalization of obstetrics as a medical field responding to debates on post-mortem caesarean sections in the second half of eighteenth-century Mexico. Before this point, she writes, midwives handled childbirth entirely and the subject was "a private and unremarkable matter" (Jaffary 174). John Tate Lanning, in his landmark historical survey of the Protomedicato, has detailed this process of professionalization or "medicalization" of midwifery (Lanning, *Protomedicato*; Allotey). Many other such studies abound and have admirably expanded historical knowledge of obstetrics, midwifery, and the role of childbirth in the early modern Spanish Empire. These works, while useful in illustrating the important developments in obstetrics during the eighteenth century, are often exclusively limited in focus to sociopolitical dimensions of birth, particularly emphasizing legal processes and the status of colonial women.

What this historiography lacks, however, is a careful exploration of the way in which "sacred embryology" demonstrates a theoretical, fundamental relationship between theology and the natural sciences. Such a relationship is usually taken as an axiomatic given without further explanation or reduced as a mechanism for explaining political power and social control in Bourbon Spain (Johnson; Rigau-Pérez). Yet the creation of the hybrid category of "sacred embryology" – by definition part theological, part scientific – has not been sufficiently explored. What epistemological framework allowed for this overlapping field of contested territory? By considering "sacred embryology" as one peculiar instance of the broader category of the scientific-theological and medico-moral, historians may better understand the mentality of the Spanish eighteenth century, and more broadly, how early modern individuals conceived of the relationship between theology and natural philosophy (including medicine) as a cooperative dialogue between two fields of knowledge. This dialogue, in turn, helps to reconsider the way that pregnancy and birth impacted the role and responsibilities of women and how medical and theological discussions defined and engaged the concept of a "mother" (*preñada, madre*).

Science Informing Theology: New Embryology and Theological Debates over Ensoulment

Spain and Latin America benefited greatly from the scientific and medical advances of the seventeenth and eighteenth centuries.[7] Marta Vicente has argued that particular attention in the health sciences was given to obstetrics and gynaecology in eighteenth-century Spain (Vicente 77). For the study of embryology and obstetrics, progress in microscopy, microbiology, anatomy, and surgery helped to further discoveries and developments related to conception, gestation, and birth. Intellectuals were well acquainted with Continental works regarding the ongoing discussion between preformationists and epigenesists (Maienschein).[8] The development of embryology was also a secondary effect of the immense intellectual activity in the field of anatomy in the eighteenth century. Perhaps more than any other scientific enterprise, anatomical studies grew during this period in Spain. Once viewed as an auxiliary technical art better suited to barbers and surgeons than physicians, by the end of the century, anatomy was a critical part of the study of medicine and accompanied a general shift in the philosophy of science that favoured experimentalism and empirical observation (Burke 25; Granjel, *Medicina*; Pardo-Tomás and Martínez-Vidal, "In tenebris" and "Medicine ... Novator Movement"; Hervás y Panduro; Robbins; Laursen; Pagden). Lastly, embryology and obstetrics benefited from increased institutional and governmental support in the eighteenth century, which furthered the professionalization of these disciplines. New anatomical theatres and surgical colleges were opened, and scholars have connected the growth of the field of obstetrics with medical reform at the Royal College of San Carlos, charged with developing instruction and training of surgical obstetricians and midwives (Burke; Martínez-Vidal and Pardo-Tomás, "Anatomical Theaters"). As previously noted, the royal office of the Protomedicato created new standards for licensure and practice of midwives in 1750 (Lanning, *Protomedicato*).

What must be emphasized is not simply the existence of scientific practices in the eighteenth-century Hispanic world, but the close link this activity had with the theological sphere. Leading theologians and religious intellectuals across the Spanish Empire monitored and read the most recent findings of embryology and incorporated them into their work. Medicine and science prompted new theological reflection and discussion about ensoulment. For example, Francesco Cangiamila, bishop of Palermo and author of the authoritative embryological text *Sacred Embryology* (Palermo, 1745), dismissed preformationist claims, favouring instead an epigenetic account of generation (Martínez 197; Cangiamila; de Demerson; Laguña; Rodriguez).[9] He specifically credited recent scientific discoveries made by Antonie van Leeuwenhoek and Nicolaas Hartsoek in microbiology as "open[ing] the way to false opinion," favouring instead the work of Caspar Friedrich Wolff's epigenetic studies (Cangiamila 22).[10] To Cangiamila, certain fixed theological doctrines formed parameters within which to conceptualize new scientific knowledge and to help to choose between models when scientific theories suffered from underdetermination (Quine). On the basis of new embryological discoveries, Cangiamila and many other Catholic authorities rejected the Aristotelian opinions of many patristic and scholastic authorities that the final animation of the fetus occurred at the fortieth day of gestation in males and the eightieth in females (Cangiamila 22; Aristotle; Jones 27). Ultimately, he concluded that, given the motion and development of the fetus as proven by natural philosophers, the animation of the soul must occur earlier than the ancients anticipated.[11] Moreover, he reaffirmed the established doctrine that "rational souls do not exist before the creation of bodies ... but in what precise time it is, one does not know" (Cangiamila 22).[12] Cangiamila supposed that the wisest position was to argue for the earliest moment of ensoulment possible. This uncertainty did not stop Spanish theologians from ruminating about rival theories of ensoulment or animation. When they did, they nearly always invoked the testimony of the natural sciences to inform and support their postulations.[13]

Theologically Motivated Science: Intrauterine Baptisms

Continual discoveries in microscopy therefore resulted in philosophical reconsiderations regarding theories of generation and theological ideas about ensoulment and animation. The theological and philosophical conversations reaffirming early ensoulment not only directly led to increased attention to embryonic development but also created an imperative impulse to develop obstetric practices that would help to rescue and save these souls. Having reaffirmed the presence of a soul in the fetus at an indeterminate but early point, theologians next cooperated with physicians to discuss a grave issue: what could be done to administer baptism to those fetuses that were in danger of dying during pregnancy, as the result of a "bad birth" or in the case of the mother's death. Baptism, according to the magisterial teaching of the Church, was a sacramental requirement for salvation. Moreover, sacramental theology dictated that the holy water used in baptism come into direct contact with a living recipient. De la Asumpción wrote that "it is indispensable that the material, which is ordinary, natural or elemental water ... should immediately touch the subject" (de la Asumpción 69).[14]

The challenge, therefore, was to ensure that holy water could encounter a fetus, either within the womb or once removed whilst living. The idea of intrauterine baptisms answered the first half of this challenge, while the development of caesarean operations responded to the second. In his *New Aspect of Medico-Moral Theology* (Zaragoza,

1742), Antonio José Rodríguez, a Cistercian theologian and member of both the Royal Academy of Madrid and the Royal Society of Sciences of Seville, provided the simple answer to this theological quandary (Rodríguez, *Nuevo Aspecto I*). "The means," he wrote, "is with some syringes, guided by hand until they encounter the little body, and thus they disperse the water" (Rodríguez, *Nuevo Aspecto I* 89).[15] Rodríguez was aware that affirming that the sacrament of baptism could legitimately be performed in utero was contrary to a vast and hefty corpus of ecclesiastical authority and tradition, including the teachings of important theologians such as Thomas Aquinas and Francisco Suarez. It was an apparent contradiction to the testimony of scripture and went against the instruction of the codified seventeenth-century Roman Rite as outlined following the Council of Trent (1545–63). Rodríguez, knowledgeable about both obstetrics and sacred theology, performed skilled theological manoeuvring to articulate his position.

Rodríguez dismissed the first of these objections quickly by rereading and reinterpreting the intent of previous generations. Past theologians had spoken against intrauterine baptisms, "supposing that the fetus was enclosed, [and] that it was impossible to be touched by the water of Baptism" (Rodríguez, *Nuevo Aspecto I* 91).[16] If these theological authorities had known that it was possible for the water to reach the body of the fetus, Rodríguez argued, they would have had no complaint. New surgical and anatomical knowledge had gifted obstetrics the ability to effectively reach the infant in utero with water. Indeed, the procedure that Rodríguez recommended even bypassed the objection of some theologians that the water would ineffectively baptize only the caul, not the infant. He wrote that

> Surgeons and Midwives should know the means and instrument: [the instrument] is reduced to a syringe with a long nose and not too narrow; the way is to first break the caul, if they have not already been [broken], until [one can] surely touch the fetus with the hand ... to introduce the syringe full of water with the same hand, guiding with it the nose to the part of the fetus which will be washed, and having assured that the nose [of the syringe] and the same introduced hand touch the fetus on the head, or body, empty the syringe, saying at the same time as the release the form: *I baptize you in the name of the Father, and of the Son, and of the Holy Spirit.* (Rodríguez, *Nuevo Aspecto I* 96)[17]

The second, "stronger argument" against intrauterine baptisms was that many commentators of the Bible had noted that baptism, a "rebirth" (*renacimiento*), could not occur unless the subject had been already born once, pointing, for example, to Christ's affirmation of the necessity of baptism in his lesson to Nicodemus in John 3:3. From this, expositors such as Augustine had concluded that "no one can be reborn, without first being born" (Rodríguez, *Nuevo Aspecto I* 92–3). This contradiction, Rodríguez asserted, was only due to an equivocation of two terms – *natus/natum*, or "born," and *genitus/genitum*, or "begotten/created." He noted, for example, that many theologians, including Aquinas, were inconsistent with their description of baptism as alternatively "rebirth" (*renacimiento*) and "regeneration" (*regeneración*) (Rodríguez, *Nuevo Aspecto I* 93). Rodríguez pointed to an angelic message to Joseph referenced in the Gospel of Matthew, in which Mary's unborn child is described as "born [*natum*] ... of the Holy Spirit" (Matt. 1:20b), Rodríguez thus concluded that *natum* was often used as a shorthand for *genitum* in the Vulgate, comparing it to the Syriac, Arabic, and Greek versions available to him, all of which used *genitus* rather than *natus* (Rodríguez, *Nuevo Aspecto I* 95). Therefore, according to Rodríguez, a fetus was eligible for the "regeneration" of baptism, because even though it was unborn, it was created or begotten.

Lastly, Rodríguez had to address the seemingly incontrovertible directive of the Roman Ritual, which proclaimed that "No one enclosed in the mother's womb should be baptized" (Rodríguez, *Nuevo Aspecto I* 95).[18] Here, Rodríguez was reduced to fine semantics – "In the case in which we are [discussing], one is not found *enclosed*, but only detained" (Rodríguez, *Nuevo Aspecto I* 95).[19] Citing the work of the Italian theologian and canon lawyer Giacomo Pignatelli (1625–98), Rodríguez claimed that "one cannot properly call 'locked in a prison' that which is at the door – and at an open door" (Rodríguez, *Nuevo Aspecto I* 95; Pignatelli).[20] New obstetrical skill and anatomical knowledge had opened this previously closed door to theology, illuminating the way to new theological conceptions.[21] In this case, medical knowledge had led Rodríguez to not only reconceptualize a theological position, but to do so by reinterpreting magisterial teaching, reassessing the intent of traditional authorities, and rereading scriptural testimony. Rodríguez, motivated by a theological telos, urged that obstetrical surgeons and midwives be trained for the intrauterine baptismal procedure.

Cangiamila, who published his *Sacred Embryology* in the same year that Rodríguez wrote the *New Aspect*, likewise affirmed the validity of such baptisms, and he advocated for the adoption and development of the procedure by the medical community.[22] Cangiamila supported Rodríguez's claim that the major resistance by the Church to intrauterine baptisms was that a child, "wrapped in two membranes" within the womb, was incapable of being effectively reached by water (Cangiamila 160).[23]

However, since the fetus often broke these membranes in the violence of the uterine contractions or with the help of a midwife, it was quite possible to remove these barriers to baptism. "It is certain," Cangiamila concluded, "that one can physically baptize the child, as all the Doctors and Surgeons today feel" (Cangiamila 160).[24] Although there is no evidence that Cangiamila and Rodríguez knew of each other's works, Cangiamila, like Rodríguez, employed a hermeneutical approach to John 3:3 that interpreted "born" (*nacido*) as "conceived."[25] Unlike Rodríguez, Cangiamila reserved the use of a syringe for only the most difficult cases, suggesting that one could simply cup the sacramental water in one's hand or use a moistened sponge (Cangiamila 160). Summarizing his position, Cangiamila noted that the same Roman Rite that prohibited intrauterine baptisms commanded that a baptism should be immediately performed should the infant's head or any other member become present outside of the womb. "Why, therefore, should it be baptized?" Cangiamila asked, writing that, "Without a doubt ... it is because it has ... shown enough of itself to be able to be baptized" (Cangiamila 171).[26] Because of increased obstetrical knowledge, particularly with midwives, the threshold of possibility had been widened to allow for new procedures. According to Cangiamila, "One can practice [it] physically, so it makes it that [this] baptism should be theologically valid" (Cangiamila 162).[27]

Cangiamila and Rodríguez's work greatly impacted the intellectual circles of the Spanish Empire. Both were the inspiration for at least five major treatises in colonial Latin America on the subject of post-mortem caesarean sections and the importance of fetal baptism, published in Guatemala, Peru, Mexico, and Alta California (Lazcano; Laguña; Iturbide; A.J. Rodríguez; Cook).[28] Rodríguez, in particular, gained the attention of Benito Jerónimo Feijóo (1676–1764), the prolific priest-philosopher whose vast oeuvre and encyclopaedic scope earned him the epithet of the "father of the Spanish enlightenment" (Payne; Ewalt 195). Although Feijóo, as a rhetorical device, named neither Antonio José Rodríguez nor the *New Aspect*, there can be little doubt that his essay "On Some Points of Moral Theology," was written in response to Rodríguez, as he references both the subjects and passage numbers that correspond to the *New Aspect* (Feijóo).[29] Feijóo wrote that Rodríguez "without a doubt" proved that "contact is possible and easy" with the fetus (Feijóo).[30] Beyond this point, however, Feijóo countered nearly every claim Rodríguez made. First, Feijóo argued that Rodríguez's definition of *natus* as "regeneration" was unsubstantiated by the original Greek. Secondly, Feijóo objected to the idea that the Tridentine authorities and previous theologians had equivocated by using "regeneration" and "rebirth" interchangeably. They did so, according to Feijóo, because "it really is one and the other" (Feijóo).[31] The authoritative definition of baptism, Feijóo claimed, was that it was simultaneously both regeneration and rebirth. For this reason, Feijóo was piqued by Rodríguez's suggestion that Aquinas, one of the most skilled logicians of the Church, could have erred in his constructions of syllogisms by his use of a variable term. If, supposed Feijóo, Aquinas had meant "regeneration" by the term "rebirth," then the consequent forbidding intrauterine baptisms would become "the most fatuous syllogism which I have ever heard" (Feijóo).[32]

Thus, Feijóo found Rodríguez's abandonment of traditional theological sources of authority overhasty. Rather than declaring intrauterine baptisms valid or invalid, however, Feijóo suggested that such baptisms be performed conditionally (*sub conditione*) – that is, that the ritual language ought to specify that the sacrament was only effective under certain conditions. This, according to Feijóó, was more consistent with the teachings of the Church and with the practices of priests outside of Spain. Although Rodríguez had claimed that the medical and theological professionals in Paris regularly performed intrauterine baptisms, Feijóo contradicted him. "The Author," Feijóo wrote, "is very badly informed"; the pronouncement, rather than "I baptize you," would, according to Feijóo, have begun conditionally with "If you are able, I baptize you" (Feijóo)[33] Although Feijóo was one of the most popular polemicists of the eighteenth-century Hispanic republic of letters, there is some indication that his position of *sub conditione* baptisms in utero became the default practice advocated by some treatises (Lazcano 99–201). Given the amount of literature subsequently published on the importance of caesarean sections for living and deceased unborn children, most theologians remained deeply disturbed and driven by the unsaved status of a fetus's soul. By 1772, the syringed application of intrauterine baptisms had become well known and frequently employed (de la Asumpción 74). Yet this procedure was insufficient, for, as theologians such as Cangiamila noted, there were complications in birth in which "there is no way to baptize the child, nor to free the mother" (Cangiamila 161).[34] In such cases, theologians, for the sake of saving the souls and lives of both mother and child, urged that obstetrical surgeons, physicians, and midwives develop the practice of caesarean operations (Cangiamila; Rigau-Pérez; de Demerson; Valle; Warren, "An Operation for Evangelization"; Few).[35]

The Cyclical Dialogue between Science and Theology

These developments in caesarean operations and intrauterine baptisms, themselves driven by theological concerns, raised new theological queries, and the conversation between the natural sciences and philosophy and theology thus became cyclical. For example, de la Asumpción challenged theologians to consider the case of a pregnant woman, unable to undergo a caesarean section or to suffer an intrauterine baptism. Again, the limits of natural knowledge prompted theological re-evaluation and assessment. "Consider," he wrote, "the human fetus ... in which it is absolutely not possible to touch it nor to reach it by human means in order to administer baptism to it ... [where it] is physically or morally impossible to introduce the hand or other instrument that assures or makes probable the ability of the water to immediately touch the body of the fetus" (de la Asumpción 69–70).[36] Here, natural and scientific knowledge would not allow for baptism, yet theological doctrine insisted that a baptism needed to occur to save the unborn child. In these circumstances, de la Asumpción proposed a doctrine earlier advanced by Ignacio Luis Bianchi that suggested the mother should name the child and entrust it to God with a prayer, relying on "Divine mercy" (de la Asumpción 73; Bianchi; Pallavicino).[37] Such a theological stance was uncomfortably close to heterodox positions that depreciated the essential nature of baptism and was a theological corner into which de la Asumpción backed reluctantly. Still, he asserted that "at first glance it seems a bit dangerous and difficult, [but] it is certainly pious and very conformed to the spirit of the Holy Scriptures, of the Holy Fathers, and Councils" (de la Asumpción 70).[38] His position was reached after considering the theological doctrine of traditional sources of authority and the limitations of the most cutting-edge obstetrical procedures, which were themselves motivated by a theological and moral imperative to save souls.

The dialogue between science and theology did not occur as frequently nor was it as widespread as many would have wished. De la Asumpción complained in his address to the Royal Society of Medicine in Seville that the fields of embryology and obstetrics were hampered by a lack of effective communication in which he blamed theologians and physicians alike. He wrote condemningly that

> Since this controversy started to become public, the suppositions which have become muddled in it, the new lights which have been lent by the advanced Anatomy and Obstetric art ... One cannot refrain from looking with disdain at the confidence with which some Systematics [theologians] still pretend to enforce contrary doctrine, criticizing as of little importance

> the resources which they have taken from the aforementioned Arts for their Theological decision ... without [these] sources and notices, the subject would still be living in the chaos of irresolution ... Oh, how I wish the day would arrive when the Courts would take account, and no Doctor, Surgeon, or Midwife would be approved without having given on this important moral point of their practice! (de la Asumpción 74–5)[39]

In this lament, de la Asumpción affirmed that Spanish theologians had relied upon anatomical and obstetrical advancements to make decisions and yet depreciated their importance; similarly, however, he fervently wished that medical professionals would take greater notice of the theological and moral dimensions of their work. For every Rodríguez and Cangiamila, it appears that there were far more theologians and physicians who persisted in their own opinions, working myopically within their own sphere.

Getting Back to Basics: Taking Theology Seriously in the Eighteenth-Century Hispanic World

It is important to understand that the motivation given by these authors for the development of intrauterine baptisms was fundamentally theological. As Adam Warren has rightly argued for the development of post-mortem caesarean operations in eighteenth-century Peru, it was "an operation for evangelization" that resulted in a new field of "priestly surgery" (Warren, "An Operation for Evangelization" 673). The development of procedures such as intrauterine baptisms and caesarean operations certainly had other ramifications, for example, in marginalizing the role of midwives (Ortiz). It is worthwhile, however, to study how the religious beliefs of these authors grounded their production of scientific and medical knowledge by providing parameters for their epistemology, methods, and practices.

The examples of Rodríguez, de la Asumpción, and Cangiamila reinforce this point. It is impossible to understand the public policies promoted by the Protomedicato or the reforms that took place within surgical colleges and universities without understanding the epistemic model that Spanish intellectuals had. This model, as seen in the case study of sacred embryology, was one which posited that theology and the natural sciences, although distinct fields of knowledge, were two territories that were in constant relation and dialogue with one another – indeed, that *ought* to be integrated. Science could expand the knowledge of the natural world, opening new possibilities or defining natural limitations that could prompt theological reconsideration and reflection. This occurred, for example, when embryological studies invited the reassessment of preformationism and ensoulment. Advances made in the natural sciences could even be convincing enough to question and destabilize long-standing religious authorities, as was the case when Rodríguez reinterpreted traditional religious teachings in favour of intrauterine baptisms. The relationship was mutual, however, and theology impacted scientific practice regularly. Theology inspired and created motivation for scientific enquiry and practices, as when the theological aim of saving souls and lives stirred interest in intrauterine baptisms. Theological considerations could also act as an arbiter between equally undetermined scientific theories, for example, between preformationists and epigenesists on the generation of the soul. Moreover, theology provided an overarching conceptual and moral backdrop in which the medical and scientific professions could exist. To understand the eighteenth-century Hispanic world, indeed, to understand the early modern mind "on its own terms," the fundamental relationship between science and theology must be explored. The example of Spanish embryology suggests some models that historians of science and religion can use to understand the way that the early modern mind viewed the relationship between these two fields. One analogy in the eighteenth century borrowed from Augustine's notions of "two books" – that is, that God revealed truth in two principle formats: the book of Nature, and the book of Scripture. In the Hispanic world, these books were *tête-bêche*, twin-bound, and meant to be read in conjunction. Within embryological discussions, one author, writing on ensoulment, stated that "All are interested in the subject ... the point is without a doubt Physical, but it has a lot of connections with the Theological" (Custodio 4).[40] Cangiamila's description of his subject of study as "sacred embryology" was, then, aptly named. The fields of natural philosophy and theology existed in an inextricably close epistemic relationship in eighteenth-century Spain.

At the same time, Rodríguez described science and theology as distinct epistemic areas, noting that they "ask to be treated separately ... there is a point that is only incumbent for Medicine to solve, and outside of this, there is another within the same case which Theology must solve" (Rodríguez, *Nuevo Aspecto I* 114).[41] Rodríguez conceived of the faculties of Medicine and Theology as separate entities that had their own problems to answer. In the case of sacred embryology, Medicine could determine whether a procedure was feasible or possible, while Theology could answer if such a procedure was morally required or permissible. The model of an integrative dialogue between two distinct fields, as described by scholar Ian Barbour, seems appropriate for describing the way in which science and theology engaged one another in the early modern world (Griffin; Cantor and Kenny). Ultimately, these models, crafted and imposed upon the past, are unable to wholly account for the historical mentality, but they remain useful lenses for interpreting and understanding early modernity. Likewise, the historical testimony of sacred embryology in the eighteenth-century Hispanic world may suggest new possible ways in which contemporary theologians and scientists may reconceptualize the relationship between these two fields.

A Gendered Perspective on Intrauterine Baptisms

In a volume of essays exploring health practices of the early modern Iberian world with a particular eye towards the application of gender as a category of analysis, it is worth noting that several scholars have argued that the development of intrauterine baptisms and caesarean sections accelerated the professionalization of the fields of embryology, gynaecology, and obstetrics, shifting the care and supervision of female bodies by females (midwives) to male health professionals and paraprofessionals (obstetric surgeons, physicians, priests, and barbers). Following Joan Scott's assertion that "gender is a primary way of signifying relationships of power," the work of scholars such as Jaffary, Few, and Warren has demonstrated that the medicalization of obstetrics and embryology could signify a shift of power, as a field previously practised by midwives became the domain of the obstetric surgeon (Scott 1067). Indeed, Few has argued that "a woman's uterus became at once a political, religious, and medicalized space apart from the female subject, and as such an independent object of surveillance and surgical intervention" (Few 98).

This is more clearly seen with the development of post-mortem caesarean sections, especially following the royal *cedula* (pragmatic command) of Charles IV in 1804 mandating the performance of such operations (Rigau-Pérez; Warren, "An Operation for Evangelization"; Few). For intrauterine baptisms, however, the pregnant mother was alive and an important part of the medical considerations. Moreover, despite the increased attention of male medical professionals, the role of the midwife continued to have an important role, particularly for births that experienced no complications. Both Rodríguez and de la Asumpción specifically expressed the view that midwives should learn and understand their instructions regarding intrauterine baptisms (Rodríguez, *Nuevo Aspecto I* 96; de la Asumpción 74–5). Previous theologians had affirmed that it was the privilege of the pregnant woman "to choose one or another midwife for the good success of the birth," as well as the wet nurse or nanny of the child (Fontecha; Usera et al. 110), and the testimony of numerous birthing treatises attest to the fact that the midwife (*comadre, partera*) was still a regular presence in eighteenth-century childbirths, particularly for those areas of the Spanish Empire where physicians were scarce to be found.[42] Reconstructing the testimony of these midwives remains a historical challenge, as treatises of Spanish midwifery authored by female midwives are, regrettably, non-existent.

One fruitful area of enquiry would be a detailed analysis of the vocabulary employed by birthing treatises, midwife guides, anatomical textbooks, and other medical works. Many scholars have noted, for example, the variation in word choice to describe a growing fetus in embryological literature of the period – the referent in question is alternatively labelled "creature" (*criatura*), "unborn child" (*niño no-nacido*), "enclosed child" (*niño encerrado*), fetus (*feto*), child or son (*hijo*), or in some cases, the aborted one (*aborto*). Similar attention and sensitivity could be given to the words used to describe the pregnant woman, often labelled "pregnant" (*preñada*), but just as often described anticipatorily as the "mother" (*madre*). Anatomical language also suffered this terminological instability with many authors employing "womb" (*vientre*) and "uterus" (*utero*) interchangeably. It is suggestive that the anatomist Martín Martínez defined the purpose of the uterus as "the only fertile field of generation" (Martínez 184).[43] Indeed, the terms for the uterus in Spanish (*vientre, utero, matriz*) include the word "mother" (*madre*). This is seen, for example, in Joseph Manuel Rodriguez's 1799 treatise, *The Charity of the Priest for the Enclosed Children in the Wombs of their Deceased Mothers*, when he offered as a vernacular anatomical definition: "the uterus [is] the *madre*" (J.M. Rodriguez 43).[44] Certainly, shifting understandings of what occurred in the "dark, inaccessible place ... the enigmatic space" of the womb impacted the way in which women in particular related to Hispanic society (Park 25, 35).

In medico-moral considerations, the mother was the conjunction of two (or more) individual concerns: two bodies, two souls, and two lives. Intrauterine baptisms were advocated as a means of using increased anatomical and medical knowledge to discharge the theological responsibility to care for the immortal soul of the fetus without endangering the mortal life of a woman. While most theologians agreed that a living woman was not obliged to a caesarean operation in order to baptize a child, it is unclear whether an intrauterine baptism, as a far safer procedure, was considered the moral duty of an expectant mother who experienced difficulties in pregnancy or labour. What is clear, however, is that as medical knowledge advanced about embryology and obstetrics, new theological concerns were raised and old questions re-evaluated. Within this field of "sacred embryology," defining and understanding the concept of "mother," both medically and theologically, was a central concern.

NOTES

1 All translations in this essay are my own, unless otherwise noted.
2 "Disertacion Theologica. Del Baptismo del Feto dentro del Utero ..." (de la Asumpción 66).
3 The work, Francesco Cangiamila's *Embriologia sacra* (Palermo, 1745), was printed in Latin, French, Italian, and Spanish and enjoyed multiple editions within the eighteenth century.
4 José Antonio Rodríguez defined medico-moralism in 1742 as "a parallel between two medicines: bodily and spiritual" ("paralelo entre las dos medicinas corporal, y espiritual"). This definition was "entirely prohibited" ("prohibida enteramente") by the Inquisition (Rodríguez, *Nuevo Aspecto I* 1).
5 Commonly defined, ensoulment refers to the occasion when a human is thought to receive a rational soul, while animation could refer more broadly to the motion of a human fetus, which had yet to receive the rational guidance of a human soul (for example, in the Aristotelian conception of a growing, soulless fetus until the age of forty or eighty days).
6 For further reading, consult: Lanning and *Protomedicato*; Burke; Granjel, *Real Academia* and *Medicina*; Ortiz; Pardo-Tomás and Martínez-Vidal, *The Ignorance of Midwives*; Fernández; Jaffary; Few.
7 Contrary to the "polemic of Spanish science," which has long shadowed the history of science in Spanish studies (Menéndez y Pelayo; Granjel, *Medicina*; Piñero et al.; Nieto-Galan).
8 There were many theories regarding fetal development in early modern medicine. Preformationism, the idea that humans (as well as other living things) grew from smaller versions of themselves in perfect, miniscule proportion, and epigenesis, the idea that organisms grew from an embryo dissimilar to the final form that became differentiated and perfected as it grew, were two popular embryological concepts.
9 Sicily was a Spanish kingdom under the rule of Charles VII of Naples and Sicily, future king of Spain (1759–88).
10 "Las observaciones microscópicas de Lowehoek y de Hartzoeker sobre los animales, han abierto el camino á esta falsa opinion" (Cangiamila 22).
11 Even in translated editions, this section on generation was deliberately written in Latin, "as this chapter [VIII] should explain so delicate a matter" (Cangiamila 28; see also McClelland).
12 "las almas racionales no existian antes de la creacion de los cuerpos. Es indubitable que el alma es criada para cada cuerpo quando está todavía

en el seno de su madre, pero en qué tiempo preciso sea esto, no se sabe" (Cangiamila 22).

13 See, for example, the debates following Manuel Custodio's 1779 publication (Custodio 3; Santiago; Alvarez and Teresa 222).

14 "es indispensable, que la materia, que es el agua usual, natural, ò elemental ... deben tocar inmediatamente al sujeto" (de la Asumpción, 69)

15 "El modo es, con unas geringuillas, guiadas con la mano, hasta encontrar el cuerpecito, y entonces disparar el agua" (Rodríguez, *Nuevo Aspecto I* 89).

16 "suponiendo, que el feto por su clausura, esta impossibilitado a ser tocado por el agua del Baptismo" (Rodríguez, *Nuevo Aspecto I* 91).

17 "que los Cirujanos, y Parteras sepan el modo, y el instrumento: este se reduce à una geringuilla de pico largo, y no muy estrecho: el modo es, romper lo primero las secundinas, si yà no lo estan, hasta tocar seguramente el feto con la mano ... introducir la geringa llena de agua con la misma mano, guiando con ella el pico à la parte del feto que se ha de lavar; y en haviendose asegurado, que el pico, y la misma mano introductora tocan al feto en cabeza, ò cuerpo, descargar la geringa, diciendo al mismo tiempo del disparo la forma: *Yo te baptizo en el nombre del Padre, y del Hijo, y del Espiritu Santo*" (Rodríguez, *Nuevo Aspecto I* 96).

18 "*Nemo in utero matris clausus baptizari debet, &c*" (Rodríguez, *Nuevo Aspecto I* 95).

19 "porque en el caso en que estamos, no se halla *cerrado*, sino detenido" (Rodríguez, *Nuevo Aspecto I* 95).

20 "no se puede llamar con propriedad cerrado en la carcel el que esta en la puerta, y la puerta abierta" (Rodríguez, *Nuevo Aspecto I* 95).

21 Although Benedict XIV reformed the Roman Ritual in 1752, the prohibition to which Rodríguez referred, "Nemo in utero matris clausus baptizari debet," remained unchanged (Benedict XIV; Baruffaldi). Cangiamila stated that Benedict XIV "is of this opinion," but provided no concrete references to support this claim (Cangiamila; Rodríguez, *Nuevo Aspecto IV* 138).

22 His work was explicitly addressed to "priests, confessors, doctors, midwives, and other persons for the cooperation for the salvation of children who are not yet born"(Cangiamila title page).

23 "envuelto en dos membranas" (Cangiamila 160).

24 "es cierto que se puede bautizar físicamente el niño, como lo sienten el dia de hoy todos los Médicos y Cirujanos" (Cangiamila 160).

25 He provided the original Greek in his textual analysis: "El primer verbo τ[ὸ] γεγεννημενον puede significar no solamente, *nacido*, sino también, *hecho, engendrado, formado, concebido*" (Cangiamila 168). This is contradictory to Feijóo's claims in his work, *Cartas Eruditas II (1773)*, Carta XXVII §49.

26 "¿Porqué, pues, se le bautiza? Sin duda ... porque ha empezado ya á manifestarse lo que basta para poder ser bautizado en alguna parte de su cuerpo" (Cangiamila 171).

27 "se puede practicar físicamente, hace que el bautismo sea teológicamente válido" (Cangiamila 162).

28 This essay has examined all of these works except Pedro Mariano Iturbide's, the only extant copy of which can be found in the Museo del Libro, Antigua, Guatemala (Few 101).

29 There is nothing to suggest that Feijóo had read Cangiamila's work at this time.

30 "el Autor impugna sin duda eficacísimamente, haciendo ver, que este contacto es posible, y fácil" (Feijóo, §45).

31 "Realmente es uno, y otro" (Feijóo §50).

32 "sale el silogismo más fatuo, que jamás se oyó en las Aulas" (Feijóo §56).

33 "que el Autor está muy mal informado ... es constante, y universal en París la práctica de la forma condicional concebida en esta voces: *Si eres capaz, yo te bautizo en el nombre del Padre*" (Feijóo §62).

34 "entonces no hay camino alguno para bautizar al niño, ni para librar á la madre, sino por medio de la operación cesárea" (Cangiamila 161–2).

35 Nearly all of the research on caesarean sections focuses exclusively on post-mortem operations. My research has indicated that by the end of the eighteenth century, a shift was occurring in the medical community that gradually favoured the use of caesarean operations. Like intrauterine baptisms, theologians were instrumental in popularizing and encouraging the development of caesarean sections in Spain, both on living patients and as a post-mortem operation designed to save fetuses whose mothers died. Though this procedure was developed in the Spanish world in tandem with intrauterine baptisms, this essay, for the purpose of scope, is concerned only with the latter.

36 "Considera al feto humano dentro del claustro materno en varios estados: uno, en que absolutamente no se puede tocar, ni alcanzar por medio humano, para administrarle el baptismo ... es physica, ó moralmente imposible introducir la mano, ú otro instrumento, que segure, ò probabilize, poder el agua tocar inmediatamente al cuerpo del feto" (de la Asumpción 69–70).

37 "misericordia Divinia" (de la Asumpción 73).

38 "à primera vista parece algo espínosa, y dificil; es ciertamente piadosa, mui conforme al espíritu de las Santas Escripturas, de los Santos Padres, y Concilios" (de la Asumpción 70).

39 "Si se examina el tiempo, que ha corrido desde que empezo à ventilarse esta controversia; las suposiciones, que en ella se mezclan; las nuevas lueces, que le ha prestado lo adelantado de la Anatomia, y arte Obstetricia; el christiano, y fervoroso empeño, con que han sostenido la parte afirmativa los mas insignes Theologos del siglo pasado, y actual; el zelo, y aplicacion, con que varios Prelados han mandado su observancia; y la certeza practica, con que se executa muchos años hà; no puede dejar de mirarse con algun desden la confianza, con que algunos

Systematicos aùn pretenden esforzar la doctrina contraria; criticando de poco importantes los recursos, que se han tomado à las Artes referidas para la decisión Theologica: siendo indisputable, y cierto, que sin sus fundamentos, y noticias, aun subsistiría la materia en el Caos de la irresolución ... ¡Ojala llegue el dia de tomarlo los Tribunales por su quenta, y que no se aprueben Medico, Cirujano, ni Comadre, sin que dèn razón de este importante ramo moral de su practica" (de la Asumpción 74–5).

40 "Todos son interesados en la materia ... El punto es sin duda Fisico; pero de mucho enlace con lo Teologico" (Custodio 4).

41 "Hay en él dos partes, que siendo distintas, piden tratarse con separacion, y hacer que conste á todos que se distinguen, para que la confusión entre ellas no haga precipitar las resoluciones. Una pertence á la facultad Médica, otra á la Teología. Esto es, hay un punto, que solo incumbe á la Medicina resolverlo; y fuera de este, hay otra dentro del mismo caso, que debe resolverlo la Teología" (Rodríguez, *Nuevo Aspecto I* 114).

42 "Previlegio octavo ... la preñada puede elegir esta, o la otra comadre, para el buen successo del parto" (Fontecha xv).

43 "El primero, y principal uso del Utero es, ser único, y fecundo campo de la generacion" (Martínez 184).

44 "*Utero*: la madre" (Rodríguez, *Nuevo aspecto I* 43).

WORKS CITED

Allotey, Janette C. "English Midwives' Responses to the Medicalisation of Childbirth (1671–1795)." *Midwifery*, vol. 27, no. 4, Aug. 2011, pp. 532–8.

Alvarez, Cristina Gómez, and Guillermo Tovar de Teresa. *Censura y revolución: Libros prohibidos por la Inquisición de México (1790–1819)*. Trama Editorial, 2009.

Aristotle. *Aristotle's History of Animals: In Ten Books*. Edited by Richard Cresswell, George Bell and Sons, 1897. http://archive.org/details/aristotleshisto00schngoog.

Baruffaldi, Girolamo. *Ad rituale romanum commentaria*. Editio altera Veneta, Aucta [et] à mendis expurgata cum indice locupletissimo., Ex Typographia Balleoniana, 1752. http://hdl.handle.net/2027/ucm.5319068813.

Benedict XIV. *Rituale romanum, caeremoniale episcoporum ac pontificale romanum*. Giovanni Generoso Salomoni, 1752. https://hdl.handle.net/2027/ucm.531797663x?urlappend=%3Bseq=5.

Bianchi, Ignacio Luis. *De remedio aeternae salutis pro parvulis in utero clausis sine baptismate morientibus*. s.n., 1768.

Burke, Michael E. *The Royal College of San Carlos: Surgery and Spanish Medical Reform in the Late Eighteenth Century*. Duke UP, 1977.

Cangiamila, Francesco. *Embriologia sagrada, o tratado de oa Obligacion que tienen los curas, confesores, médicos ... de cooperar á la salvacion de los niños que aun no han nacido*. Translated by Joaquín Castellot, La Imprenta de Pedro Marin, 1774. http://hdl.handle.net/2027/ucm.5310802280.

Cantor, Geoffrey, and Chris Kenny. "Barbour's Fourfold Way: Problems with His Taxonomy of Science-Religion Relationships." *Zygon: Journal of Religion and Science*, vol. 36, no. 4, Dec. 2001, pp. 765–81.

Cook, Sherburne F. "Sarría's Treatise on the Cesarean Operation, 1830." *California and Western Medicine*, vol. 47, no. 2, Aug. 1937, pp. 107–9.

Custodio, Manuel. *Disertacion fisico-teologica, en que se establece el preciso instante de la animación racional del feto en el cuerpo humano*. Josef Padrino, 1779. http://hdl.handle.net/2027/ucm.531654100x.

de Demerson, Paula. "La cesarea post mortem en la España de la Ilustración." *Asclepio: Revista de historia de la medicina y de la ciencia*, vol. 28, 1976, pp. 185–233.

de la Asumpción, Vicente. "Disertacion theologica: Del baptismo del feto dentro del utero." *Memorias académicas de la Real Sociedad de Medicina y Demás Ciencias de Sevilla*, edited by Bonifacio Juan Ximenez de Lorite, vol. 2, Impreso en casa de D. Eugenio Sanchez Reciente, 1772. https://hdl.handle.net/2027/ucm.5326679020?urlappend=%3Bseq=106.

Ewalt, Margaret R. *Peripheral Wonders: Nature, Knowledge, and Enlightenment in the Eighteenth-Century Orinoco*. Bucknell UP, 2008.

Feijóo, Benito Jerónimo. *Cartas eruditas y curiosas*. 1777 reprint, vol. I, carta XXVII, en la Imprenta Real de la Gazeta, 1777. http://www.filosofia.org/bjf/bjfc227.htm#c227.

Fernández, Enrique. "Tres testimonios del control y desplazamiento de las comadronas en España (siglos XIII al XVII)." *Revista Canadiense de Estudios Hispánicos*, vol. 32, no. 1, 2007, pp. 89–104.

Few, Martha. *For All of Humanity: Mesoamerican and Colonial Medicine in Enlightenment Guatemala*. U of Arizona P, 2015.

Fontecha, Juan-Alonso de. *Diez previlegios para mugeres prenadas*. Luys Martynez Grande, 1606.

Granjel, Luis S. *Historia de la Real Academia Nacional de Medicina*. Real Academia Nacional de Medicina, 2006.

– *La medicina española del siglo XVIII*. Ediciones Universidad de Salamanca, 1979.

Griffin, David Ray. "On Ian Barbour's Issues in Science and Religion." *Zygon: Journal of Religion and Science*, vol. 23, no. 1, Mar. 1988, pp. 57–81.

Hervás y Panduro, Lorenzo. *El hombre físico, o Anatomia humana fisico-filosofica*. Vol. I, En la Imprenta de la Administracion del Real Arbitrio de Beneficencia, 1800.

Iturbide, Pedro Mariano. *Breve y diminuto compendio de la obligación que hay de bautizar los fetos*. Oficina de Don Ignacio Beteta, 1788. Museo del Libro, Antigua, Guatemala, fol. 23.

Jaffary, Nora E. *Reproduction and Its Discontents in Mexico: Childbirth and Contraception from 1750 to 1905*. U of North Carolina P, 2016.

Johnson, Rhi. "Birthing an Epistemological Shift: The Discursive Function of Eighteenth-Century Obstetrics Manuals." *Dieciocho: Hispanic Enlightenment*, vol. 39, no. 1, 2016, pp. 83–106.

Jones, David Albert. *The Soul of the Embryo: Christianity and the Human Embryo*. Continuum, 2004.

Laguña, Francisco González. *El zelo sacerdotal para con los niños no-nacidos*. En la imprenta de los Niños Expositos, 1781. http://archive.org/details/9317877.nlm.nih.gov.

Lanning, John Tate. *Academic Culture in the Spanish Colonies*. Oxford UP, 1940.

– *The Royal Protomedicato: The Regulation of the Medical Profession in the Spanish Empire*. Edited by John Jay TePaske, Duke UP, 1985.

Laursen, John Christian. "Medicine and Skepticism: Martín Martínez (1684–1734)." *The Return of Scepticism: From Hobbes and Descartes to Bayle*, edited by Gianni Paganini, Springer Science + Business Media, 2003, pp. 305–26.

Lazcano, Francisco Xavier. *Indice practico moral, para los sacerdotes, que auxilian moribundos*. En la Imprenta del Colegio Rl. de S. Ildefonso, 1754. John Carter Brown Library. http://archive.org/details/indicepracticomo00lazc.

Maienschein, Jane. "Epigenesis and Preformationism." *The Stanford Encyclopedia of Philosophy*, edited by Edward N. Zalta, Spring 2017. *Stanford Encyclopedia of Philosophy*, https://plato.stanford.edu/archives/spr2017/entries/epigenesis/.

Martínez, Martín. *Anatomia completa el hombre, con todos los hallazgos, nuevas doctrinas y observaciones raras hasta el tiempo presente, y muchas advertencias necessarias para la cirugia: Segun el methodo con que se explica en nuestro theatro de Madrid*. En la Imprenta Real, por Don Miguel Francisco Rodriguez, 1745. http://hdl.handle.net/2027/ucm.5325111688.

Martínez-Vidal, Àlvar, and José Pardo-Tomás. "Anatomical Theatres and the Teaching of Anatomy in Early Modern Spain." *Medical History*, vol. 49, no. 3, July 2005, pp. 251–80.

McClelland, Ivy Lilian. *Ideological Hesitancy in Spain 1700–1750*. Liverpool UP, 1991.

Menéndez y Pelayo, Marcelino. *La ciencia española : Polémicas, indicaciones y proyectos*. 1879. www.cervantesvirtual.com; http://www.cervantesvirtual.com/obra-visor/la-ciencia-espanola-polemicas-indicaciones-y-proyectos--0/html/.

Nieto-Galán, Agustí. "The Images of Science in Modern Spain." *The Sciences in the European Periphery during the Enlightenment (New Studies in the History and Philosophy of Science and Technology)*, edited by K. Gavroglu, vol. 2, Springer, 1999, pp. 73–94.

Ortiz, Teresa. "From Hegemony to Subordination: Midwives in Early Modern Spain." *The Art of Midwifery: Early Modern Midwives in Europe*, edited by Hilary Marland, Routledge, 1993, pp. 95–114.

Pagden, Anthony. "The Reception of the 'New Philosophy' in Eighteenth-Century Spain." *Journal of the Warburg and Courtauld Institutes*, vol. 51, 1988, pp. 126–40.

Pallavicino, Sforza. *Istoria del Concilio di Trento*. Vol. 3, Tipografia della Minerva ticinese, 1836.

Pardo-Tomás, J., and A. Martínez-Vidal. "In tenebris adhuc versantes. The Response of Spanish Novatores to the Invective by Pierre Régis." *Dynamis (Granada, Spain)*, vol. 15, 1995, pp. 301–40.

Pardo-Tomás, José, and Àlvar Martínez-Vidal. *The Ignorance of Midwives: The Role of Clergymen in Spanish Enlightenment Debates on Birth Care*. 2007.

– "Medicine and the Spanish Novator Movement: Ancients vs. Moderns, and Beyond." *Beyond the Black Legend: Spain and the Scientific Revolution/Mas allá de la leyenda negra: España y la revolución científica*, edited by William Eamon and Victor Navarro Brotóns, Universidad de Valéncia, 2007, pp. 323–46.

– Park, Katharine. *Secrets of Women: Gender, Generation, and the Origins of Human Dissection*. Zone Books, 2010.

Payne, Stanley G. *A History of Spain and Portugal*. Vol. 2, U of Wisconsin P, 1973.

Pignatelli, Giacomo. *Consultationes canonicae, in quibus praecipuae controversiae* ... Vol. 1, sumptibus Gabrielis [et] Samuelis de Tournes, 1700. Piñero, José María López, et al. "Selección bibliográfica de estudios sobre la ciencia en la España de los siglo XVI y XVII." *Anthropos: Boletín de información y documentación*, no. 20, 1982, p. 28.

Quine, Willard Van Orman. "Two Dogmas of Empiricism." *The Philosophical Review*, vol. 60, 1951, pp. 20–43.

Reid, Anne Marie. *Medics of the Soul and the Body: Sickness and Death in Alta California, 1769–1850*. U of Southern California P, 2013.

Rigau-Pérez, José G. "Surgery at the Service of Theology: Postmortem Cesarean Sections in Puerto Rico and the Royal Cedula of 1804." *The Hispanic American Historical Review*, vol. 75, no. 3, Aug. 1995, pp. 377–404.

Robbins, Jeremy. *Arts of Perception: The Epistemological Mentality of the Spanish Baroque, 1580–1720*. Routledge, 2013.

Rodríguez, Antonio José. *Nuevo aspecto de theologia medico-moral y ambos drechos o paradoxas physico-theologico legales, obra ritica, provechosa a parrocos, confessors, y professors de ambos derechos, y util a medicos, philosophos, y eruditos*. Vol. I, Francisco Moreno, 1742.

– *Nuevo aspecto de theologia medico-moral y ambos drechos o Pparadoxas physico-theologico legales, obra ritica, provechosa a parrocos, confessors, y professors de ambos derechos, y util a medicos, philosophos, y eruditos*. Tercera edición (original 1769), vol. IV, Madrid, 1787. http://hdl.handle.net/2027/ucm.5320780974.

Rodriguez, Joseph Manuel. *La caridad del sacerdote para con los niños encerrados en el vientre de sus madres difuntas, y documentos de la utilidad, y necesidad de su práctica*. F. de Zuñiga y Ontiveros, 1799. http://archive.org/details/b29315499.

Rodríguez, Martha Eugenia. "Costumbres y tradiciones en torno al embarazo y al parto en el México virreinal." *Anuario de Estudios Americanos*, vol. LVII, no. 2, 2000, pp. 501–22.

Santiago, Juan Wenceslao de. *Carta censoria: Contra la disertacion del Doctor D. Manuel Custodio, que intentó establecer el preciso instante de la animacion Rracional del feto en el cuerpo humano*. En la Oficina de D. Manuèl Nicolás Vazquez y Compañia, 1780.

Scott, Joan W. "Gender: A Useful Category of Historical Analysis." *The American Historical Review*, vol. 91, no. 5, Dec. 1986, pp. 1053–75.

Usera, Gabriel, et al. *Historia bibliográfica de la medicina española, ó coleccion de las mejores obras de esta ciencia*. Vol. IV, Imprenta de la Viuda de Jordán e Hijos, 1846.

Valera Candel, Manuel, and Carlos López Fernández. "Giuseppe Cervi, Guillaume Jacobe y las relaciones entre la 'Regia Sociedad de Medicina y Demás Ciencias de Sevilla' y la 'Royal Society of London' en 1736." *Dynamis : Acta Hispanica Ad Medicinae Scientiarumque. Historiam Illustrandam*, vol. 18, 1998, pp. 377–426.

Valle, Rosemary Keupper. "The Cesarean Operation in Alta California during the Franciscan Mission Period (1769–1833)." *Bulletin of the History of Medicine*, vol. 48, no. 2, Summer 1974, pp. 265–75.

Vicente, Marta V. *Debating Sex and Gender in Eighteenth-Century Spain*. Cambridge UP, 2017.

Warren, Adam. "Between the Foreign and the Local: French Midwifery, Traditional Practitioners, and Vernacular Medical Knowledge about Childbirth in Lima, Peru." *História, Ciências, Saúde: Manguinhos*, vol. 22, no. 1, Mar. 2015, pp. 179–200.

– "An Operation for Evangelization: Friar Francisco González Laguna, the Cesarean Section, and Fetal Baptism in Late Colonial Peru." *Bulletin of the History of Medicine*, vol. 83, no. 4, Winter 2009, pp. 647–75.

– *Piety and Danger: Popular Ritual, Epidemics, and Medical Reforms in Lima, Peru, 1750–1860*. U of California P, 2004.

Contributors

Margaret E. Boyle is Associate Professor of Romance Languages and Literatures at Bowdoin College. Her research focuses on the literature and culture of early modern Spain and colonial Latin America, with particular interest in the history of gender. She is the author of the award-winning *Unruly Women: Performance, Penitence and Punishment in Early Modern Spain* (2014). She has published articles recently in postmedieval, gender and history, and *comedia* performance. For 2020, she was awarded a Fulbright Senior Scholar for Spain to be in residence at the López Piñero Institute for the History of Science and Medicine in Valéncia.

Emily Colbert Cairns is Associate Professor of Spanish in the Department of Modern Languages at Salve Regina University. She has held research fellowships at the Bancroft Library, University of California, Berkeley, in the Biblioteca Nacional in Madrid, and has worked in the archives in the Archivo Histórico Nacional in Madrid, Spain, and Newport, RI. She has published on *converso* and crypto-Jewish identity in the early modern period in *eHumanista, Chasqui, Cervantes Journal,* and *La corónica.* Her monograph *Esther in Early Modern Iberia and the Sephardic Diaspora: Queen of the Conversas* was published in 2017.

George A. Klaeren is a doctoral candidate in the Faculty of Theology and Religion at the University of Oxford. His research examines the category of natural theology in the eighteenth-century Iberian world, and he is more broadly interested in the history of knowledge in early modern Europe, especially in the Spanish Empire, and the intersection of religion, science, and magic during the long-eighteenth century. He holds a previous PhD in Early Modern European History from the University of Kansas, and his research has received support from the Fulbright Program, the American Catholic Historical Association, the John Carter Brown Library, and the Latin American and Iberian Institute of the University of New Mexico.

Kathleen M. Kole de Peralta is Assistant Professor of environmental health history at Idaho State University. Her research examines early modern Iberia and Peru to 1) capture the intrinsic and historical relationship between environment and health in urban areas; 2) demonstrate the evolution of health as a fluid, changing concept depending on the social and cultural context within which it was produced; and 3) use the digital humanities and open-access platforms to make enviro-health history accessible to English- and Spanish-speaking audiences.

Maríaluz López-Terrada is Senior Researcher (Investigadora científica) at INGENIO (CSIC-Universitat Politècnica e València). She has published more than one hundred books, articles, and book chapters on the history of science in early modern Spain. Her research focuses on the social history of medicine, particularly hospitals, medical practice, medial pluralism, and popular practice related to health and disease. She also works natural history of the same period, especially the introduction of American plants into Europe.

Patricia W. Manning is Associate Professor in the Department of Spanish and Portuguese at the University of Kansas. She has a wide range of research interests in early modern Spanish literary and cultural studies, including the *novela cortesana*, Cervantes, book and visual culture, the Inquisition, emblems, and the Society of Jesus. She has published on Jesuit departure protocols in *Renaissance and Reformation/ Renaissance et Réforme* and the *Bulletin of Spanish Studies*. Her book *Voicing Dissent in Seventeenth-Century Spain: Inquisition, Social Criticism and Theology in the Case of El Criticón* (2009) examines the manner in which clerics like Baltasar Gracián negotiated inquisitorial strictures.

Bárbara Mujica is Professor Emerita at Georgetown University. She has published and lectured widely on Teresa de Ávila and her followers, on Spanish theatre, and on women's writing. Her most recent scholarly books are *Women Writers of Early Modern Spain: Sophia's Daughters* (2004), *Teresa de Jesús: Espiritualidad y feminismo* (2006), *Teresa de Ávila, Lettered Woman* (2008), *Shakespeare and the Spanish Comedia* (ed.) (2013), and *A New Anthology of Early Modern Spanish Theater: Play and Playtext* (2014).

Sarah E. Owens is Professor of Spanish and Director of First Year Experience at the College of Charleston. She specializes in the writings of colonial and early modern Spanish nuns. Her research has taken her to the archives of Mexico, Spain, Chile, Peru, and the Vatican. She is editor and translator of the award-winning *Journey of Five Capuchin Nuns* (2009) and co-editor of the award-winning *Women of the Iberian Atlantic* (2012). Her latest book, *Nuns Navigating the Spanish Empire* (2017), was supported by a Fellowship from the National Endowment for the Humanities.

Carolin Schmitz is based at the Department of History and Philosophy of Science, University of Cambridge, where she is conducting her Wellcome Trust–funded research project on medical encounters and social order in early modern Spain (2018–2021). She holds a degree in history, Spanish philology, and ethnology (Trier, Germany), and a master in history of science and scientific communication (Valéncia, Spain). After completing her PhD on the history of the patient in early modern Spain, she held a Max Weber Fellowship at the European University Institute (2017–2018).

Karen Stolley is Professor of Spanish at Emory University. She is the author of *Domesticating Empire: Enlightenment in Spanish America* (2013) and *El lazarillo de ciegos caminantes: un itinerario crítico* (1992). She has published articles in journals including *Dieciocho, Guaranguao, Revista de Estudios Hispánicos, Latin American Literary Review*, and *Revista de crítica literaria latinoamericana*.

Sherry Velasco is Professor of early modern Spanish literature and culture in the Department of Latin American and Iberian Cultures and the Department of Gender and Sexuality Studies at the University of Southern California. She is the author of four monographs and one edited collection: *Lesbians in Early Modern Spain* (2011); *Male Delivery: Reproduction, Effeminacy, and Pregnant Men in Early Modern Spain* (2006); *The Lieutenant Nun: Transgenderism, Lesbian Desire, and Catalina de Erauso* (2000); and *Demons, Nausea and Resistance in the Autobiography of Isabel de Jesús (1611–1682)* (1996). Velasco's current book project is tentatively titled "Listening to Algerian Women and Moriscas from Spain to Algiers."

Index

Page numbers in *italics* denote illustrations or tables.

Toronto Iberic

1 Anthony J. Cascardi, *Cervantes, Literature, and the Discourse of Politics*
2 Jessica A. Boon, *The Mystical Science of the Soul: Medieval Cognition in Bernardino de Laredo's Recollection Method*
3 Susan Byrne, *Law and History in Cervantes'* Don Quixote
4 Mary E. Barnard and Frederick A. de Armas (eds), *Objects of Culture in the Literature of Imperial Spain*
5 Nil Santiáñez, *Topographies of Fascism: Habitus, Space, and Writing in Twentieth-Century Spain*
6 Nelson Orringer, *Lorca in Tune with Falla: Literary and Musical Interludes*
7 Ana M. Gómez-Bravo, *Textual Agency: Writing Culture and Social Networks in Fifteenth-Century Spain*
8 Javier Irigoyen-García, *The Spanish Arcadia: Sheep Herding, Pastoral Discourse, and Ethnicity in Early Modern Spain*
9 Stephanie Sieburth, *Survival Songs: Conchita Piquer's* Coplas *and Franco's Regime of Terror*
10 Christine Arkinstall, *Spanish Female Writers and the Freethinking Press, 1879–1926*

11 Margaret Boyle, *Unruly Women: Performance, Penitence, and Punishment in Early Modern Spain*
12 Evelina Gužauskytė, *Christopher Columbus's Naming in the* diarios *of the Four Voyages (1492–1504): A Discourse of Negotiation*
13 Mary E. Barnard, *Garcilaso de la Vega and the Material Culture of Renaissance Europe*
14 William Viestenz, *By the Grace of God: Francoist Spain and the Sacred Roots of Political Imagination*
15 Michael Scham, Lector Ludens*: The Representation of Games and Play in Cervantes*
16 Stephen Rupp, *Heroic Forms: Cervantes and the Literature of War*
17 Enrique Fernandez, *Anxieties of Interiority and Dissection in Early Modern Spain*
18 Susan Byrne, *Ficino in Spain*
19 Patricia M. Keller, *Ghostly Landscapes: Film, Photography, and the Aesthetics of Haunting in Contemporary Spanish Culture*
20 Carolyn A. Nadeau, *Food Matters: Alonso Quijano's Diet and the Discourse of Food in Early Modern Spain*
21 Cristian Berco, *From Body to Community: Venereal Disease and Society in Baroque Spain*
22 Elizabeth R. Wright, *The Epic of Juan Latino: Dilemmas of Race and Religion in Renaissance Spain*
23 Ryan D. Giles, *Inscribed Power: Amulets and Magic in Early Spanish Literature*
24 Jorge Pérez, *Confessional Cinema: Religion, Film, and Modernity in Spain's Development Years, 1960–1975*
25 Joan Ramon Resina, *Josep Pla: Seeing the World in the Form of Articles*
26 Javier Irigoyen-García, *"Moors Dressed as Moors": Clothing, Social Distinction, and Ethnicity in Early Modern Iberia*
27 Jean Dangler, *Edging toward Iberia*
28 Ryan D. Giles and Steven Wagschal (eds), *Beyond Sight: Engaging the Senses in Iberian Literatures and Cultures, 1200–1750*
29 Silvia Bermúdez, *Rocking the Boat: Migration and Race in Contemporary Spanish Music*
30 Hilaire Kallendorf, *Ambiguous Antidotes: Virtue as Vaccine for Vice in Early Modern Spain*
31 Leslie Harkema, *Spanish Modernism and the Poetics of Youth: From Miguel de Unamuno to* La Joven Literatura
32 Benjamin Fraser, *Cognitive Disability Aesthetics: Visual Culture, Disability Representations, and the (In)Visibility of Cognitive Difference*
33 Robert Patrick Newcomb, *Iberianism and Crisis: Spain and Portugal at the Turn of the Twentieth Century*

34 Sara J. Brenneis, *Spaniards in Mauthausen: Representations of a Nazi Concentration Camp, 1940–2015*
35 Silvia Bermúdez and Roberta Johnson (eds), *A New History of Iberian Feminisms*
36 Steven Wagschal, *Minding Animals in the Old and New Worlds: A Cognitive Historical Analysis*
37 Heather Bamford, *Cultures of the Fragment: Uses of the Iberian Manuscript, 1100–1600*
38 Enrique García Santo-Tomás (ed), *Science on Stage in Early Modern Spain*
39 Marina Brownlee (ed), *Cervantes'* Persiles *and the Travails of Romance*
40 Sarah Thomas, *Inhabiting the In-Between: Childhood and Cinema in Spain's Long Transition*
41 David A. Wacks, *Medieval Iberian Crusade Fiction and the Mediterranean World*
42 Rosilie Hernández, *Immaculate Conceptions: The Power of the Religious Imagination in Early Modern Spain*
43 Mary Coffey and Margot Versteeg (eds), *Imagined Truths: Realism in Modern Spanish Literature and Culture*
44 Diana Aramburu, *Resisting Invisibility: Detecting the Female Body in Spanish Crime Fiction*
45 Samuel Amago and Matthew J. Marr (eds), *Consequential Art: Comics Culture in Contemporary Spain*
46 Richard P. Kinkade, *Dawn of a Dynasty: The Life and Times of Infante Manuel of Castile*
47 Jill Robbins, *Poetry and Crisis: Cultural Politics and Citizenship in the Wake of the Madrid Bombings*
48 Ana María Laguna and John Beusterien (eds), *Goodbye Eros: Recasting Forms and Norms of Love in the Age of Cervantes*
49 Sara J. Brenneis and Gina Herrmann (eds), *Spain, World War II, and the Holocaust: History and Representation*
50 Francisco Fernández de Alba, *Sex, Drugs, and Fashion in 1970s Madrid*
51 Daniel Aguirre-Oteiza, *This Ghostly Poetry: Reading Spanish Republican Exiles between Literary History and Poetic Memory*
52 Lara Anderson, *Control and Resistance: Food Discourse in Franco Spain*
53 Faith Harden, *Arms and Letters: Military Life Writing in Early Modern Spain*
54 Erin Alice Cowling, Tina de Miguel Magro, Mina García Jordán, and Glenda Y. Nieto-Cuebas (eds), *Social Justice in Spanish Golden Age Theatre*

55 Paul Michael Johnson, *Affective Geographies: Cervantes, Emotion, and the Literary Mediterranean*
56 Justin Crumbaugh and Nil Santiáñez (eds), *Spanish Fascist Writing: An Anthology*
57 Margaret E. Boyle and Sarah E. Owens (eds): *Health and Healing in the Early Modern Iberian World: A Gendered Perspective*